# Progress
# in Motor Control

## Volume Three

## Effects of Age, Disorder, and Rehabilitation

**Mark L. Latash, PhD**
**The Pennsylvania State University**

**Mindy F. Levin, PhD, PT**
**The University of Montreal**

**Editors**

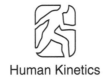

Human Kinetics

Library of Congress Cataloging-in-Publication Data

Progress in motor control / Mark L. Latash, Mindy F. Levin, editors.
    p.    cm.
    Includes bibliographical references and index.
    Contents: v. 3. Effects of age, disorder, and rehabilitation.
    ISBN 0-7360-4400-0
    1. Human locomotion. 2. Motor ability. 3. Bernshteîn, N.A.
(Nikolaî Aleksandrovich), 1896-1966. I. Latash, Mark L., 1953-
II. Levin, Mindy F., 1953-
QP301.P767    1998
612.7'6—DC21

**QP**
**301**
**.P767**
**v.3**

97-44950
CIP

ISBN: 0-7360-4400-0

Copyright © 2004 by Mark L. Latash and Mindy F. Levin

**Acquisitions Editor:** Judy Patterson Wright, PhD; **Managing Editor:** Amy Stahl; **Assistant Editors:** Amanda Gunn, Derek Campbell; **Copyeditor:** Karen Bojda; **Proofreader:** Jim Burns; **Indexer:** Marie Rizzo; **Permission Manager:** Dalene Reeder; **Graphic Designer:** Fred Starbird; **Graphic Artist:** Kathleen Boudreau-Fuoss; **Photo Manager:** Dan Wendt; **Cover Designer:** Jack W. Davis; **Photographer (cover):** Courtesy of *Fizkultura i Sport*; **Art Manager:** Kelly Hendren; **Printer:** Bang Printing

Printed in the United States of America    10  9  8  7  6  5  4  3  2  1

**Human Kinetics**
Web site: www.HumanKinetics.com

*United States:* Human Kinetics
P.O. Box 5076
Champaign, IL 61825-5076
800-747-4457
e-mail: humank@hkusa.com

*Canada:* Human Kinetics
475 Devonshire Road Unit 100,
Windsor, ON N8Y 2L5
800-465-7301 (in Canada only)
e-mail: orders@hkcanada.com

*Europe:* Human Kinetics
107 Bradford Road, Stanningley,
Leeds LS28 6AT, United Kingdom
+44 (0) 113 255 5665
e-mail: hk@hkeurope.com

*Australia:* Human Kinetics
57A Price Avenue
Lower Mitcham
South Australia 5062
08 8277 1555
e-mail: liaw@hkaustralia.com

*New Zealand:* Human Kinetics
Division of Sports Distributors NZ Ltd.
P.O. Box 300 226 Albany
North Shore City
Auckland
0064 9 448 1207
e-mail: blairc@hknewz.com

# Contents

# Preface

All three volumes in the *Progress in Motor Control* series are united by a common theme: understanding the basic mechanisms of the control and coordination of voluntary movements. The first volume, *Progress in Motor Control: Bernstein's Traditions in Movement Studies,* commemorated the centenary of Nikolai Alexandrovich Bernstein's birth and addressed the impact of Bernstein's contribution to the field now defined as motor control. The second volume, *Progress in Motor Control: Structure-Function Relations in Human Movements*, emphasized the biomechanical and neurophysiological aspects of motor control that participate in the production of coordinated movements.

This third volume, *Progress in Motor Control: Effects of Age, Disorder, and Rehabilitation*, explores recent progress in theoretical and experimental studies, presenting cutting-edge research and experimental findings in motor control literature, including sensorimotor disorders and rehabilitation, and provides insights for clinical applications. Studies of disordered motor control have both practical and theoretical importance. First, they contribute to the understanding of mechanisms of motor disorders and help evaluate and optimize therapies. Second, they provide valuable information about the range of control strategies that the central nervous system can use to produce voluntary movements following pathological changes. Bernstein appreciated both aspects of clinical movement studies. A few of his clinical papers have recently been translated into English and published in the journal, *Motor Control*. This current volume can be seen as continuing that particular aspect of Bernstein's heritage. In particular, the volume focuses on several topics whose roots can be traced back to the seminal studies by Bernstein, Hughlings Jackson, Gelfand, Tsetlin, Von Holst, and other great researchers who laid the foundation of motor control. Among these topics are the relationship between posture and movement, the role of motor variability, kinematic redundancy, and the relationship between neurophysiological structures and mechanics of voluntary movements.

## Organization

The current volume bridges the gap between theory and practice for professionals working with individuals with problems in the control of movement and coordination. It is organized into four parts. Part I, "Sensorimotor Integration" includes three chapters. Chapter 1 presents an update and new developments along a line of research that started with the inauguration of the equilibrium-point hypothesis in 1965 by Anatol Feldman. This chapter revisits the classic question of the relationship between posture and movement. The notions of shifting reference frames are applied to complex whole-body movements requiring the control of multiple muscles and offer a dynamic resolution to the problems of muscle and joint redundancy. It is suggested that muscle and joint synergies may not be planned by the central nervous system but emerge as a result of a particular organization of the neural control. This is a provocative and novel approach to the problem of motor redundancy. Chapter 2 addresses the problem of redundancy at the kinematic level for multijoint arm movements. Current motor control theories based on mathematical principles that underlie trajectory planning of multijoint arm movements are reviewed. This chapter accepts a traditional approach to the problem of motor redundancy assuming that it is indeed a problem to be solved by the controller, the central nervous system. Chapter 3 addresses kinematic redundancy during development and shows how the relationships between posture and movement change between 4 and 9 months of age. This reveals the changing coordination patterns and mastery of the redundant kinematic degrees of freedom during motor maturation. The problem of kinematic redundancy is viewed from the dynamic system perspective, as a problem of central organization of the many degrees of freedom into a coordinative structure.

The chapters in part II, "New Approaches to Motor Variability," present computational models that work at different levels of the neuromotor hierarchy. Chapter 4 describes the most recent developments of the idea of neural fields as a way of controlling voluntary movements within the dynamic field model. This model addresses how previous information and prior motor history are integrated with current multimodal perceptual information to plan movement that continually evolves in time. Chapter 5 describes a new computational approach to the notion of synergies, the origin of which can be traced back to classic papers by Gelfand and Tsetlin. This approach avoids the famous Bernsteinian problem of the elimination of redundant degrees of freedom by suggesting that systems participating in the production of voluntary movements should be viewed not as redundant but rather as abundant. The final chapter in this part, chapter 6, summarizes a series of recent studies aimed at building a coherent model of motor cortical functioning in terms of muscle-based encoding. According to this model, motor cortical neurons activate muscle groups while taking into account the state-dependence of muscle force production and effects of multijoint mechanics. The different approaches to motor variability described in the three chapters of part II underscore the importance and controversy of this phenomenon. They all suggest that motor variability is not simply a consequence of noise within the system for movement production, but it is a consequence of purposeful control strategies.

Part III of this volume, "Changes in Motor Control with Age or Neurological Disorder," contains chapters that address issues of control of posture and locomotion in healthy individuals and in individuals with neurological deficits. Chapter 7 analyzes reactions of healthy people to unexpected postural perturbations during stance and walking. The results illustrate the task-specificity of kinematic responses. Chapter 8 reviews changes in postural control with age, with particular emphasis on the role of protective arm movements for fall prevention. Chapter 9 analyzes the question of redundancy as it relates to adaptation to permanent brain damage seen in children with spastic hemiparesis resulting from cerebral palsy. This chapter describes how the damaged nervous system adapts patterns of reaching and grasping by exploiting the redundancy of the neuromuscular system. All three chapters emphasize the importance of adaptive changes in movement patterns in people with an impaired central nervous system, and this theme continues in part IV.

Part IV, "Motor Rehabilitation After Stroke or Spinal Cord Injury," summarizes the principles and techniques of new therapies for recovery after central nervous system injury. Chapter 10 reviews the vast experience of the authors on the use of functional electrical stimulation and partial unloading (weight support) to improve locomotor function in neurological patients. Chapter 11 describes the use of stimulators implanted in the spinal cord of children with clinically complete and incomplete spinal lesions. Besides presenting truly unique clinical material, the data provide strong support for the existence of spinal pattern generators within the lumbar enlargement of the human spinal cord. The final chapter of the volume, chapter 12, reviews principles of motor control and learning after stroke-related brain damage and summarizes recent research on the control and recovery of arm movements in stroke survivors who are treated with different motor retraining approaches.

In keeping with the traditions of the *Progress in Motor Control* series, the chapters in this volume were written for the reader who is well educated in the different subfields that comprise the area of motor control. They present state-of-the-art accounts and the interpretation of the authors on a variety of issues, including new approaches to motor rehabilitation, especially after stroke or spinal cord injury. This reference volume will be appreciated by a wide range of professionals working in both basic and applied areas of motor control such as neurophysiology, biomechanics, psychology, kinesiology, motor disorders, motor rehabilitation, physical therapy, and others. Graduate and postdoctoral students in these areas can also use the book as additional reading.

## Acknowledgments

The organization of the "Progress in Motor Control III" conference would not have been possible without the generous support of the Quebec Ministry of Science and Technology, the Canadian Institutes of Health Research, the Quebec Health Research Fund, the Network of Rehabilitation Researchers of Quebec, the Centre for Interdisciplinary Research in Rehabilitation, the Whitaker Foundation, and Human Kinetics Publishers. We are very grateful to Anatol Feldman, John Kalaska, David Ostry, and Philippe Archambault, who shared the load of organizing and running the meeting.

# Credits

**Figure 1.2**

Adapted, by permission, from F.G. Lestienne and A.G. Feldman, 2001, "Du schéma corporel au concept de Configuration de Référence: Une approche théorique de la production du mouvement," *Evolutions Psychomotrices* 53: 127-143.

**Figure 1.3**

Adapted, by permission, from F.G. Lestienne, B. Le Goff, and P.H. Liverneaux, 1995, "Head movement trajectory in three-dimensional space during orienting behavior toward visual targets in rhesus monkeys," *Experimental Brain Research* 102(3): 393-406.

**Figure 1.4**

Adapted, by permission, from P. Perrin and F.G. Lestienne, 1994, *Méchanismes de l'équilibration humaine* (Paris: Masson).

**Figure 1.7**

Reprinted from Journal of Electromyograph & Kinesiology, Vol 8, Feldman, et al., "Multi-muscle control in human movements," pp 383-390, Copyright 1998, with permission of Elsevier Science.

**Figure 1.8**

Adapted from *Neuroscience Letters* Vol. 283, Lestienne et al., "Multi-muscle control of head movements in monkeys: The referent configuration hypothesis." pp. 65-68, Copyright 2000, with permission of Elsevier Science.

**Figure 1.9**

Adapted, by permission, from F.G. Lestienne and A.G. Feldman, 2002, "Une approche théorique de la production du mouvement: Du modèle lambda au concept de 'Configuration de Référence Productrice d'Actions.'" *Science et Motricité* 45: 63-84.

**Figure 6.1, a and b**

Reprinted, by permission, from E. Todorov, 2000a, "Direct cortical control of muscle activation in voluntary arm movements: A model," *Nature Neuroscience* 3: 391-398; and 2000b, Reply to "One motor cortex, two different views," *Nature Neuroscience* 3: 963-964.

**Figure 6.2, c** *(left)* **and e**

Reprinted, by permission, from E. Todorov, 2000a, "Direct cortical control of muscle activation in voluntary arm movements: A model," *Nature Neuroscience* 3: 391-398.

### Figure 6.3, a and c

Reprinted, by permission, from E. Todorov, 2000a, "Direct cortical control of muscle activation in voluntary arm movements: A model," *Nature Neuroscience* 3: 391-398.

### Figure 6.4, c and f

Reprinted, by permission, from E. Todorov, 2000b, Reply to "One motor cortex, two different views," *Nature Neuroscience* 3: 963-964; and 2000a, "Direct cortical control of muscle activation in voluntary arm movements: A model," *Nature Neuroscience* 3: 391-398.

### Figure 6.5

Reprinted, by permission, from E. Todorov, 2002, "Cosine tuning minimizes motor errors," *Neural Computation* 14: 1233-1260.

### Table 11.4

Reprinted, by permission, from E. Shapkova, A. Mushkin, and K. Kovalenko, 1999, "Motor rehabilitation for children with neurological complications of thuberculous spondylitis," *Problems of Tuberculosis* 3: 27-30.

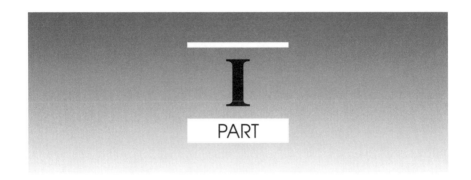

# Sensorimotor Integration

# 1

# Action-Producing Frames of Reference for Motor Control

*Francis G. Lestienne and Francine Thullier*
Laboratoire de Neurosciences
de l'Homme en Mouvement
University of Caen

*Anatol G. Feldman*
Neurological Science Research Center
University of Montreal

Mechanically, the human body is very flexible due to hundreds of bony segments connected by numerous elastic structures: skeletal muscles. How does the nervous system control so many muscles in a coherent way to maintain either a stable body posture or to produce multijoint movements (figure 1.1)? This fundamental question of motor control provokes lively debates among scientists; yet, despite over a century of intensive studies of different aspects of motor performance (the kinematics of body segments, electromyographic [EMG] patterns, synaptic connections, and the activity of neurons and afferents), we have only begun to comprehend the nature of multimuscle control. In this chapter, we outline some possible answers to the question of how the nervous system controls multiple joints and muscles. In particular, it is necessary to explain how the nervous system selects a specific set of muscles and joints to produce a desired goal-directed movement. Since the same motor goal can be achieved using different muscles and joints, how does the nervous system recruit muscles in a unique way for each movement, thereby solving the redundancy problem?

We think it is essential to address motor control problems within a physiologically feasible theoretical framework. The existence of different, often conflicting, theories of motor control does not facilitate this task. Nevertheless, the number of useful theories is sharply reduced if we consider their capacity to solve the classic problem of the relationship between posture and movement. Von Holst and Mittelstaedt (1950/1973) emphasized the necessity of explaining why there is no resistance from posture-stabilizing mechanisms when a person intentionally moves away from an initial posture. We illustrate an empirically well-founded solution to this problem, a solution that underlies the $\lambda$ model for motor control (Asatryan and Feldman, 1965). We also show that force control models, the currently dominant theories of motor control, are fundamentally unable to incorporate the empirical solution of the posture–movement problem or to offer a new solution to this problem. We conclude that such theories have no physiological ground.

Interestingly, the empirical solution of the posture–movement problem provides an answer to the question of how the nervous system organizes and uses frames of reference (FRs) or systems of coordinates in movement production. It appears that the activity of central, reflex, and mechanical components of the neuromuscular system is frame dependent in that a change in some parameter of the FR, such as its origin, metrics, geometric characteristics, and orientation in other FRs, influences the activity of all components of the neuromuscular system. Therefore, by manipulating parameters of the FRs, control signals may guide motor actions. Respectively, any brain areas that issue signals that influence the parameters (determinants) of FRs are called control levels. In this chapter, we give several examples of such action-producing FRs. One such FR is related to the body scheme, as illustrated by experimental data on postural control in weightlessness (Clément et al., 1984; Lestienne and Gurfinkel, 1988a, 1988b) and in normal conditions on the Earth's surface (Feldman et al., 1998; Lestienne and Feldman, 2001). We explore the relationship between the body scheme and the referent configuration of the body. These notions are inherent in the theoretical framework of the $\lambda$ model (Feldman et al., 1999; Feldman and Levin, 1995; Lestienne and Feldman, 2001, 2002; Lestienne, Ghafouri, and Thullier, 1995). Some conclusions stemming from the concept of the referent body configuration have been tested experimentally by analyzing the EMG activity of multiple muscles during head movements by monkeys (Lestienne et al., 2000), leg movements by ballet dancers (Thullier and Plotkin, 2001), and sitting-to-standing-to-sitting movements by humans (Feldman et al., 1998). Finally, we illustrate the point that in the framework of the $\lambda$ model, movements can be guided without redundancy problems at the levels of both joints and muscles.

## Task-Specific Spatial and Temporal Patterns of Muscle Activation

The recruitment of muscles and gradation of muscle activity are task specific, making motor actions adequate, smooth, and elegant (Flash and Hogan, 1985; Hasan

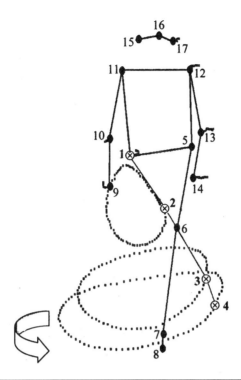

**Figure 1.1** *Rond de jambe* of a classical ballet dancer. A ballet dancer moved the tip of the right foot along an ellipsoidal curve in the horizontal plane. Four digital cameras recorded the positions of 17 markers on the leotard of the dancer. Each marker was seen simultaneously by at least two cameras. These data were used to reconstruct the movement in three-dimensional space.

Adapted from Thullier and Plotkin (2001).

and Karst, 1989; Henneman, 1981; Koshland and Hasan, 1994; Lacquaniti, 1992; Liverneaux and Lestienne, 1989; Loeb and Levine, 1990; Nichols, 1994; Tax et al., 1989; Weijs et al., 1999). The efficiency of a muscle depends on its anatomical arrangement (e.g., its length, cross-sectional area, or moment arm) and on the biomechanical and biochemical properties of its motor units. The recruitment and activation patterns of muscles are constrained biomechanically and, in part, by natural laws. For example, any movement, whether it is produced passively or intentionally by the nervous system, obeys the laws of mechanics. Therefore, to move a body segment (e.g., the arm) from one posture to another, it is necessary first to accelerate and then to decelerate the segment. By activating agonist muscles more strongly than the antagonist muscles, the nervous system accelerates the body segment. Then antagonist muscles overpower the agonist muscles to decelerate the segment. This results in an approximately bell-shaped graph of movement velocity and a smooth transition from one posture to another (Gribble and Ostry, 1996; Hogan and Flash, 1987; Lestienne, 1979). The described pattern of agonist–antagonist activation is called *reciprocal* and is considered fundamental for movement production (Sherrington, 1906/1947). The reciprocal pattern does not necessarily imply that one group of muscles is active while the other is silent. The activation periods can overlap so that the two groups are active simultaneously, a phenomenon called *coactivation*. Coactivation can be produced not only during reciprocal activation but also in isolation, which occurs, for example, when a person intentionally stiffens all muscles of the elbow joint while maintaining the same joint angle.

Muscle coactivation and reciprocal activation result from appropriate changes in the membrane potentials of motoneurons. Sometimes these changes are subthreshold and do not result in activation of motoneurons and muscles. These cases should not be considered unimportant. Quite the contrary, subthreshold influences can dramatically influence the response of the system to unexpected perturbations. For example, previously facilitated motoneurons react to an unexpected stretch of the muscle more quickly and strongly than the same motoneurons in the absence of facilitation. The subthreshold changes in membrane potentials thus exemplify *feedforward* processes that, in particular, prepare the neuromuscular system for unexpected perturbations. In fact, changes in the membrane potential of motoneurons precede the generation of EMG activity and muscle force, and therefore, all movements are produced in a feedforward manner.

It is important to integrate theoretically the cases of both supra- and subthreshold changes in the state of motoneurons of a muscle or group of muscles. It has been experimentally observed that active movements of the arm from one position to another result from changes in the activation thresholds of appropriate muscles (Asatryan and Feldman, 1965). By definition, the activation threshold of a muscle is its specific length or the joint angle at which motor units of this muscle begin to be recruited. Many descending and segmental systems are involved in the specification of activation thresholds (Feldman and Orlovsky, 1972; Matthews, 1959), supporting the notion that shifts in the activation thresholds underlie the control of movements. This notion is also supported by the recent finding that deficits in the central regulation of thresholds result in dramatic problems in posture and movement regulation in subjects with neurological impairments such as deafferentation, hemiparesis, and cerebral palsy (Cirstea and Levin, 2000; Jobin and Levin, 2000; Levin et al., 2000; see also Levin, chapter 12 in this volume).

These empirical findings, especially the finding of the central regulation of muscle activation thresholds, were used to introduce the notions of reciprocal (R) and coactivation (C) commands underlying sub- and suprathreshold changes in the state of agonist and antagonist muscles (figure 1.2). We would like to emphasize that, unlike the traditional notions of reciprocal activation and coactivation described in terms of respective changes in the EMG activity of agonist and antagonist muscles, R and C commands are described in terms of shifts in the activation thresholds of these muscles and, like the thresholds, are spatially dimensional variables. These commands divide the biomechanical

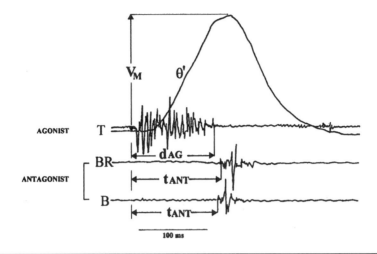

**Figure 1.2** Fast elbow flexion in a human subject. Curve θ' shows the movement velocity ($V_M$ is its maximum value). The movement is initiated and accelerated by activation of agonist muscles (triceps brachii, T) and decelerated by activation of antagonist muscles (brachioradialis, BR, and biceps brachii, B). Abbreviations: dAG is the duration of the antagonist EMG burst; tANT is the time between the onsets of EMG activity in the agonist and antagonist muscles.

Adapted from Lestienne and Feldman (2001).

range of the joint angle into zones. In particular, with the same specific choice of the commands, two opposing groups of muscles may be active simultaneously in one zone but separately in other zones (Levin and Dimov, 1997; see figure 1.2). Thus, the actual pattern of muscle activation depends not only on these commands but also on the current joint angle. It is also possible that, depending on the specific values of the R and C commands, all muscles of the joint may be silent either in the whole or in a part of the biomechanical range of the joint. Additional factors determine whether or not muscles are activated or silent. These factors are the dependence of muscle activation thresholds on the rate of change in muscle length, proprioceptive feedback to a given muscle from afferents of other muscles, and history or time-dependent properties of motoneurons (Feldman and Levin, 1995; Nichols, 1994). While generalizing the notion of the R command to multiple skeletal muscles and joints, we will arrive at the concept of the referent configuration of the body, which is essential for the identification of global factors used by the nervous system to control multiple muscles in a coherent way without a redundancy problem.

Although there is a consensus that muscle activation patterns are task specific, the answer to the question of how this specificity is achieved by the nervous system is a matter of controversy. This situation might result, in part, from the absence of a consensus regarding the basic, elementary principles underlying the control of movement, as illustrated in the next two sections.

# Debates on Reflexes and Central Pattern Generators

Sherrington (1906/1947) suggested that movements are generated as a chain of reflexes, each resulting from the afferent pattern elicited by the preceding reflex. The notion of "reflex" has undergone a substantial evolution. The initial view that reflexes are involuntary, stereotypic responses to external stimuli is highly outdated. There is now a growing understanding that reflexes are organized in a very flexible way, allowing the nervous system to tune their properties (parameters) to meet the task demands. The stretch reflex is especially illustrative in this respect. Its threshold is identical to the previously described muscle activation threshold. Therefore, the notion that the activation thresholds of muscles are broadly regulated by control levels to produce intentional movements applies equally to stretch reflex thresholds. In addition, the sensitivity of the stretch reflex to position and velocity is regulated in a task-specific way (Houk and Rymer, 1981). Thus, according to the contemporary view, reflexes are adjustable neuromuscular actions that appear to play a much more essential role in movement production than previously thought.

Many researchers have hypothesized that movements can be initiated and guided entirely endogenously, by a central pattern generator (CPG; Beevor, 1904). This view became dominant after the findings that walking and scratching can be produced in deafferented animals (Brown, 1911). Since then, the number of movements that are known to be preserved after proprioceptive deafferentation has substantially increased (e.g., Bizzi et al., 1976; Bossom, 1974; Taub, 1976). The issue of how the CPG is adjusted to specific task demands or to changing external conditions has been investigated by many researchers (for a recent review, see Orlovsky et al., 1999).

Some modifications of the CPG concept imply the existence of schemes of action (Piaget, 1936), generalized motor programs (Schmidt, 1975, 1988), action schemes (Turvey, 1977), or abstract memory of families of movements (Pailhous and Bonnard, 1989). Bernstein's (1967) notion of the engram is reminiscent of the scheme of action presented by Piaget (1936), Lashley (1951), or Turvey (1977), implying that the nervous system has at its disposal central commands that are organized before the onset of movement (see also Bossom, 1974; Keele, 1968; Seashore, 1938; Taub, 1976). A common assumption underlying the modifications of the CPG model is that actions are represented in the nervous system in a virtual (abstract) form and are transformed into a real form by adjusting certain parameters according to the desired action and available sensory signals.

Although the results of deafferentation experiments clearly showed that some movements can be produced in the absence of proprioceptive signals, they contributed little to the understanding of how central control processes and afferent signals are integrated in actions of the *intact* neuromuscular system. In addition, the interpretation of results of deafferentation experiments is complicated by the fact that humans and animals compensate for the loss of proprioceptive afferents by learning to use remaining sensory signals from unimpaired, especially vestibular and visual, sensory systems to produce efficient movements. Nevertheless, even after many years of training, deafferented patients are unable to stand or walk without strong assistance and cannot maintain a steady-state position of the arm without seeing it (Levin et al., 2000).

Indeed, the importance of proprioceptive signals has been revealed in many movements, even in those that traditionally were considered in essence centrally programmed (e.g., scratching). It has been shown that a deafferented limb in cats produces functionally inefficient scratching movements: It "scratches" in the air, near the irritated site of the ear (Deliagina et al., 1975). In humans, it has been shown that cutaneous information plays a critical role in typing (Terzuolo and Viviani, 1980). The suggestion that proprioceptive reflexes play an insignificant role in the generation of EMG activity in the fastest movements, especially in the timing of the initial agonist EMG burst (Higgins and Angel, 1970), has also been questioned: Adamovich et al. (1997) demonstrated by perturbation methods that not only the magnitude but also the timing of the initial and subsequent EMG bursts depends on the proprioceptive inputs. Adamovich et al. (1997) suggested that rather than suppressing proprioceptive reflexes, control levels rapidly decrease the thresholds of reflexes, resulting in the agonist EMG bursts. Thus, according to this hypothesis, the nervous system takes advantage of resetting reflex thresholds to produce even the fastest movements. By resetting the thresholds at a maximal rate, the nervous system compels muscles to work almost at their full capacity, making them relatively insensitive to additional, external perturbations.

This brief review shows that some movements can be produced in the absence of proprioceptive feedback, especially after relearning based on the remaining sensory feedback (see chapter 12 in this book). The deafferentation experiments, however, initially gave the false impression that proprioceptive afferent signals play a minor role in movement production. These experiments could not help in addressing the fundamental question of how central control and afferent signals are integrated in the production of movements in intact organisms. Simple observations of motor deficits in deafferented patients point to a fundamental role of proprioceptive signals in movement production.

## Different Theories of Motor Control

In the past, attempts to integrate central control and afferent (in particular, proprioceptive) signals in a theory of motor control were made by several researchers. In particular, Von Holst and Mittelstaedt (1950/1973) emphasized the necessity of explaining how the body is able to move to a new posture without provoking the resistance of posture-stabilizing mechanisms to the deviation from the initial posture. They were fully aware of the results of deafferentation experiments that imply the existence of a CPG but emphasized that the CPG hypothesis does not solve the posture–movement problem. They also emphasized that the reflex theory, in which reflexes were considered as rigid, stereotypic structures, also failed to solve the posture–movement problem. To solve this problem, Von Holst and Mittelstaedt formulated the reafference principle, which states that, to produce a movement, control levels influence sensory feedback to motoneurons and thus reset the spatial coordinates at which a stable posture can be established. This idea is considered in detail in the next section.

In his approach to the problem of integration of central control signals and sensory feedback, Bernstein (1967) emphasized that the muscle is characterized not by a single force–length relationship but by a family of such relationships. As a result, control levels can select, at best, a single force–length relationship from this family but not a specific combination of muscle force and length. Specific values of muscle force and length eventually emerge following the interaction of the muscle with other muscles and with external, including gravitational, forces. Bernstein (1967) also noticed that central control and sensory signals converge at the level of motoneurons and concluded that EMG patterns cannot be predetermined by a central program. In other words, the relationship between the central control signals and the motor output is undetermined; the same set of central commands can result in different actions, depending on, for example, external forces. Bernstein (1967) suggested that to get the desired motor output, control levels should monitor sensory signals to produce appropriate continuous and discrete corrections to get the desirable action (the principle of sensory corrections).

Although Bernstein and Von Holst strongly argued against the hypothesis of direct programming of the motor output, it was revived comparatively recently, with some modifications, in force control models. These models were inspired by advances in computer science and the theory of adaptive systems successfully used in robotics (Hannaford and Winters, 1990; Raibert, 1986). According to these models, the nervous system directly programs and specifies muscle activations, forces, and torques computed for the desired movement trajectory of the effector. To make this strategy work, the brain should have some knowledge of the physical properties of the body and the environment. Our everyday experience shows that, while making a movement, we unconsciously rely on gravity acting on the body, inertia of body segments, elasticity and viscosity of muscles, and even interactive torques resulting from the relative rotations of different body segments (Bernstein, 1967). Indeed, the nervous system is also skillful in anticipating and neutralizing the undesirable effects of mechanical distortions resulting from changes in the physical properties of the body and environment during movements (Berthoz, 1996).

Knowledge of the physical properties of the body and environment in itself is insufficient to compute muscle torques. Therefore, force control models postulate a mathematical procedure called *inverse dynamics,* the ability of the brain to compute the muscle forces and torques required for the generation of the desired movement trajectory. The term *inverse* in the context of force control models implies that the computations, in a sense, invert cause–effect relationships determined by the natural dynamic laws that govern the peripheral part of the neuromuscular system. For example, according to the laws of mechanics, acceleration and changes in other kinematic variables are effects, not causes, of acting forces. In the inverse dynamics method, forces are computed as if they were caused by kinematic variables.

The concept of inverse dynamics was borrowed from robotics, where torques are computed according to the planned kinematics of robots' movements (Hollerbach and Atkeson, 1987; Slotine and Li, 1991). Applied to the neuromuscular system, this method implies that, while computing muscle torques, the nervous system may take into account the complex dynamic behavior of mechanical, reflex, and central components of the neuromuscular system. These inverse computations can be made only with some neural representation of the equations describing the input–output interactions of these components and the environment. Force control models thus postulate the existence of neural structures that imitate, at least approximately, the dynamic properties of these components and are used for inverse dynamic computations. The postulated structures are called *internal models* (Kawato et al., 1987; Shadmehr and Mussa-Ivaldi, 1994; Wolpert et al., 1995). It is also postulated that internal models may be used not only for inverse but also for straightforward computations to prevent possible movement errors.

In these postulated internal models, individual muscle forces and EMG activity are further computed based on the values of joint torques. To overcome the problem associated with a redundant number of muscles, the computations employ some optimization criteria, such as the minimization of overall muscular activity.

It should be noted that any computation of variables, whether made by a computer or the nervous system, is a mathematical process that yields only symbolic values of these variables and does not result in a physical action unless the appropriate transformation (physical interface) is made. Force control models have not addressed the strategy by which the computed (i.e., virtual) values characterizing the motor output (muscle forces and EMG activity) are transformed into a real motor output. It is doubtful that force control models can overcome this drawback: The assumption that the motor output is directly specified by control signals conflicts with Bernstein's (1967) illustrations that the relationship between control signals and the motor output is undetermined.

Force control models have other problems that point to their fundamental failures. Studies of neural, biomechanical, and afferent components of the neuromuscular system leave no doubt that these components obey dynamic laws that prescribe cause–effect relationships in the system. What happens if control levels impose on these components the values of variables computed according to inverse cause–effect relationships? We will show that the system resists such interference. To reach the goal despite the resistance, the control levels would be required to amplify their action. This means that, instead of taking advantage of the natural dynamics of the neuromuscular system, control levels would struggle with it, making the control strategy extremely inefficient in terms of energy costs, EMG activity, and force production. We illustrate these failures of force control strategy by analyzing the classic problem in motor control of the relationship between posture and movement.

Von Holst and Mittelstaedt (1950/1973) stated that powerful neuromuscular mechanisms (postural reflexes) generate EMG activity and forces in order to resist perturbations that deflect the body from an initial posture. At the same time it is clear that the organism can intentionally adopt different postures. Each new posture adopted can be considered a deviation from the initial one. Resistance to the deviation would tend to return the organism to its initial position. How then is an intentional movement from the initial posture to a new posture possible without resistance?

One possible answer to this question is that postural reflexes are completely or partially suppressed by a central pattern generator during the transition to a new posture. Von Holst and Mittelstaedt (1950/1973) correctly rejected this suggestion as conflicting with experimental observations. Specifically, any posture of the body is maintained by resisting reactions similar to the response to perturbations seen in the restoration of the initial posture.

Von Holst and Mittelstaedt (1950/1973) outlined the reafference principle, a solution to the posture–movement problem; they suggested that the nervous system influences afferent systems in some way to reset the initial postural state so that the same postural mechanisms that stabilize the initial posture would act to produce movement to a new posture.

A specific solution to the posture–movement problem was suggested by Merton (1953), who assumed that the activity of gamma motoneurons projecting onto muscle spindle receptors sets the desired muscle length, whereas the stretch reflex acting as a servo regulator compels the neuromuscular system to follow up the set position with a minimal positional error. To actualize this strategy, the gain (stiffness) of the muscle-reflex system would have to be higher than is experimentally observed, and therefore the hypothesis has been rejected.

Another form of the reference principle that is free from the deficiency of Merton's (1953) hypothesis is the $\lambda$ model for motor control (Asatryan and Feldman, 1965; Feldman and Levin, 1993, 1995; Latash, 1993), a version of the equilibrium-point hypothesis (Bizzi et al., 1992; Feldman, 1966, 1986). Specifically, the model is based on the experimental finding that the postural resetting is produced by changing the length-dimensional muscle activation thresholds (Asatryan and Feldman, 1965; Feldman and Orlovsky, 1972; Matthews, 1959). By changing the thresholds ($\lambda$s), the nervous system shifts the spatial coordinates at which an equilibrium posture can be reached and maintained. In this way, the initial posture appears to be a deviation from the newly specified posture. Therefore, the same neuromuscular mechanisms that produce EMG signals and forces in response to deviation from the initial position produce, without any programming or computation, EMG signals and forces tending to eliminate the deviation from the new posture and thus move the system to it (Feldman and Levin, 1995). The model was also supported by findings that many descending systems, including corticospinal ones, have the capacity to regulate the activation thresholds (Feldman and Orlovsky, 1972). Further support stemmed from recent studies that showed dramatic movement problems following deficits in the regulation of activation thresholds in neurological patients (Levin and Dimov, 1997; Levin et al., 2000). From these data, one can say that the posture-resetting mechanism in the $\lambda$ model is not a hypothesis, it is a fact.

Thus, the empirical evidence that resetting muscle activation thresholds underlies active movement production implies that the basic postulate of force control models—central programming of kinematic variables, EMG patterns, and forces—is fundamentally incorrect (cf. Todorov, 2000; see also Todorov, chapter 6 in this volume). It is not difficult to see the root of the problem in force control models: They failed to answer the basic question posed by Von Holst and Mittelstaedt (1950/1973) of how the system can actively move from an initial posture without triggering the resistance of posture-stabilizing mechanisms. By disregarding the empirical mechanism of postural resetting (shifts in muscle activation thresholds), force control models postulate movements produced by overcoming such resistance. For example, Schweighofer et al. (1998) simulated planar point-to-point arm movements using a force control strategy. Their equations 6 and 8 show that after the movement offset, muscles generate tonic activity in proportion to the distance between the initial and the final muscle lengths. This implies that the final position is reached by overcoming the resistance to the deviation of the arm from the initial position. Thus, at the final position, the muscle activity cannot be minimized without driving the limb back to the initial position. This prediction of the force control model obviously conflicts with the common observation that, after the transition of the arm to a new position, muscle activation can be minimized without arm motion. Control strategies that tolerate the resistance to deflections from the initial posture each time an active movement is produced are highly inefficient in terms of EMG activity, force production, and energy costs.

Can force control models overcome these deficiencies by incorporating the postural resetting that underlies intentional movements? It is doubtful that this can be done in a logically consistent way; the empirical data show that EMG signals, muscle forces, and movement emerge as a dynamic response of the system to postural resetting. By definition, a response is dynamic if, after an initial input, it evolves in time following the natural, physical laws governing the system, like the trajectory of a flying stone. It would be inappropriate to say that computations of forces and trajectories underlie the behavior of the stone. Similarly, the basic computational principles underlying force control models are incompatible with natural dynamic laws governing the production of EMG activity, force, and movement in the neuromuscular system.

# Multijoint and Multimuscle Control: Redundancy Problems and Synergies

Movements typically involve multiple muscles and a substantial number of segments of the body (figure 1.1). Due to the biomechanical linkage between segments, forces and torques generated at one degree of freedom (DF) influence many other DFs. Control levels may also relate the motions at different DFs in different ways to adjust them to external conditions (e.g., obstacles) and achieve the motor goal. It is puzzling, however, how the system makes a choice of a specific movement out of many possible movements to produce an action. This puzzle is called the redundancy problem in multijoint control. A similar redundancy problem is associated with the control of multiple skeletal muscles. One approach to the redundancy problem was suggested by Bernstein (1935, 1967). He assumed that the nervous system has the capacity to interrelate the central influences guiding different DFs and thus coordinate their motions. These interrelationships can be imposed in a task-specific way and coexist with the biomechanical constraints associated, in particular, with the body geometry and limitations in the range of joint motion. Thus, coordinated, multiple DFs of the body are controlled as if they were reduced to a single joint. Such coordination is called a unit or a synergy. Each synergy is a flexible structure that can be adjusted to specific task demands by modifying a comparatively small number of controlled parameters (one or two). It was assumed that the system organizes several synergies and employs them in isolation or in combination depending on task demands. This idea has obtained substantial empirical support. Figure 1.3 illustrates synergies utilized during head movements that accompany shifts in the gaze. Head movements in three-dimensional (3D) space involve seven vertebrae. This biomechanical complexity is especially striking at the level of the upper cervical vertebral column, which includes the atlantooccipital and lateral atlantoaxial joints with six DFs controlled by four pairs of muscles (Liverneaux and Lestienne, 1989). Kinematic and EMG analysis revealed that the nervous system employed a comparatively simple strategy in dealing with the number of redundant DFs of the neck–head plant. Lestienne, Le Goff, and Liverneaux (1995) identified four functional units or synergies that can be orchestrated by the nervous system to account for the remarkable variety of trajectories and head–neck positions in 3D space (figure 1.3). The EMG patterns of each unit are unique for each subject, but in all cases only four units are effectively employed to manage the number of redundant DFs of the neck–head system.

A somewhat different approach to the problem of joint redundancy can be developed in the theoretical framework of the $\lambda$ model based on the empirical solution of the posture–movement problem. This solution implies that control levels guide movement by changing specific neurophysiological parameters and modifying them if the resulting action is in error. This parametric control strategy releases control levels from the burden of solving redundancy problems in terms of output, mechanical, and EMG variables. In response to changes in control parameters, appropriate values of mechanical variables and their transformations (e.g., from hand kinematics to joint angles) emerge automatically, following the natural tendency of the neuromuscular system to reach an equilibrium state. This approach does not reject the notion of synergies but suggests that synergies might be an emergent property resulting from the parametric control strategy (see the section "Guiding Movements Without Redundancy Problems").

## Sensorimotor Integration and the Body Scheme

The spatial orientation and the configuration of the body can be described in appropriate frames of reference (FRs) or systems of coordinates. It is likely that the nervous system uses these FRs to guide motor actions. An FR associated with the

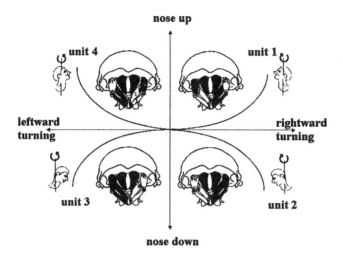

**nose up**

unit 4                                    unit 1

leftward                                  rightward
turning                                   turning

unit 3                                    unit 2

**nose down**

**Figure 1.3**  Biomechanical complexity of the upper cervical vertebral column and functional units of coordination. Four units or synergies combine head rotations (left/right) with its tilts (up/down). The muscles activated during functioning of these units are shown in black. This diagram shows the suboccipital muscles controlling the first two vertebrae (the axis and the atlas): the rectus capitis posterior minor and major and the obliquus capitis inferior and superior.

Adapted from Lestienne, Le Goff, and Liverneaux (1995).

environment is called *allocentric*. In this FR, the direction of gravity represents the objective vertical that is perceived by the vestibular system. Paillard (1971) suggested that the vertical is the "external plumb line" that is essential in the identification of stationary points in the environment by the visual and auditory systems. Indeed, our perception of the vertical direction can be affected, for example, by centrifugal forces arising in an airplane during turns. These forces together with the gravitational force act on the otolith organs and determine the subjective vertical.

Another FR, called the egocentric FR, is associated with the body. In this FR, the system localizes its own articulators and objects of the external world relative to the body surface. Geometrically, the location of objects in this FR can be described in polar coordinates as distances and angles or in Cartesian coordinates as distances from the anatomically determined frontal and sagittal planes.

Different somatosensory systems are involved in the organization of FRs as well as in postural stabilization, reflexes, movement control, and perception (figure 1.4; Perrin and Lestienne, 1994). Head movements in relation to the environment can be detected by changes in the optical flow but, more directly, by the vestibular sensors located in the inner ear and forming a gravito-inertial "powerhouse" that is sensitive to angular and linear head movements. Afferent signals from some of these sensors (otolith organs) detect the gravitational vertical and, together with the other vestibular sensors (semicircular channels), form the allocentric FR.

Signals related to movements and muscle forces are conveyed by muscle and joint afferents. Together with afferent signals from cutaneous receptors sensitive to touch, pressure, friction, pinning, and so on, they contribute to the formation of the egocentric FR. Signals from muscle and cutaneous afferents are also responsible for perception of the weight, size, volume, shape, texture, compliance, and rigidity of objects. These signals are used to form an intrinsic representation of objects—haptic sensation that cannot be obtained from vision alone (Jeannerod, 1997). The combined sensory array can thus be used to fill in the internal egocentric FR with objects from the environment (Berthoz, 1996; Ghafouri and Lestienne, 1996, 2000).

In his book *Science and Hypothesis* [La science et l'hypothèse], Poincaré (1902/ 1968) discussed the role of movement in the perception of space. He pointed out that although movements physically are produced in 3D space, the organism does not necessarily picture them in that space but rather picks up the sensations, or motor impressions, that accompany movements. Even the vestibular system that detects both the gravitational force and the accelerations resulting from rotations and translations of the head in space does not tell us that space is three-dimensional. Poincaré emphasized that the function of the sense organs is to signal changes in the external environment. He also suggested that visual images represent only one aspect of our feeling of space and that only through motor experiences can we recognize that space is three-dimensional. In this context, Poincaré assumed that adequate perception of the orientation of the body in the environment is based on the integration of signals from different sensory systems. If this assumption holds, deficits in this integration can cause substantial errors in the perception of body orientation.

This hypothesis was confirmed in studies of the control of posture in weightlessness (Clément et al., 1984; Lestienne and Gurfinkel, 1988a, 1988b; see also the acknowledgments at the end of this chapter). In these experiments, astronauts on a space station wore a head-mounted optical device in which they could see an unstructured surface stabilized with respect to the head. Thus, they could not detect the orientation of the body in the space station. When asked to stand vertically to the floor with their feet attached to it, astronauts leaned their bodies forward by more than 30° while reporting that their body was perpendicular to the floor. In weightlessness, the vestibular system is dysfunctional, and its afferent output cannot be used to identify the vertical direction. Tactile perception from the feet is also distorted compared with that elicited by body weight during standing on the Earth. Therefore, the natural visual, vestibular, and tactile clues allowing one to identify the vertical direction on the Earth were not available to subjects in these experiments. EMG analysis (figure 1.5) showed that, rather than relaxing the leg muscles, astronauts actively specified the posture that they considered vertical. During standing on the Earth, the activity of ankle extensors dominates over flexor activity (Clément et al., 1984), whereas in weightlessness the activity of ankle flexors becomes dominant. With adaptation to weightlessness, the deviation of the body from vertical to the floor of the spaceship progressively decreased, and

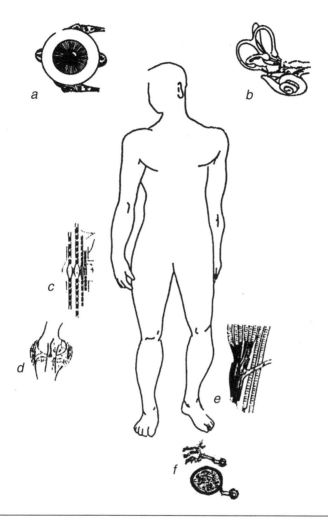

**Figure 1.4** *(a)* Visual, *(b)* vestibular, and *(c-f)* proprioceptive afferent systems involved in the control of posture and movement. The vestibular system includes three semicircular canals and two otolith organs. *(c)* Muscle spindles, *(d)* tendon receptors, *(e)* articular receptors, and *(f)* tactile receptors belong to the proprioceptive system.

Adapted from Perrin and Lestienne (1994).

the body orientation and the projection of the body's center of gravity approached those observed during standing in normal weight conditions on the Earth (figure 1.5; Lestienne and Gurfinkel, 1988a).

We cannot rule out the possibility that the vestibular and visual systems in this experiment elicited some bias in sensing the body orientation that diminished with the adaptation to weightlessness. Alternatively, in the beginning of the flight, subjects might have used the same sensory cues to identify body orientation that they

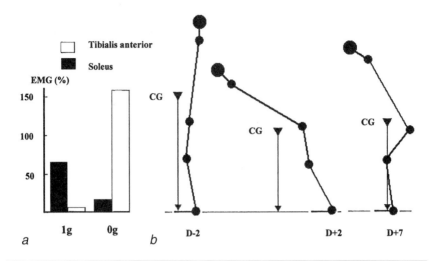

**Figure 1.5**  EMG activity of leg postural muscles and the body orientation of an astronaut in weightlessness. *(a)* EMG activity of the tibialis anterior (flexor) and soleus (extensor) muscles of the ankle joint on the surface of the Earth (1*g*) and during space flight (0*g*). *(b)* The astronaut's head was covered with an optical system that was lit inside and fixed in relation to the head (stabilized vision). The feet were attached to the floor of the spacecraft. The astronaut was instructed to stand upright, that is, perpendicular to the floor. The diagrams show the postural orientation 2 days before the flight (D – 2) and 2 and 7 days after the beginning of the flight (D + 2; D + 7). The vertical lines mark the projection of the body's center of gravity (CG) onto the floor.

Adapted from Lestienne and Gurfinkel (1988a, 1988b).

use in everyday life on the Earth's surface. Specifically, deprived of vestibular and visual cues, they might have sensed orientation based on proprioceptive signals from antigravitational muscles, in particular, ankle extensors. On the Earth's surface, these muscles are active and balance the weight of the body. In the absence of weight in the spacecraft, the unbalanced extensor torque could elicit a backward deviation of the body, which, according to the sensory cues perceived on the Earth's surface, is associated with the feeling of instability and falling backward. To prevent this feeling, the astronauts may have felt it necessary to suppress the activity of extensor muscles. Simultaneously, the astronauts activated the flexor muscles. They thus leaned their bodies forward and stretched the passive extensors. This process continued until the afferent flow from the extensors reached the level associated with normal standing on the Earth. The astronauts might have felt this comfortable proprioceptive flow from extensors with reaching a vertical position, even though the body was actually leaning forward. With adaptation to weightlessness over several days of flight, subjects gradually decreased the dependence of their sense of direction on the earthly cues and thus diminished the subjective error. This explanation suggests that, in the absence of usual vestibular and visual signals identifying the orientation of the body in the environment, subjects change the body configuration until the proprioceptive signals from antigravitational muscles resemble those associated with the normal standing on the Earth, resulting in an error in the perception of the body's orientation in the environment.

Sensory integration is necessary not only for correct perception of the vertical but also for an internal representation of the body geometry called the *body scheme* (Head and Holmes, 1911). Adrian (1947) suggested that the body scheme is internally represented in relation to the external world. More recently, in his book *Descartes' Error*, Damasio (1994) paraphrased the same idea: "The body, as represented in the brain, may constitute the indispensable frame of reference for the neural processes that we experience as the mind. . . . " He also suggested that in the domain of human action "the body is used as a yardstick."

Several studies favor the existence of an internal body scheme that is preserved as a coherent whole in changing external conditions (Lestienne and Gurfinkel, 1997). In particular, it has been shown that, when asked to draw ellipses in different planes during flight in a spaceship, subjects orient them in relation to the longitudinal axis of the body, regardless of the orientation of the body in the environment (Gurfinkel, Lestienne, Levik, Popov, and Lefort, 1993). The interpretation of complex tactile stimuli on the body surface is also preserved in these conditions, and the stimuli are correctly identified in relation to the longitudinal axis of the body (Gurfinkel, Lestienne, Levik, and Popov, 1993).

Although the existence of an internal body scheme seems well justified empirically (see also Fukson et al., 1980), the absence of a rigorous definition of this concept in neurophysiological terms has limited its utility in motor control studies. This problem has been overcome in the $\lambda$ model of motor control by advancing a related but more explicitly defined concept: that of the referent configuration of the body. This new concept of the referent configuration simultaneously addresses the question of how multiple muscles are controlled in a coherent way. It also strengthens the basic idea of the $\lambda$ model that action-producing frames of reference are pre-existing neural structures with key parameters (such as the origin points) modified by control levels to produce motor actions directly, without computation or transformation of intermediate or output variables. The referent configuration concept also illustrates the idea that the natural tendency of the neuromuscular system to reach an equilibrium state is a manifestation of a more general principle, the principle of minimal interaction, by which the interactions in the system are minimized. These points are clarified in the remaining sections.

## The Referent Configuration of the Body

The empirical solution of the posture–movement problem suggests that the activation of each muscle depends on the difference between the actual ($x$) and the threshold length ($\lambda$). It becomes obvious that the posture–movement problem and the problem of FRs are directly related: The threshold length represents the referent value or the origin of the spatial FR in which the muscle is activated. As a consequence, changes in the origins of the FRs of appropriate muscles result in EMG signals, kinematic values, and force values without programming and computations, which in turn result in a motor action. To emphasize this aspect of FRs, we call them action-producing FRs (Feldman and Levin, 1995; cf. Colby, 1998). In the theoretical framework of the $\lambda$ model, many action-producing FRs can be defined in a physiologically feasible way. In this section, we introduce an FR dealing with possible configurations of all skeletal muscles of the body.

The activation threshold can be defined not only for a single muscle (the threshold length, $\lambda$) but also for the group of muscles spanning a joint (the threshold joint angle) and even for all skeletal muscles of the body. In the latter case, we are talking about the configuration of the body described by a set of threshold values of all joint angles of the body. This is a particular configuration of the body at which all skeletal muscles reach their activation thresholds simultaneously. This configuration can be considered the referent (R) configuration, with which actual configurations of the body (Q) are compared. The notion of the referent configuration is a natural extension of the notion of the reciprocal command previously defined for muscles of single joints to all skeletal muscles of the body. Any Q is described by a respective set of actual joint angles. Since R is the threshold configuration, the difference between the Q and R configurations is a global factor that, together with local biomechanical and reflex factors, determines how strongly appropriate neurons and muscles are activated or deactivated. This factor makes all skeletal muscles of the body function as a coherent whole. The R configuration plays the role of the origin of the spatial FRs representing all possible configurations Q of the body. The activity in the neuro-muscular system is determined automatically, depending on the proximity of the actual configuration to the referent configuration. Since the origin of this FR is a particular configuration of the whole body (R), it makes no sense to associate the origin with a point on the body, contrary to the usual assumption that internal FRs should be centered on the shoulders, head, arms, or eyes. The feasibility of the R concept has been confirmed experimentally (see the next section).

Given a referent configuration, different body configurations become nonequivalent in terms of resistance to external forces and muscle forces and the patterns of EMG activity associated with them. Based on this property, the proximity of any actual configuration to the R configuration and to other configurations can be defined. Mathematically, this means that the configurational space has a metric. In other words, given a specific R configuration and the biomechanical and neuronal constraints, we can determine the distance $(d_{12})$ between any two body configurations: $d_{12} = f(Q_1, Q_2)$. Note that the notion of distance is defined in a neurophysiological rather than geometrical sense: It characterizes the cost of the transition from one posture to another in terms of overall EMG activity, energy required, and so on. A more specific description of the metric is an experimental, rather than theoretical, question. Regardless of the specific answer to this question, the metrics of the configurational space determine the posture to which the body will move in response to a change in external conditions (forces) or central resetting of the R configuration. For example, by changing the R configuration, control levels alter the distance between the initial and the referent configurations. As a consequence, the activity in the neuromuscular system changes, resulting in an intentional movement or, if the movement is prevented, isometric forces (Feldman and Levin, 1995). When movement is not obstructed, the body will move until it reaches a configuration at which all forces and torques (muscular and external) become balanced and neural interactions in the system become minimal within the limits determined, in particular, by biomechanical constraints.

Thus, following the metric, the body moves to a posture at the shortest distance from the initial posture; this implies the existence of a minimization principle that, together with all constraints, determines how the system moves. Because the distance depends on biomechanical constraints, the posture that is geometrically closest to the initial posture may not be the closest in the neurophysiological sense, especially in the presence of obstacles or external forces. For example, in the presence of the gravitational force, the body will reach an equilibrium posture $(Q_e)$ but not the R posture, since the balance of all forces at the latter cannot be established. It is also important that, constrained by the metrics and external conditions, the motor response of the system to a change in the R configuration is produced without any redundancy problems. Redundancy problems would exist only if all body postures were equivalent and it would be necessary to intentionally choose between them each time the system moves.

The referent configuration can be considered a virtual geometrical image of the body (cf. Decety, 1996; Decety and Ingvar, 1990) with which the actual configuration is compared to generate motor actions. In this strategy, the goal of the system is not to reach the R configuration; in most cases this may be physically impossible because of gravitational force. Regardless of the specific R configurations used for action, what is essential for the system is whether or not the resulting, actual configuration of the body, Q, is consistent with reaching the goal in the environment, for example, grasping an object. If the Q configuration is not adequate, the system corrects the R configuration until the resulting Q configuration is satisfactory.

The notion of the referent body configuration is reminiscent of the idea of Rosenbaum et al. (1993) that the nervous system produces movements by changing the body posture, combined with memorized (but weighted) body postures. The postural control in Rosenbaum and colleagues' hypothesis was not described in terms of specific neurophysiological variables, such as muscle activation thresholds in the referent configuration hypothesis. Therefore, in its present form, Rosenbaum and colleagues' hypothesis does not address the issue of how postural control is related to EMG patterns. In addition, in some mechanical conditions, the actual posture cannot be changed by control levels. For example, the elbow angle cannot be changed in isometric conditions. Rosenbaum and colleagues' hypothesis does not explain how the system is controlled in such cases. These deficiencies of the hypothesis can easily be corrected by assuming that the nervous system memorizes and specifies an appropriate not actual but virtual R configuration of the body, in response to which the actual body postures emerge. In isometric conditions, the actual configuration remains the same, but the distance between Q and R is modified by changes in the R configuration, resulting in isometric muscle forces.

How does the nervous system specify the appropriate referent configurations of the body? Before addressing this question, we describe the results of experiments confirming the existence of such configurations.

## Experimental Testing of the Referent Body Configuration

As mentioned earlier, the necessity of balancing gravitational torques prevents the body from reaching the referent configuration at which the active joint torques are zero. Consider, however, movements with reversal in direction. Such movements are produced by reversing the changes in the R configuration. Initially, the body follows the changes in the R configuration, with some delay determined, in particular, by the inertia of the body. Due to this delay, for some time after the changes in the R configuration are reversed, the body follows the preceding R configuration. Moving toward each other, the actual and the referent configurations temporarily match ($Q = R$). This is illustrated schematically for sit-to-stand-to-sit movements in figure 1.6. In the absence of a coactivation command, the R configuration is, by definition, the configuration of the body at which the activation thresholds of all muscles are reached simultaneously. Thus, the matching of the two configurations is associated with a global minimum of muscle activity, with the depth of the minimum limited by the coactivation command.

Unexpectedly, a global activity minimum can be observed in many body movements with reversal. We illustrate this phenomenon for several movements in figures 1.7 through 1.9: sit-to-stand-to-sit movements (figure 1.7; Feldman et al., 1998),

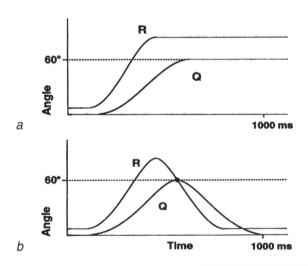

**Figure 1.6**   Theoretical diagrams showing the referent (R) and the resulting actual (Q) head positions for sit-to-stand movements *(a)* without and *(b)* with reversal. The referent and the actual positions temporarily match each other at the intersection point in *b* when the R configuration is reversed.

head movements following reversible shifts in a visual target (figure 1.8; Lestienne et al., 2000), and leg movements produced by ballet dancers (figure 1.9; Thullier and Lestienne, 2002; Thullier and Plotkin, 2001). In sit-to-stand-to-sit movements in humans (figure 1.7), the EMG activity recorded from 16 functionally diverse muscles of the arm, trunk, and legs was minimized during the transition from rising to lowering the body.

During totally free head rotations about a vertical axis from a neutral position toward and away from a lateral position by monkeys, the intramuscular EMG activity recorded from seven pairs of functionally diverse neck muscles was also minimized

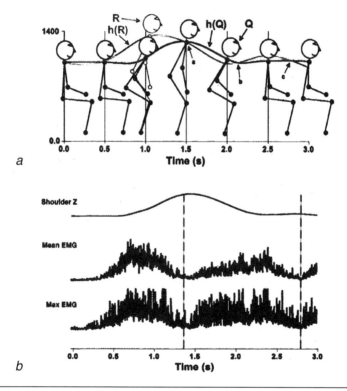

**Figure 1.7** Sit-to-stand movement with reversal by humans. *(a)* Configuration of the body (sagittal plane) when the subject stands up while pointing to a target and then returns to the sitting position. The time interval between each image is 500 ms. The hypothetical referent body configuration and the referent shoulder position are shown in gray. *(b)* EMG activity of each muscle was normalized (according to the amplitude) to compute the mean and maximal EMG activity of 16 muscles involved in the movement (deltoideus anterior, pectoralis major, latissimus dorsi, dorsal extensors of the thorax, dorsal extensors of the lumbar vertebrae, obliquus internus, rectus abdominis, obliquus externus, tensor fasciae latae, gluteus maximus, medial hamstring, lateral hamstring, quadriceps femoris, vastus medialis, tibialis anterior, and lateral gastrocnemius).

Adapted from Feldman et al. (1998).

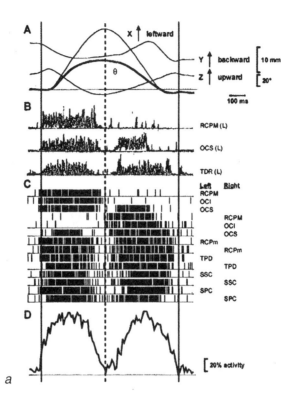

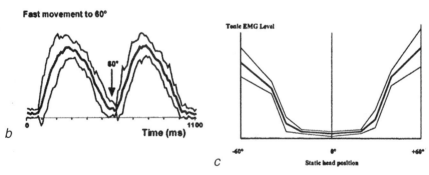

**Figure 1.8** Horizontal head rotation with reversal by monkeys. *(a)* Kinematic variables and EMG activity of seven pairs of dorsal neck muscles (rectus capitis posterior minor and major, obliquus capitis inferior and superior, trapezius pars descendens, semispinalis capitis, and splenius capitis) during fast head movement from neutral (resting) position to 60° left and back. *(b)* Mean of the normalized EMG activities of the seven pairs of neck muscles for 10 rapid repetitions of the movement described in *a*. *(c)* Ensemble tonic EMG levels at the right (–60°), left (60°), and intermediate (0°) head positions to which the head moved and then stayed after the movement.

Adapted from Lestienne et al. (2000).

during reversals of the movement at the two positions where the lateral deviation of the head from the neutral position became maximal (figure 1.8, *a* and *b*). In contrast, at the same lateral positions, the EMG activity of neck muscles was maximal if these positions were reached and maintained (figure 1.8*c*). When the position was maintained, EMG activity at the appropriate muscles was apparently necessary to counterbalance the gravitational torque acting on the unrestrained head as well as the elastic torque of the stretched contralateral muscles. Thus, a global EMG minimum occurred only in dynamic situations, when the head movements were reversed.

In expert ballet dancers, a global minimum in the EMG activity of muscles of the right leg was observed when they moved the toe of the right foot along a straight line with reversal (figure 1.9). To make this movement, it was necessary to stabilize the body while standing on the left leg, and therefore muscles of the

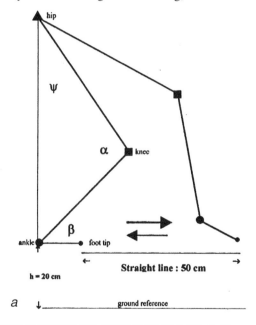

**Figure 1.9**   Leg movement in which the toe of the right leg traveled along the straight line, with reversal, by a ballet dancer standing on the left leg. *(a)* Stick diagram of movement. *(b)* The upper 10 traces show the EMG activity of 8 muscles of the right leg (GL, BF, S, VL, VM, P, TA, GM) and 2 muscles of the back (RAbd, LBE) on the right side of the body in one of 10 repetitions of the movement. The lower 3 traces show EMG activity of muscles (RF, BF, GL) of the left leg. (c) The rectified, normalized, and averaged activity of the 8 muscles of the right leg (solid line). Dotted lines show ± standard deviation. Arrows mark the instants when the integral activity of these muscles becomes minimal. Abbreviations for muscles: BF – biceps femoris; GL – gastrocnemeus lateralis; GM – gluteus maximus; LBE – lumbar back extensor; P – psoas; RAbd – rectus abdominis; RF – rectus femoris; S – soleus; TA – tibialis anterior; VL – vastus lateralis; VM – vastus medialis.

Adapted from Lestienne and Feldman (2002).

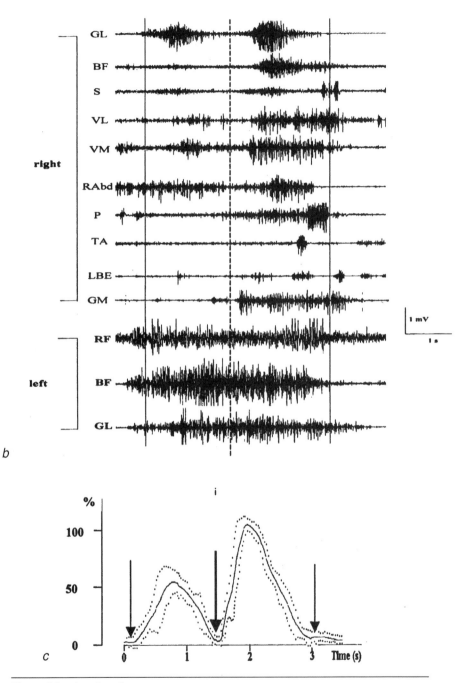

*b*

*c*

**Figure 1.9** *(continued)*

left leg remained tonically active. In addition, experienced ballet dancers tended to make this movement in an elegant way by stabilizing the head, pelvis, and the trunk. The EMG activity of 14 muscles of the trunk, pelvis, and both legs was recorded. Despite the functional and anatomical diversity of muscles of the right leg, their activity was minimized at the reversal phase of the movement (figure 1.9).

It has been found (e.g., Bernstein, 1967) that the nervous system often takes advantage of different external forces as well as of both passive elastic muscle forces and those accumulated by preceding activation. It was unclear, however, how the neuromuscular system is controlled to achieve this effect. The referent configuration hypothesis gives an example of how this might be done: By reversing the changes in the R configuration, the system minimizes the muscles' EMG activity and lets the external and elastic forces come into play.

Indeed, the existence of global minima in the overall EMG activity of skeletal muscles is not the only prediction of the referent configuration hypothesis. An immediate consequence of the hypothesis is that the EMG patterns should be direction dependent, a phenomenon known as directional tuning of muscles. This is because the changes in the R configuration, for example, of the arm used to produce arm movements are different for different movement directions. As a consequence, the emergent EMG patterns are also direction specific. Direction-specific changes in the R configuration are also produced to grade isometric forces, so the emergent EMG patterns in isometric tasks are also direction specific. Indeed, directional tuning applies not only to muscles and motoneurons but also to any spinal or supraspinal neurons involved in movement or isometric force generation. The directional tuning of motoneurons and neurons has been observed in numerous studies (Georgopoulos et al., 1982, 1992; Hasan and Karst, 1989; Sergio and Kalaska, 1998; Weijs et al., 1999).

## Guiding Movements Without Redundancy Problems

The problem of multimuscle redundancy has been solved in the theoretical framework postulating that all muscles of the body generate their activity constrained by the difference between the actual and the referent configurations. This global factor in combination with individual anatomical and biomechanical properties of muscles diversifies their EMG patterns. The efficiency of such a multimuscle control strategy has been illustrated by simulation of movements of the spinal column produced by 160 muscles (Beauséjour et al., 1999).

The reason that numerous theoretical solutions of redundancy problems have been unsuccessful, to our view, is that they were based on the mistaken assumption that the nervous system solves these problems by dealing directly with output variables.

Thus, a solution to the problem of joint redundancy should be sought in terms of control parameters, an approach that has been successful in the solution of the problem of muscle redundancy (as discussed earlier). That solution was based on the assumption that individual FRs for activation of muscles are embedded into a hierarchically higher FR: the FR for body configuration in which all muscles are controlled as a coherent whole. A similar idea might help to solve the problem of joint redundancy. Specifically, consider all possible R configurations and appropriate configurational FRs used by the nervous system. We can assume that the configurational FRs are embedded in a higher FR associated with the body surface and the environment in which goal-directed actions are produced. We clarify this idea by applying it to pointing movements, although it is applicable to many actions in the environment, including locomotion.

It seems natural to suggest that there are neurons at spinal and supraspinal levels that project onto motoneurons of skeletal muscles and integrate proprioceptive signals from different muscles and joints as well as skin afferent signals, thus receiving influences that depend on the coordinates of the effector (e.g., the tip of the index finger in pointing movements). By analogy with motoneurons, independent control influences on these neurons can be interpreted as specifying the threshold (referent) coordinates of the endpoint. Control levels may shift these referent coordinates in an FR associated with the environment to produce a referent trajectory for the effector. The difference between the actual and the referent coordinates determines whether or not such neurons are activated and eventually influence motoneurons of arm and trunk muscles to produce an actual trajectory.

The control signals that change the referent coordinates of the arm endpoint result in a change in the neural activity that perturbs the initial interactions between different components of the neuromuscular system: neurons, muscles, external forces, and proprioceptive loops. The whole hierarchical structure is guided by a minimization principle following from the rule that, in each FR, the activity of different components of the neuromuscular systems depends on the difference between the actual and referent (threshold) values of appropriate variables, and the emergent muscle activity drives the system in the direction that tends to diminish the difference and thus minimize the activity, within the limits determined by task constraints. The muscle-reflex system clearly shows this tendency: In response to activation, muscles shorten, allowing homonymous and heteronymous proprioceptive feedback to diminish the activity. Moreover, proprioceptive systems contribute to this minimization in two ways: by changing the activity of motoneurons depending on output (i.e., mechanical variables) and by changing their thresholds depending on the speed of changes in muscle length (Feldman and Levin, 1995) and afferent influences from synergists and antagonists (Feldman and Orlovsky, 1972; Matthews, 1959). Thus, the minimization of activity in the system is achieved not only by moving the body in the appropriate direction but also by adjusting the values of control parameters at subordinate levels, a self-regulatory process reminiscent of the principle of minimal interaction postulated for neuronal ensembles by Gelfand and Tsetlin (1971; see also chapter 5 by Latash and colleagues in this book).

In the framework of the $\lambda$ model, the principle of minimal interaction is described by the following points.

1. Activity of each component of the neuromuscular system depends on the difference between the actual (physical) and the referent (threshold) values

of appropriate variables. The values of the physical variables are transmitted to the elements by appropriate afferent systems, whereas independent control signals determine the referent values for these variables.

2.  Active movements or isometric torques are produced by shifting the referent values of physical variables.

3.  The afferent feedback to each element and the interactions between different elements are specifically organized to drive the system to a state in which the difference between the physical and actual variables, and thus the overall activity in the system, is minimized, within the limits determined by task constraints.

In the theoretical framework outlined here, pointing movements are produced in the following way. Control levels shift the referent coordinates of the effector in an external FR along a referent trajectory. The response of the system is guided by the principle of minimal interaction that imposes changes in the referent configuration of the body and in individual activation thresholds of muscles. As a consequence, the actual configuration of the body will change, and the effector will move along an actual trajectory until a final arm configuration associated with minimal activity in the system is reestablished. The actual and referent trajectories of the effector may not coincide due to several biomechanical factors. In particular, in movements in a horizontal plane, the weight of the arm segments deflects the actual hand trajectory downward relative to the referent one. One can produce referent trajectories rising at some angle from a horizontal plane to make the resulting actual trajectory horizontal. In general, if the final position of the effector is different from its desired target position, control levels may adjust the referent shifts so that the movement error is nullified. In the same framework, different physiological mechanisms—in particular, coactivation commands—diminish the sensitivity of the actual hand trajectory to mechanical perturbations, arm inertia, or velocity-dependent torques acting between adjacent segments (Feldman and Levin, 1995).

We have thus outlined noncomputational, dynamic solutions to the problems of multimuscle and multijoint redundancy. These solutions do not reject the notion of synergies or the recently proposed classification of multijoint coordination into two types (controlled and uncontrolled manifolds) that are more essential and less essential, respectively, for reaching the motor goal (for details see Latash and colleagues' chapter 5 in this volume). Rather, our solutions suggest that synergies or manifolds, like trajectories and forces, may be emergent properties of the neuromuscular behavior resulting from the response of the system to changes in control parameters in specific environmental conditions.

## Conclusions

Our analysis illustrates several points important for the understanding of perception and action. First, mechanical terminology (force, position, velocity, acceleration, stiffness, viscosity, resting muscle length, inertial and interactive torques, etc.) is a necessary part of any description of movement production. It is time to acknowledge, however, that Bernstein, Von Holst, and many others were right in suggesting that the question of how movements are controlled by the brain cannot be answered in a mechanical framework. Nor can it be answered in a mechanical framework complemented by the notion of the brain's direct involvement in the programming of EMG patterns. These researchers' ideas should especially be stressed when the dominant theories (inverse dynamic computations based on internal models) reduce the problem of motor control to the programming of mechanical variables and EMG activity.

Second, deafferentation experiments were successful in demonstrating that movements can be produced in the absence of proprioceptive signals. However, these experiments failed to address the question of how these signals are integrated with independent control signals in intact organisms.

Third, the explanation of how movements can be produced without triggering the resistance of posture-stabilizing mechanisms to deviations from the initial posture (the posture–movement problem) might be the first criterion in establishing the validity of a theory of motor control. For such an explanation, it is necessary but not sufficient to postulate a mechanism of shifts in the equilibrium position of the neuromuscular system. For example, in force control models, it is typically assumed that shifts in the equilibrium position of the arm are produced by changing the activity of arm muscles, an assumption that does not solve the posture–movement problem.

Fourth, the posture–movement problem has been solved in experimental studies showing that postural resetting and the resulting movements are produced by shifts in muscle activation thresholds, an empirical fact underlying the $\lambda$ model for motor control. It has been demonstrated that the $\lambda$ model has the capacity to explain these phenomena: the movement kinematics and EMG patterns of pointing movements, adaptation of these movements to different force fields and inertial and interactive torques, and the appearance of positional errors in the presence of Coriolis forces, that is, inequifinality, a phenomenon that was mistakenly considered to conflict with the model. (Although the $\lambda$ model predicts the possibility of equifinal behavior in some conditions, it does not claim that equifinality is a universal phenomenon that should be observed in all cases of intermittent perturbations.)

Fifth, we generalized the model by introducing the concept of action-producing frames of reference. In particular, all possible configurations of the body can be considered as points in a frame in which a referent configuration specified by brain control levels acts as origin. Each muscle's activation depends on the difference between the actual and the referent body configurations. The concept of action-producing frames of reference in combination with the principle of minimal interaction of neuromuscular systems explains how control levels may guide multimuscle and multijoint systems without redundancy problems.

# Acknowledgments

This work was supported by the CIHR, NSERC, and FCAR (Canada) and DAT/793/CNES/99/7694 and 793/CNES/2000/8202 (France). We thank Mindy Levin for helpful comments on the manuscript. The studies of postural control in weightlessness described here that suggest the existence of a postural body scheme (Lestienne and Gurfinkel, 1988a; 1988b) were carried out at the Centre National d'Etudes Spatiales during several space flights, in close collaboration with Professor Victor Gurfinkel from the Institute for Information Transmission Problems (Russian Academy of Science).

# References

Adamovich, S.V., Levin, M.F., and Feldman, A.G. (1997) Central modification of reflex parameters may underlie the fastest arm movement. *J Neurophysiol* 77: 1460-1469.

Adrian, M. (1947) *The physiological background of perception.* Oxford: Clarendon Press.

Asatryan, D.G., and Feldman, A.G. (1965) Functional tuning of the nervous system with control of movement or maintenance of a steady posture: I. Mechanographic analysis of the work of the limb on execution of a postural task. *Biophysics* 10: 925-935.

Beauséjour, M., Aubin, C.É., Feldman, A.G., and Labelle, H. (1999) Simulations de tests d'inflexion latérale à l'aide d'un modèle musculo-squelettique du tronc. *Ann Chir* 53: 742-750.

Beevor, C.E. (1904) *The Croonian lectures on muscular movements and their representation in the central nervous system.* London: Adlar.

Bernstein, N.A. (1935) The problem of interrelation between coordination and localization [in Russian]. *Arch Biol Sci* 38: 1-35.

Bernstein, N.A. (1967) *The coordination and regulation of movements.* London: Pergamon Press.

Berthoz, A. (1996) *Le sens du mouvement.* Paris: Odile Jacob.

Bizzi, E., Hogan, N., Mussa-Ivaldi, F.A., and Giszter, S. (1992) Does the nervous system use equilibrium-point control to guide single and multiple joint movements? *Behav Brain Sci* 15: 603-613.

Bizzi, E., Polit, A., and Morasso, P. (1976) Mechanisms underlying achievement of final head position. *J Neurophysiol* 39: 435-444.

Bossom, J. (1974) Movement without proprioception. *Brain Res* 71: 285-296.

Brown, T.G. (1911) The intrinsic factors in the act of progression in the mammal. *Proc R Soc Lond B Biol Sci* 84: 308-319.

Cirstea, M.C., and Levin, M.F. (2000) Compensatory strategies for reaching in stroke. *Brain* 123: 940-953.

Clément, G., Gurfinkel, V.S., Lestienne, F.G., Lipshits, M.I., and Popov, K.E. (1984) Adaptation of postural control to weightlessness. *Exp Brain Res* 57: 61-72.

Colby, C.L. (1998) Action-oriented spatial reference frames in cortex. *Neuron* 20: 15-24.

Damasio, A.R. (1994) *Descartes' error.* New York: Putnam.

Decety, J. (1996) The neurophysiological basis of motor imagery. *Behav Brain Res* 77: 45-52.

Decety, J., and Ingvar, D.H. (1990) Brain structures participating in mental simulation of motor behavior: A neurophysiological interpretation. *Acta Psychol* 73: 13-34.

Deliagina, T.G., Feldman, A.G., Gelfand, I.M., and Orlovsky, G.N. (1975) On the role of central program and afferent inflow in the control of scratching movements in the cat. *Brain Res* 100: 297-313.

Feldman, A.G. (1966) Functional tuning of the nervous system with control of movement or maintenance of a steady posture: II. Controllable parameters of the muscle. *Biophysics* 11: 565-578.

Feldman, A.G. (1986) Once more on the equilibrium point hypothesis ($\lambda$-model) for motor control. *J Mot Behav* 18: 17-54.

Feldman, A.G., Archambault, P., and Lestienne, F.G. (1999) Multi-muscle control is based on the specification of referent body image. In Gantchev, G.N., Mori, S., and Massion, J. (Eds.), *Motor control, today and tomorrow,* pp. 163-179. Sofia: Academic Publishing House "Prof. M. Drinov."

Feldman, A.G., and Levin, M.F. (1993) Control variables and related concepts in motor control. *Concepts Neurosci* 4: 21-51.

Feldman, A.G., and Levin, M.F. (1995) Positional frames of reference in motor control: The origin and use. *Behav Brain Sci* 18: 723-806.

Feldman, A.G., Levin, M.F., Mitnitski, A., and Archambault, P. (1998) Multi-muscle control in human movements. Keynote lecture. *J Electromyogr Kinesiol* 8: 383-390.

Feldman, A.G., and Orlovsky, G.N. (1972) The influence of different descending systems on the tonic reflex in the cat. *Exp Neurol* 37: 481-494.

Flash, T., and Hogan, N. (1985) The coordination of arm movements: An experimentally confirmed mathematical model. *J Neurosci* 5: 1688-1703.

Fukson, O.I., Berkinblit, M.B., and Feldman, A.G. (1980) The spinal frog takes into account the scheme of its body during the wiping reflex. *Science* 209: 1261-1263.

Gelfand, L.M., and Tsetlin, M.L. (1971) Some methods of controlling complex systems. In Gelfand, L.M., Gurfinkel, V.S., Fomin, S.V., and Tsetlin, M.L. (Eds.), *Models of structural-functional organization of certain biological systems,* pp. 329-345. Cambridge: MIT Press.

Georgopoulos, A.P., Ashe, J., Smyrnis, N., and Taira, M. (1992) The motor cortex and the coding of force. *Science* 233: 1416-1419.

Georgopoulos, A.P., Kalaska, J.F., Caminiti, R., and Massey, J.T. (1982) On the relations between the direction of two-dimensional arm movements and cell discharge in primate motor cortex. *J Neurosci* 2: 1527-1537.

Ghafouri, M., and Lestienne, F.G. (1996) Gesture orientation and trajectory deformation in the three dimensional space. In Harling, P.H., and Edwards, A. (Eds.), *Progress in gestural interaction,* pp. 227-234. New York: Springer-Verlag.

Ghafouri, M., and Lestienne, F.G. (2000) Altered representation of egocentric peripersonal space in elderly. *Neurosci Lett* 289: 193-196.

Gribble, P.L., and Ostry, D.J. (1996) Origins of the power law relation between movement velocity and curvature: Modeling the effects of muscle mechanics and limb dynamics. *J Neurophysiol* 76: 2853-2860.

Gurfinkel, V., Lestienne, F., Levik, Y., and Popov, K.E. (1993) Egocentric references and human spatial orientation in microgravity: 1. Perception of complex tactile stimuli. *Exp Brain Res* 95: 339-342.

Gurfinkel, V., Lestienne, F.G., Levik, Y., Popov, K.E., and Lefort, L. (1993) Egocentric references and human spatial orientation in microgravity: 2. Body centered coordinates in the task of drawing ellipses with prescribed orientation. *Exp Brain Res* 95: 343-348.

Hannaford, B., and Winters, J.M. (1990) Actuators properties and movement control: Biological and technological models. In Winters, J.M., and Woo, S.L.-Y. (Eds.), *Multiple muscle systems: Biomechanics and movement organization,* pp. 101-119. New York: Springer-Verlag.

Hasan, Z., and Karst, G.M. (1989) Muscle activity for initiation of planar two-joint arm movements in different directions. *Exp Brain Res* 76: 651-655.

Head, H., and Holmes, G. (1911) Sensory disturbances from cerebral lesions. *Brain* 34: 102-244.

Henneman, E. (1981) Recruitment of motoneurons: The size principle. In Desmedt, J.E. (Ed.), *Progress in clinical neurophysiology: Vol. 9. Motor unit types, recruitment and plasticity in health and disease.* Basel: Karger.

Higgins, J.R., and Angel, R.W. (1970) Correction of tracking errors without sensory feedback. *J Exp Psychol* 84: 412-416.

Hogan, N., and Flash, T. (1987) Moving gracefully: Quantitative theories of motor coordination. *TINS* 10: 170-174.

Hollerbach, J.M., and Atkeson, C.G. (1987) Deducing planning variables from experimental arm trajectories: Pitfalls and possibilities. *Biol Cybern* 56: 279-292.

Houk, J.C., and Rymer, W.Z. (1981) Neural control of muscle length and tension. In Brookhart, J.M., Mountcastle, V.B., and Geiger, S.R. (Eds.), *Handbook of physiology: Section 1. The nervous system: Vol. 2. Motor control.* Bethesda, MD: American Physiological Society.

Jeannerod, M. (1997) *The cognitive neuroscience of action.* Oxford: Blackwell.

Jobin, A., and Levin, M.F. (2000) Regulation and stretch reflex threshold in elbow flexors in children with cerebral palsy: A new measure of spasticity. *Develop Med Child Neurol* 42: 531-540.

Kawato, M., Furukawa, K., and Susuki, R. (1987) A hierarchical neural network model for control and learning of voluntary movements. *Biol Cybern* 57: 169-185.

Keele, S.W. (1968) Movement control in skilled motor performance. *Psychol Bull* 70: 387-403.

Koshland, G.F., and Hasan, Z. (1994) Selection of muscles for initiation of planar three joint arm movements with different final orientations of the hand. *Exp Brain Res* 98: 157-162.

Lacquaniti, F. (1992) Automatic control of limb movement and posture. *Curr Opin Neurobiol* 2: 807-814.

Lashley, K.S. (1951). The problem of serial order in behavior. In Jeffress, L.A. (Ed.), *Cerebral mechanisms in behavior.* New York: Wiley.

Latash, M.L. (1993) *Control of human movement.* Champaign, IL: Human Kinetics.

Lestienne, F.G. (1979) Effects of inertial load and velocity on the braking process of voluntary limb movements. *Exp Brain Res* 35: 407-418.

Lestienne, F.G., and Feldman, A.G. (2001) Du schéma corporel au concept de Configuration de Référence: Une approche théorique de la production du mouvement. *Evolutions Psychomotrices* 53: 127-143.

Lestienne, F.G., and Feldman, A.G. (2002) Une approche théorique de la production du mouvement: Du modèle lambda au concept de "Configuration de Référence Productrice d'Actions." *Sci Motricité* 45: 63-84.

Lestienne, F.G., Ghafouri, M., and Thullier, F. (1995) What does body configuration in microgravity tell us about the contribution of intra and extrapersonal frames? *Behav Brain Res* 18: 766-767.

Lestienne, F.G., and Gurfinkel, V.S. (1997) Réflexions sur le concept de représentation interne: Le contrôle du mouvement et de l'attitude posturale. In Petit, J.L. (Ed.), *Les neurosciences et la philosophie de l'action,* pp. 177-198. Paris: Librairie Philosophique J. Vrin.

Lestienne, F.G., and Gurfinkel, V.S. (1988a) Postural control in weightlessness: A dual process underlying adaptation to an unusual environment. *TINS* 11: 359-363.

Lestienne, F.G., and Gurfinkel, V. (1988b) Posture as an organizational structure based on a dual process: A formal basis to interpret change of posture in weightlessness. *Prog Brain Res* 76: 307-313.

Lestienne, F.G., Le Goff, B., and Liverneaux, P. (1995) Head movement trajectory in three-dimensional space during orienting behavior towards visual targets in rhesus monkeys. *Exp Brain Res* 102: 393-406.

Lestienne, F.G., Thullier, F., Archambault, P., Levin, M.F., and Feldman, A.G. (2000) Multi-muscle control of head movements in monkeys: The referent configuration hypothesis. *Neurosci Lett* 283: 65-68.

Levin, M.F., and Dimov, M. (1997) Spatial zones for muscle coactivation and the control of postural stability. *Brain Res* 757: 43-59.

Levin, M.F., Selles, R.W., Verheul, M.H., and Meijer, O.G. (2000) Deficits in the coordination of agonist and antagonist muscles in stroke patients: Implications for normal motor control. *Brain Res* 853: 352-369.

Liverneaux, P.A., and Lestienne, F.G. (1989) Morpho-anatomy and muscle synergies of the cervical spine during head orienting movements. In Louis, R., and Wiedner, A. (Eds.), *Cervical spine II,* pp. 112-116. New York: Springer.

Loeb, G.E., and Levine, W.S. (1990) Linking musculoskeletal mechanics to sensorimotor neurophysiology. In Winters, J.M., and Woo, S.L.-Y. (Eds.), *Multiple muscle systems: Biomechanics and movement organization,* pp. 121-130. New York: Springer-Verlag.

Matthews, P.B.C. (1959) The dependence of tension upon extension in the stretch reflex of the soleus muscle in the decerebrated cat. *J Physiol (Lond)* 147: 521-546.

Merton, P.A. (1953) Speculation on the servo-control of movement. In *The spinal cord: A Ciba foundation symposium,* pp. 247-260. London: Churchill.

Nichols, T.R. (1994) A biomechanical perspective on spinal mechanisms of coordinated muscular action: An architecture principle. *Acta Anat* 151: 1-13.

Orlovsky, G.N., Deliagina, T.G., and Grillner, S. (1999) *Neural control of locomotion: From mollusk to man.* New York: Oxford University Press.

Pailhous, J., and Bonnard, M. (1989) Programmation et contrôle du mouvement. In Bonnet, C., Ghiglione, R., and Richard, J.-F. (Eds.), *Traité de psychologie cognitive,* pp. 129-197. Paris: Dunod.

Paillard, J. (1971). Les déterminants moteurs de l'organisation spatiale. In Jeddi, J. (Ed.), *Le corps en psychiatrie*, pp. 53-69. Paris: Masson.

Perrin, P. and Lestienne, F.G. (1994) *Mécanismes de l'équilibration humaine*. Paris: Masson.

Piaget, J. (1936) *La naissance de l'intelligence chez l'enfant*. Neuchâtel, Switzerland: Delachaux and Niestlé.

Poincaré, H. (1968) *La science et l'hypothèse*. Paris: Flammarion. (Original work published in 1902)

Raibert, M.H. (1986) *Legged robots that balance*. Cambridge: MIT Press.

Rosenbaum, D.A., Engelbrecht, S.E., Bushe, M.M., and Loucopoulos, L.D. (1993) Knowledge model for selecting and producing reaching movements. *J Mot Behav* 25: 217-227.

Schmidt, R.A. (1975) A schema theory of discrete motor skill learning. *Psychol Rev* 82: 225-260.

Schmidt, R.A. (1988) *Motor control and learning: A behavioral emphasis*. Champaign, IL: Human Kinetics.

Schweighofer, N., Arbib, M.A., and Kawato, M. (1998) Role of the cerebellum in reaching movements in humans: I. Distributed inverse dynamic control. *Eur J Neurosci* 10: 86-94.

Seashore, C.E. (1938) *Psychology of music*. New York: Academic Press.

Sergio, L.E., and Kalaska, J.F. (1998) Changes in the temporal pattern of primary motor cortex activity in a directional isometric force versus limb movement task. *J Neurophysiol* 80: 1577-1583.

Shadmehr, R., and Mussa-Ivaldi, F. (1994) Adaptive representation of dynamics during learning of a motor task. *J Neurosci* 14: 3208-3224.

Sherrington, C.S. (1947) *The integrative action of the nervous system*. New Haven, CT: Yale University Press. (Original work published in 1906)

Slotine, J.-J., and Li, W. (1991) *Applied nonlinear control*. Englewood Cliffs, NJ: Prentice Hall.

Taub, E. (1976) Movement in nonhuman primates deprived of somatosensory feedback. *Exerc Sports Sci Rev* 4: 335-374.

Tax, A.A.M., Denier van der Gon, J.J., Gielen, C.C.A.M., and van den Tempel, C.M.M. (1989) Differences in the activation of m. biceps brachii in the control of slow isotonic movements and isometric contractions. *Exp Brain Res* 76: 55-63.

Terzuolo, C., and Viviani, P. (1980) Determinants and characteristics of motor patterns used for typing. *Neurosci* 5: 1085-1103.

Thullier, F., and Lestienne, F.G. (2002) Multi-joint coordination during drawing ellipsoidal figures with leg in ballet dancers. *Arch. Physiol. & Biochem.*, 110:23.

Thullier, F., and Plotkin, E. (2001) Orientation du geste graphique dans l'espace tridimensionnel: Coordination pluri-articulaire au cours de l'exécution du "rond de jambe" chez le danseur. *Sci Motricité* 43-44: 115-116.

Todorov, E. (2000) Direct cortical control of muscle activation in voluntary arm movements: A model. *Nature Neurosci* 3: 391-398.

Turvey, M.T. (1977) Preliminaries to a theory of action with reference to vision. In Shaw, R., and Hillsdale, J., *Perceiving, acting and knowing: Toward an ecological psychology*. Hillsdale, NJ: Erlbaum.

Von Holst, E., and Mittelstaedt, H. (1973) The reafference principle: Interaction between the central nervous system and the periphery. In Martin, R. (Ed.), *The collected papers of Erich von Holst*, pp. 139-173. Coral Gables, FL: University of Miami. (Original work published in 1950)

Wallace, S.A. (1981) An impulse-timing theory for reciprocal control of muscular activity in rapid, discrete movements. *J Mot Behav* 13: 144-160.

Weijs, W.A., Sugimura, T., and van Ruijven, L.J. (1999) Motor coordination in a multi-muscle system as revealed by principal component analysis of electromyographic variation. *Exp Brain Res* 127: 233-243.

Wolpert, D.M., Gharamani, Z., and Joardan, M.J. (1995) An internal model for sensorimotor integration. *Science* 269: 1179-1182.

# 2

# Computational Models and Geometric Approaches in Arm Trajectory Control Studies

*Tamar Flash*
Weizmann Institute of Science

*Magnus E. Richardson*
Ecole Normale Superieure

*Amir A. Handzel*
University of Maryland

*Dario G. Liebermann*
Tel-Aviv University

The control of human goal-directed motor behavior requires that the nervous system carry out extremely complicated computations. While these computations are still poorly understood, over the last decade research has been conducted to gain better understanding of the information-processing and control mechanisms subserving human movement generation.

There are many hypotheses concerning the nature of the motion-planning and control strategies that underlie movement generation in biological systems in general and in humans in particular. These theoretical hypotheses have been based on experimental studies of particular motor tasks. Although the strategies employed by the nervous system may vary among different tasks, the planning and control principles that we seek to unravel should be as widely applicable as possible while at the same time as computationally simple as possible. Mathematical models to investigate and analyze human motor control strategies are therefore needed, with the goal of simplifying and unifying current theories. In this chapter, the plausibility of this approach is demonstrated for the arm in a wide variety of motor tasks and movements. In particular, the models presented here focus on attempts to unravel the strategies subserving the nervous system in overcoming or utilizing the excess degrees of freedom that exist at both the task and articulator levels during hand trajectory generation. The main premise of our approach is that the brain makes intelligent and efficient use of the abundant possibilities available to perform any motor task by selecting the optimal performance strategies for that particular task. This possibility of optimal selection of particular motor actions among the large number of possible ones might be one of the sources of the flexibility and richness of natural motor behavior in biological systems, which are unmatched by any current artificial system.

In general, the area of motor control research is strongly interrelated with robotics, which shares a similar goal of translating perception into action (Hollerbach, 1982). Over the last two decades, a rich exchange of ideas has taken place between the research fields of biological motor control and robotics (Atkeson et al., 2000; Schaal, 1999). In particular, robotics has proven to be a useful medium for suggesting and testing ideas about biological motor control. Likewise, since human capabilities far surpass those of artificial systems, insights gained from the study of biological motor control can provide useful ideas on how to design and control robotic systems.

Thus, in addition to the basic goal in human motor control research of unraveling the principles that underlie movement generation by the brain, a further important goal is to identify and characterize those algorithms for their possible future use in both rehabilitation and robotics. In particular, there is recent interest in designing robotic systems (e.g., humanoid robots) that can operate in unaltered human environments (Atkeson et al., 2000; Schaal, 1999). Such robots should be able to move and manipulate objects in the same fashion as humans. For this to be possible, it is necessary first to gain a better understanding of how humans move and then to develop models that describe in a mathematically concise way the principles that underlie the generation of such movements.

However, it is not generally clear if it is always advantageous for artificial manipulators or even humanoid robots to use the same motion planning strategies as humans use. It is widely assumed that humans perform movements that are optimal in some sense, but what is optimal for the human arm and nervous system might well be suboptimal or overly restrictive for a robotic arm and its controller. For example, researchers recently suggested that humans plan reaching movements that minimize the errors in achieving the final target, which are caused by the noise existing in different biological components (Harris, 1998; Harris and Wolpert, 1998). Although this hypothesis predicted trajectories that were in excellent agreement with experimental results, the underlying principle does not translate well to robots. In digital systems, noise is not a significant issue, and hence movements based on this hypothesis would indeed be rather restrictive.

In this chapter, some current formulations of human motor control strategies are reviewed. In particular, we present a group of models that focus on the kinematic characteristics of hand trajectories expressed in terms of spatial coordinates during the generation of point-to-point and curved movements. This group of models assumes that the motor system selects hand trajectories that maximize motion smoothness. The concept of smoothness here relates to reducing the magnitude of higher-order derivatives of position with respect to time. It is possible therefore to consider alternative smoothness criteria, each associated with a different order of differentiation of position with respect to time. We also briefly compare the success of such models in accounting for the behavior observed during both reaching and drawing movements. We then describe an alternative model, the so-called two-thirds power law, for curved and drawing movements and present our attempts to unify this law with optimization models, in particular with the smoothness maximization models.

A fundamental question concerning movement representation within the brain is what metrics are used for these representations. We describe in this chapter a mathematical framework involving the use of affine differential geometry that we have recently developed for the description of human movements. As summarized here, this framework can serve as a powerful tool for the description of both two-dimensional (2D) and three-dimensional (3D) hand trajectories.

In the first few sections of the chapter, we focus on kinematic analysis and modeling of hand trajectories expressed in terms of spatial coordinates. However, the generation of multijoint motor behavior also requires the nervous system to specify the trajectories of individual joints and to coordinate different joint rotations. Hence, another level with excess degrees of freedom is that of joint planning. Consequently, another fundamental question in upper-limb motor control research is what principles dictate the selection and specification of the kinematic features of joint rotations and the temporal coupling and coordination of those different rotations. To address these questions, the next sections focus on the analysis of motion-planning strategies for 3D arm movements and the similarities and differences that exist between eye and arm movement generation. Here we briefly review recent studies in which Lie algebra was used to model 3D arm movements. Finally, conclusions from the studies presented here as well as possible future extensions are described.

# Experimental and Neurophysiological Studies of Reaching and Drawing

When humans perform motor actions such as pointing toward an object or reaching a visual target, one might easily be puzzled by the contrast between the complexity associated with the generation of the movements and the apparent ease and simplicity with which they are performed. This contrast is especially notable in light of the very large number of possible ways available to the nervous system to achieve the same goal. Bernstein (1967) suggested that the selection of particular movement primitives and the rules according to which they are assembled into more complex motor actions act as constraints that enable the motor system to resolve the excess degrees of freedom problem (i.e., the motor redundancy problem) in such a way that only a finite number of solutions are used by the system. Kinematic invariance is thought to reflect the existence of such motion primitives and laws of motion. Evidence for the plausible existence of such primitives or templates can be found in the typical kinematic features of the hand paths and tangential velocity profiles observed during multijoint reaching movements. For example, reaching for an object is carried out along a nearly straight-line hand path (Flash and Hogan, 1985) for movements directed toward different target locations (Haggard and Richardson, 1996; Hollerbach and Flash, 1982), even in the absence of vision during the movement, as long as the starting and final positions are known (Rossetti et al., 1994). The hand velocity profiles start and end at rest and are characteristically bell-shaped (Morasso, 1981). Task conditions or the instructions to the subject may change the symmetry of the velocity profile or its scale, but on the whole the basic shape is preserved (Atkeson and Hollerbach, 1985; Morasso, 1981). This invariance may imply that unique generalized solutions are internally represented within the neural circuitries of higher-level central nervous system (CNS) structures, such as the motor cortex and the cerebellum, as well as within lower-level neural structures, such as the spinal cord (Bizzi et al., 1991; Bizzi and Mussa-Ivaldi, 1995).

A heated debate surrounds the question of what motor variables are possibly represented within different brain areas. Earlier neurophysiological studies showed that the direction of arm movements during reaching is coded by neurons whose firing rate varies as a cosine function of the angle between a cell's preferred direction and the movement direction (Georgopoulos, 1986). Cosine tuning was found to be ubiquitous in the brain. Assuming that motor cortical neurons code for muscle force, Todorov (2002) argued that this form of tuning is optimal in the sense that it minimizes the net effect of neuromotor noise, resulting in minimal motor errors. Zhang and Sejnowski (1999) proposed an alternative model that showed that cosine tuning may result from geometric constraints. Based on their interpretation of neural populations, Georgopoulos et al. (1982) concluded that the motor cortex codes for high-level parameters, such as the direction and magnitude of hand velocity. Alternatively, others have argued that the cortex specifies low-level parameters, such as muscle force or mechanical power (Scott, 2000; Scott et al. 2001).

Recently, Todorov (2000) attempted to resolve the conflict between these alternative interpretations by suggesting that cortical neurons code for the force level generated by groups of muscles. Since muscle force depends on a muscle's length and velocity of shortening, however, to produce a desired force level within a group of muscles, cortical neurons issue signals that are intended to compensate for this dependency. This argument would account for many phenomena, including the coding of hand direction and speed by the population vector. Another phenomenon that was accounted for by Todorov's model is the discrepancy in direction between the population vector and movement direction in the presence of external loads. The time lag between the neural activity (as expressed by the population vector) and the movement it codes for has been found to increase with increases in the path curvature (Schwartz and Moran, 1999). An explanation for this observation has also been suggested by Todorov (2000). Several authors later debated the validity of several of the assumptions underlying Todorov's model as well as some of its implications (Georgopoulos and Ashe, 2000; Moran and Schwartz, 2000).

## Theories of Human Motor Control

No direct experimental means are available to infer the algorithms used by the CNS to plan movements. The experimental approach has been to consider the moving human as a "black box" and to set simple motor tasks for human subjects and record the generated arm trajectories. However, by examining the invariants and qualities of the recorded motion, researchers hope that some general strategies of motor planning can be inferred. Because of the variations among subjects and their tendency to alter strategies depending on task instructions (Desmurget et al., 1997), there are a number of competing hypotheses in the literature, each supported by substantial experimental evidence. For example, it has been proposed that the CNS plans multijoint arm movements using the coordinates of the joint angles (Soechting and Lacquaniti, 1981) or the coordinates of the hand's position (Flash and Hogan, 1985; Morasso, 1981). More recently it has been suggested that the movements planned are robust against the inherent errors in the motor system (Harris and Wolpert, 1998). Several of these theories were expressed in the form of a cost function associated with the production of the movement trajectory; the prediction of these theories is a trajectory that minimizes the corresponding cost. Because the cost is a function of the whole trajectory, it can be called a global minimization. In contrast to these are the motor planning strategies that are functions of local geometric features. An example is the well-studied two-thirds power law (Lacquaniti et al., 1983) that has been used to predict velocity profiles from local curvature relations. Despite the apparent difference in the underlying principles of these local and global theories, we will show their predictions to be remarkably similar. In this chapter, we analyze the two motor control hypotheses in light of these similarities.

A series of studies, briefly described later in this chapter, were aimed at investigating the principles that underlie trajectory planning of 2D and 3D human arm movements. Several fundamental questions arise in this context: (1) In what coordinate systems (joint, hand) are natural movements planned? (2) What rules govern the selection of particular movements among the infinite number of possible ones? (3) What types of constraints or rules are used to resolve the existing kinematic redundancies in order to limit (or take advantage of) the excess degrees of freedom that exist at all the different levels of motor specification?

# Trajectory Planning: Hand Level

In this section, several of the mathematical frameworks and models developed for the description of the trajectory planning principles underlying the generation of hand movements are described. We first describe optimization models for reaching and curved movements. This is followed by a description of the two-thirds power law, which captures the observed relationship between the curvature of the path followed by the hand, and the hand speed. We then describe several more recent studies that were aimed at unifying these two alternative descriptions, namely optimization-based models and the two-thirds power law. Finally, we present a recently developed mathematical framework, based on affine differential geometry, which was aimed at investigating the metrics used for the planning and for the internal representations of drawing movements.

## *Optimization Models*

In this subsection, optimization models for the description of reaching and curved movements are described. These models assume that motion planning and the selection of particular trajectories among the large number of possible ones is based on the wish to optimize a certain cost function which is associated with the production of the entire trajectory. In particular, the models we discuss assume the maximization of motion smoothness, which was assumed to be equivalent to the minimization of hand jerk.

### Reaching Movements

Earlier observations of planar horizontal arm movements by Morasso (1981) and by Hollerbach and Flash (1982) showed that point-to-point hand trajectories in the horizontal plane are essentially straight with bell-shaped velocity profiles. In curved movements in the horizontal plane, although the hand paths appeared smooth, movement curvature was not uniform and the hand trajectories typically displayed two or more curvature maxima. The hand velocity profiles also had two or more peaks, and the minima between adjacent peaks corresponded to the maxima in curvature (Abend et al., 1982; Flash and Hogan, 1985).

To account for these experimental observations, Flash and Hogan (1985, 1995) suggested a mathematical model of the organization of voluntary arm motions. According to this model, a major objective of motor coordination is to achieve the smoothest possible movements under the circumstances. This objective was equated with the minimization of hand jerk (rate of change of acceleration). The unique trajectories that yield the best performance were mathematically determined and compared with measured movements. In particular, this cost function was defined in terms of the time course of the hand's position $r(t) = (x(t), y(t))$ as follows:

$$C_n = \int_0^T \left( \left( \frac{d^3 x}{dt^3} \right)^2 + \left( \frac{d^3 y}{dt^3} \right)^2 \right) dt \qquad (2.1)$$

where $T$ is the duration of the movement and $x$ and $y$ are the horizontal and vertical coordinates of the hand, respectively. The cost function can be used for obtaining the full trajectory, that is, the path as well as the time profile, given the position, velocity, and acceleration boundary conditions specified at the beginning and end of the movement. The model succeeded in accounting for the qualitative features and quantitative details of the observed trajectories, including the invariance of the trajectory of the hand during reaching movements with respect to translation and rotation in the work space, as well as to amplitude and time scaling.

While the minimum-jerk model assumes the minimization of the rate of change of acceleration (which corresponds to the third-order derivative of hand position with respect to time), other smoothness criteria involving different orders of differentiation with respect to time might be considered. These cost functions, which have become known as mean squared derivative (MSD) cost functions, favor smoothness by minimizing the average value of the squared $n$th derivative of the hand position vector **r** with respect to time and are expressed as follows:

$$C_n = \int_0^T \left( \left( \frac{d^n x}{dt^n} \right)^2 + \left( \frac{d^n y}{dt^n} \right)^2 \right) dt \qquad (2.2)$$

Here again the quantity $T$ has been introduced to specify the duration of the movement in question. Although these theories predict the shapes of movements in time and space, they are scalable in time, so the value $T$ must be supplied from experiment. The value $n$ can take any positive integer value, each corresponding to a different theory of motor control. These theories have been named minimum acceleration, minimum jerk, and minimum snap for $n = 2$, $3$, and $4$, respectively. It was recently argued that all such models are equally good (Harris, 1998). However, different smoothness criteria give rise to different predicted trajectories. Namely, the order of the time-dependent polynomial predicted by minimizing a particular smoothness criterion depends on the order $n$ of the time derivative of position appearing in the cost function (equation 2.2). This in turn, however, dictates the shape of the velocity profile that characterizes the predicted trajectory (figure 2.1). We have recently demonstrated that only the models based on $n = 3$ and $n = 4$ are acceptable for reaching movements (Richardson and Flash, 2000). This conclusion was arrived at

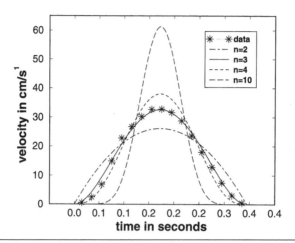

**Figure 2.1**    The MSD profiles for $n = 2, 3, 4,$ and 10 with a specified duration $T$. The profiles became narrower and taller as $n$ increases. The experimental curve for reaching movements is best fitted by minimum jerk ($n = 3$) and minimum snap ($n = 4$).

by analyzing the velocity profiles predicted by the alternative smoothness criteria and comparing the success of the different MSD cost functions in accounting for the experimentally observed values of $V_{peak}$/(average velocity), where $V_{peak}$ is the magnitude of the maxima of the velocity profile and the average velocity is equal to $L/T$, where $L$ is the movement amplitude and $T$ is the movement duration.

The predicted values of $V_{peak}$/(average velocity) for the different MSD cost functions are as follows:

$$\frac{V_{peak}}{L/T} = \frac{1}{4^{n-1}} \frac{(2n-1)!}{(n-1)!^2} \tag{2.3}$$

The resulting values are 1.5 for minimum acceleration ($n = 2$), 1.875 for minimum jerk ($n = 3$), and 2.186 for minimum snap ($n = 4$). Since the experimentally observed ratio is 1.6 to 1.9, this implies that $n = 3$ gives the best fit, but $n = 4$ is also acceptable.

It should be stated that all the preceding cost functions are expressed in terms of the time derivatives of the position vector of the hand and not in terms of joint positions or joint torques. Theories analogous to the minimum-jerk model, expressed in terms of the rate of change of joint torques or motor commands, were developed and compared with experimental data (Uno et al., 1989). While it was claimed that these theories are more successful in accounting for the experimental data (Uno et al., 1989), Flash and Hogan (1995) presented evidence in favor of optimization models that are expressed in terms of hand position and not in terms of intrinsic variables, such as joint torques or muscle tensions.

### Curved and Obstacle-Avoidance Movements

To describe curved and obstacle-avoidance movements, the minimum-jerk model was extended by assuming that a small number of points are specified along the path through which the hand should pass (Flash and Hogan, 1985). The time of passage through those *via points* and the hand velocity at that time were not specified a priori but were predicted by the model. For the simplest case of one via point between the initial and final positions, the theory yielded explicit mathematical expressions for the hand motion that reproduced all the features of the experimental observations (Flash and Hogan, 1985): distinct maxima in the speed profile with a minimum between them that coincided temporally with a curvature maximum; trajectory shape invariance with respect to translation, rotation, amplitude, and time scaling; and nearly equal durations of movement from the initial position to the via point and from the via point to the final position. Viviani and Terzuolo (1982) referred to the latter phenomenon as the *isochrony principle,* the observation that large and small movement segments of the trajectory are characterized by roughly equal durations.

## *The Two-Thirds Power Law*

One of the most striking characteristics of drawing and curved movements in a horizontal plane is the segmentation of the hand velocity profile and the coupling between the path's curvature and the speed of the movement. The so-called two-thirds power law was formulated to describe this segmentation (Lacquaniti et al., 1983). This law captures a phenomenon typical of naturally executed drawing movements whereby angular velocity decreases with increasing curvature and is proportional to the curvature to the two-thirds power:

$$A = KC^{2/3} \qquad (2.4)$$

where $A$ is the angular velocity and $C$ is the movement curvature. The gain factor of this relationship, $K$, was demonstrated to be piecewise constant and to be determined by the linear extent of each individual segment. Given that $A = VC$ (where $V$ is the tangential velocity), this law can also be expressed as

$$V = KC^{-1/3} \qquad (2.5)$$

These observations suggest that, in spite of the apparent continuity of drawing movements, they are in fact intrinsically discontinuous and are constructed of individual segments or strokes (see figure 2.2).

Motivated by the desire to examine whether alternative descriptions of the kinematic features of hand trajectories emerge from similar organizing principles, a more recent study contrasted the two approaches to the study of movement planning (Viviani and Flash, 1995). In this paper, data on the drawing of complex 2D trajectories, including ellipses, a cloverleaf, and a figure eight, were obtained and used to test whether the covariations of the temporal and geometrical parameters of the movement formalized by the two-thirds power law and by the isochrony principle could be derived from the minimum-jerk model. Convergence of the two approaches regarding the relationship between tangential velocity and curvature was satisfactory. Scaling of velocity within movement subunits could be derived from

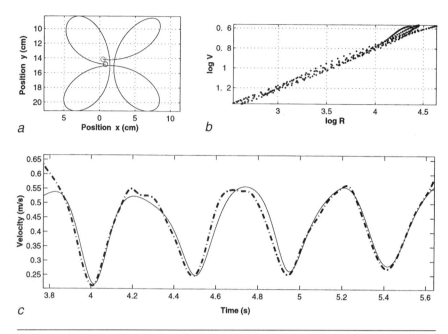

**Figure 2.2**    Measured and modeled paths and velocity profiles for drawing a figure of a cloverleaf. Shown are *(a)* the hand path, *(b)* the relationship between log $V$ and log $R$, where $V$ is the hand speed and $R$ is the radius of curvature, and *(c)* the predicted and measured velocity profiles. The predicted velocity profiles (solid curve) closely matched those of the recorded movements (dashed curves). Note that the velocity profile predicted from the minimum-jerk model (dashed line in *c*) closely matched the measured velocity profile (solid line).

the minimum-jerk hypothesis. Global isochrony, which refers to the observation that the durations of drawing movements of different lengths (e.g., small versus large ellipses) are nearly equal (Viviani and Schneider, 1999), however, could not be deduced from the optimal control hypothesis. These findings have demonstrated that the two-thirds power law and the minimum-jerk model are compatible with each other. Moreover, the conclusion from the study of Viviani and Flash (1995) was that motion plans might undergo different levels of specification, from more abstract representations of the intended movements, which may specify only locations of via points, through intermediate levels at which the entire geometrical form of the movement segments (e.g., the hand path) might be specified (Todorov and Jordan, 1998), and finally to levels that specify or represent the entire kinematic plan of the intended trajectories.

## *The Unification of Alternative Models*

In the study by Viviani and Flash (1995), the compatibility between the minimum-jerk model and the two-thirds power law was numerically demonstrated. More recently, however, in a more analytical study, we investigated what power laws between speed and curvature are predicted by the different MSD cost functions defined by the order $n$ of the time derivative of hand position (Richardson and Flash, 2000). In particular, the following power law relationship between speed and curvature was assumed:

$$V = KC^{-\beta} \tag{2.6}$$

We then demonstrated based on this assumption how the exponent of the power law can be predicted from the minimum jerk and other MSD cost functions for shapes that are similar to circles. The result is quite general, but specific examples were analyzed for the frequently studied experimental tasks of ellipse drawing, as well as the more interesting case of the cloverleaf. A mathematical method to obtain the theoretical predictions for the exponent $\beta$ was developed based on the minimization of an MSD cost function along a given path, similarly to the approach used in Todorov and Jordan (1998). The method was simply to insert the power law as expressed by equation 2.6 into the cost function, but with the exponent kept as a variable to be obtained through minimization. In this way a general form for $\beta$, as predicted by the minimization of the MSD functions, was found. However, an exact calculation was not possible due to the mathematical complexity of the problem. Perturbation theory was therefore used to obtain the exponents at the desired level of approximation. The details can be found in Richardson and Flash (2000). However, the shapes in question were generally assumed to be close to circles whose curvature and velocity were simply constants. A small expansion parameter $\varepsilon$ was then found, and perturbation calculation allowed $\beta$ to be found accurately for the ellipse and for different orders $n$ of the MSD cost functions:

$$\beta_n = \frac{1}{3} - \frac{8}{3(9^n - 1)} + \text{small corrections of order } \varepsilon \tag{2.7}$$

These calculations yielded these respective values of $\beta$ for the different cost functions: $\beta_2 = 0.3000$ (minimum acceleration), $\beta_3 = 0.3297$ (minimum jerk), and $\beta_4 = 0.3329$ (minimum snap). Thus for the ellipse, the different costs gave functions that were not simply harmonic but were experimentally indistinguishable from 1/3 (the value for simple harmonic motion) for $n > 2$. For the ellipse this method enabled a first-principles derivation of the two-thirds power law, and the result holds for all sizes, reasonable eccentricities, and periods of ellipse drawings.

This calculation was repeated also for the cloverleaf, which was used in earlier experimental studies (Viviani and Flash, 1995), yielding the following general equation for $\beta_n$:

$$\beta_n = \frac{3}{7} - \frac{8}{7} \frac{(3 + 9^n)}{(1 - 2 \cdot 9^n + 49^n)} + \text{non-negligible corrections} \tag{2.8}$$

This equation allowed predicting the following values: $\beta_2 = 0.3857$ (minimum acceleration), $\beta_3 = 0.4214$ (minimum jerk), $\beta_4 = 0.4273$ (minimum snap), and $\beta_\infty = 0.4286$. Viviani and Flash (1995) showed that the experimental values for the cloverleaf are within the range of 0.32 to 0.40. Thus, the values of $\beta$ which were obtained by the perturbative expansion do not agree well with the experimental results. Nevertheless, it was recently shown by Richardson and Flash (2002) that this is only the result of the perturbative approach; using a numerical approach to solve the optimization problem, a better agreement (e.g., $\beta = 0.36$) with the two-thirds power law and with the experimental results was achieved.

## *Affine Differential Analysis of Human Movements*

After the preceding experimental and theoretical studies, we became interested in the nature of the metrics subserving the internal neural representations of human movement. Hence, in a recent study, we developed a mathematical framework based on differential geometry, Lie group theory, and Cartan's moving frame method for the analysis of human hand trajectories (Handzel and Flash, 1999). In this work we showed that the two-thirds power law is equivalent to having the hand move at a piecewise constant affine velocity such that within each segment the unimodular affine arc length ($\sigma = \int C^{1/3} \, ds$) is proportional to movement time. We also studied the affine differential geometry of 2D curves based on Elie Cartan's moving frame approach. Textbooks dealing with affine differential geometry (e.g., Guggenheimer, 1977), as well as several recent papers (e.g., Calabi et al., 1996), discuss the fact that the trajectories of a one-parameter subgroup of unimodular affine transformations are conics or straight lines. The affine curvature $\chi$ is conserved in this process and is constant along the trajectory, and the curve has no inflection points. Thus, conics (the parabola, ellipse, and hyperbola with $\chi = 0$, $\chi > 0$, and $\chi < 0$, respectively) are the orbits of some point under the action $G = e^{\sigma v}$, where $v$ is the Cartan matrix with zero trace that depends on the affine curvature $\chi$, which is the simplest nontrivial affine differential invariant.

This framework was then used to account for the temporal characteristics of human movements. Thus, it was found that the time-scaling property of human movements is equivalent to keeping the affine arc length invariant under speed changes. In particular, for an ellipse, which is generated with a constant affine velocity, a simple relationship exists between the ellipse's perimeter and duration:

$$L = 2\pi^2 A_r^{1/3} = KT \tag{2.9}$$

where $L, A_r$, and $T$ are the ellipse's perimeter, area, and movement duration, respectively. We also explored the implications of the behaviorally observed two-thirds power law with respect to the possible internal dynamics of the neural populations that take part in neural representation and coding for arm trajectories. Georgopoulos et al. (1982) and Schwartz (1993) have shown that the movement velocity vector is represented by $N$, the neuronal population vector. In our work we succeeded in showing that a variational principle based on $N$ and $dN/dt$ leads to the two-thirds power law and is consistent with a Kepler-like law whereby

$$(d\sigma/dt)^3 = N \times dN/dt = K \tag{2.10}$$

Our current research in this direction is aimed at exploring the possibility that affine differential invariants (such as the affine curvature and its derivative) can be used to examine movement segmentation and classification. For this purpose, we are currently applying the numerical methods developed by Calabi et al. (1996). Using these methods, the affine arc length, curvature, and its first derivative were calculated for measured scribbling and human 2D drawing trajectories. This work opens up many possible new directions for future research, including the study of the interactions that may exist between human motor actions and visual perception and research on the metrics of the neural representations of arm trajectories.

Earlier investigations of 3D hand trajectories (Soechting and Terzuolo, 1987) indicated that the coupling between curvature and speed observed in 2D movements is still maintained in 3D hand trajectories. For spatial trajectories the notion of a geometrical form is expressed by the curvature and the torsion profiles. Curvature expresses the "bending" of a trajectory, while torsion expresses the "twisting" of the trajectory. Soechting and Terzuolo (1987) also reported that 3D hand trajectories are piecewise planar. That is, the local plane of the trajectory remains the same for an entire movement segment, implying that locally the torsion component is nearly zero. It then changes abruptly to a new plane within which the hand keeps moving for a while, and so on. Independently of the study by Handzel and Flash (1999) on 2D hand trajectories, Pollick and Sapiro (1997) also unraveled the relationship between affine velocity and the two-thirds power law. We extended the affine analysis to 3D movements (Pollick et al., 1997) and tested the predicted relationship between 3D Euclidean velocity ($V$), torsion ($\tau$), and curvature ($C$). Namely, for nonzero torsion, the condition for a movement to be at constant affine velocity is that $V^6 C^2 \tau$ equals a constant, and thus a one-sixth power relationship is obtained between $V$ and $1/(C^2 \tau)$. This relationship was applied to data on drawing unconstrained 3D scribbles. Entire movement sequences were divided into nearly planar parts and nonplanar parts. Data from the nearly planar regions were analyzed by fitting linear regressions between log $V$ and log($1/C$), which resulted in an average slope of 0.338 (SD = 0.041, $r^2 = 0.74$ where SD and r are the statistical descriptions of the analysis.). Data from the nonplanar regions were analyzed by fitting linear regressions between log $V$ and log $[1/(C^2 \tau)]$ and yielded an average slope of 0.164 (SD = 0.020, $r^2 = 0.79$). These results suggest that both planar and nonplanar regions of human 3D drawing motions conform to motion at constant affine velocity.

# Kinematic Constraints and 3D Trajectory Planning: Joint Level

Studies of 2D horizontal planar movements have suggested that multijoint movements are planned in hand coordinates. These, or any 2D or 3D plan, must be transformed into joint coordinates. This is the so-called inverse kinematics problem, whose solution is complicated by the existence of an excessive number of degrees of freedom at the joint level compared with the hand level. Recently, we conducted a series of studies aimed at investigating the possibility that some intrinsic constraints exist that restrict the number of degrees of freedom in the wrist, elbow, and shoulder joints during pointing, grasping, and drawing movements, thus enabling the motor controller to resolve kinematic redundancies (Gielen et al., 1997; Liebermann, 1999; Liebermann et al., 1999).

The orientation of an object after rotation along two noncolinear axes depends on the order of the rotations. This phenomenon has enormous implications for joints with three degrees of freedom, since it implies that the orientation of a limb depends on previous joint rotations if no constraints are imposed on the rotations. Yet it is well known that the orientation of the eyes in the head is unique for each gaze direction. This has been called Donders' law (Donders, 1848). Similar observations were made with respect to the orientation of the head and shoulder, although each of these joints has three degrees of freedom.

Extending these ideas to 3D arm trajectories, we examined the possibility that similar kinematic constraints operate also in the case of 3D arm pointing movements, with and without elbow flexion (Gielen et al., 1997; Liebermann, 1999; Liebermann et al., 1999). Arm movements in 3D space were recorded, using a movement recording system and virtual reality displays. In particular, we investigated the reduction in the number of rotational degrees of freedom in the shoulder and elbow during pointing movements with the fully extended arm and in movements requiring either elbow flexion or extension. The postures of both the upper arm and forearm were described by rotation vectors, which represent these postures as a rotation from a reference position to the present position. The rotation vectors for the upper arm and forearm were found to lie in a 2D (curved) surface both for the fully extended arm and for pointing with elbow flexion (Gielen et al., 1997). The orientations of the 2D surfaces fitted to the rotation vectors of the upper arm and forearm were the same for pointing with both fully extended arm and for movements with elbow flexion/extension. The scatter in the rotation vectors' torsion relative to the 2D surface was typically $3°$ to $4°$ (occasionally only $1.5°–2°$), which is rather small considering the available full range of possible torsion (Liebermann et al., 1999).

Donders' law applied to the human arm states that arm posture for pointing to a target does not depend on previous arm positions. Thus, our experimental results show that the upper arm demonstrates minimal violations of Donders' law. We also examined the movement records and found that, unlike saccadic eye movements, the recorded joint rotations in the shoulder during aiming movements were not all single-axis rotations (Liebermann, 1999). On the contrary, the direction of the angular velocity vector changed during the movement, depending on the amplitude, direction, and starting position of the movement (see figure 2.3). Gielen et al. (1997) also did not find support for single-axis rotations using a similar task. However, they reported that deviations from single-axis rotations were consistent and reproducible.

We also investigated what strategies dictate the kinematic features of 3D pointing movements (Liebermann 1999; Liebermann et al. 1999). In contrast to the straight hand paths observed during planar horizontal arm movements, movement trajectories in the vertical plane were observed to be either straight or curved, depending on the location of the movement endpoint (Atkeson and Hollerbach, 1985). This observation argues against strict control of movement in hand space but leaves open the question of why certain movements are curved while others are straight. No satisfactory explanation for this phenomenon was suggested, nor does any general model exist that suggests what principles govern the selection and generation of arm trajectories in 3D movements. This motivated us to develop a mathematical model to attempt to account for the observed path of any 3D hand movement. Our initial hypothesis was that in pointing movements the rotations about the shoulder joint obey Listing's law and the movements about the shoulder and elbow joints are single-axis rotations (Liebermann, 1999). Listing's law states that rotations of a joint in a unit-sphere space are carried out using a fixed-orientation 2D map that contains tilt and yaw coordinates only. Listing's law thus allows a unique description of the torsion component from joint elevation and horizontal rotation coordinates within the 2D map (the so-called Listing's plane; Westheimer, 1957). We further assumed that there is a fixed relationship between the shoulder and elbow angular velocities. Computer simulations of hand trajectories based on this model showed that for many movements the predicted behavior is in good agreement with the experimental data (figure 2.4). However, further efforts should be made to predict the directions of the angular velocity vectors and the hand paths in those cases in which movements about the two joints are not single-axis rotations.

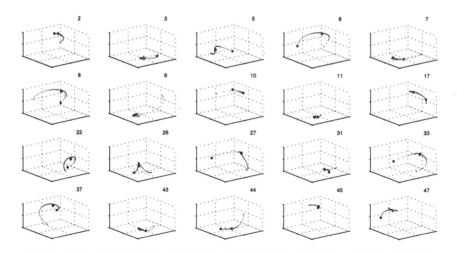

**Figure 2.3**  A 3D view of a set of the endpoints of the angular velocity vectors of shoulder joint rotations during pointing with a fully extended arm toward a series of targets in the work space. The circles plotted at the ends of the curves represent the ends of the movements. The circles placed midway along the curve represent the median locations of the endpoints of the angular velocity vectors. The directions of the vectors varied for individual movements and across trials.

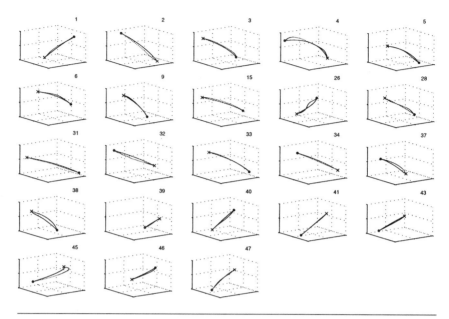

**Figure 2.4**    Predicted (solid lines) versus measured (dotted lines) 3D hand paths for one subject during a series of pointing movements with a fully extended arm toward 5-cm virtual balls located within a 1-m³ work space. The simulated paths were predicted based on the model described in the text (Liebermann, 1999; Liebermann et al., 1999).

## Theoretical Studies

In another series of studies, we attempted to develop a mathematical framework that would be appropriate for the description and analysis of both eye and arm movements (Handzel and Flash, 1999). First, we analyzed the geometry of eye rotations, in particular saccades, using basic Lie group theory and differential geometry. Various parameterizations of rotations were derived through a unifying mathematical treatment. Transformations between coordinate systems were computed using the Campbell-Baker-Hausdorff formula. Next, we showed that Listing's law can be described by means of the Lie algebra $so(3)$, which is decomposed into Listing's plane and the orthogonal axis of torsion rotations. The axes of rotation in Listing's plane generate the geometrical structure of a 2D sphere $S^2$, which corresponds to the space of gaze directions, giving direct connection to Donders' law. Although Donders' law admits many 2D submanifolds of the rotation group, only the sphere is an integral surface of the Lie algebra elements (i.e., translation invariant vector fields), which lie in Listing's plane. Finally, to rotate between two nonprimary eye positions contained in Listing's plane, the rotation axis itself lies outside the plane; this reflects the structure of the rotation group. That is, the rotations that correspond to Listing's plane do not form a subgroup of $SO(3)$.

This work was extended to suggest a unified mathematical framework for coordinate systems that represent the positions and movements of the two eyes combined during binocular eye movements (Handzel and Flash, 1997). Here the Lie algebra formalism was used to represent the kinematic aspects of the motion, namely, the tangential velocity and the time evolution of the curve traced by the end effector. We described the trajectories of single-eye rotations as geodesic paths in the space of the group $SO(3)$. Thanks to their algebraic structure, geodesic paths in Lie groups are finite compositions of one-parameter subgroups. In extending this description to binocular eye movements, we identified the binocular coordinates as the direct sum of two copies of single-eye coordinates, namely, $so(3) + so(3) = so(4)$. We then showed that different bases of the binocular Lie algebra can be used to describe either the two eyes or what we call *central demands,* that is, conjugate eye motion and antisymmetric motion (vergence). In a preliminary study using the binocular coordinates and smooth velocity functions, we have begun modeling the motion and trajectories of the two eyes in an attempt to reproduce experimentally measured data.

## Conclusions

In this chapter various theories concerning the planning and control of 2D and 3D arm movements were presented. Two distinct motor control strategies were hypothesized to reflect some level of planning by the CNS. The two strategies (global and local) were presented and mathematically analyzed with the hope of providing a simple description of human hand trajectories. One theory, the two-thirds power law, states that when the hand moves along a curved trajectory, the velocity is proportional to a power of the local curvature. The second strategy, based on optimization principles, proposes that movements are generated in order to achieve the smoothest possible trajectories. By explicit calculation, it was shown that the two-thirds power law and the minimum-jerk model produce common predictions. Two drawn forms were analyzed: the ellipse and the cloverleaf. The numerical values of the power law exponents were found to be $\beta = 0.3297$ for the ellipse and $\beta = 0.36$ for the cloverleaf, in remarkable agreement with experimental data. Together with previous results for point-to-point straight movements (Flash and Hogan, 1985) and numerical results for more complex shapes (Viviani and Flash, 1995; Todorov and Jordan, 1998), the present results suggest that the minimum-jerk cost function can be used to produce humanlike movements for a wide variety of motor tasks performed in the plane commonly used for drawing and writing. This is not to say that it is closer to the planning strategies that the CNS is actually using. Other proposals may have captured subtle aspects of human movements that the minimum-jerk model misses (Harris and Wolpert, 1998; Uno et al., 1989). However, they are considerably more complex computationally, and the minimum-jerk cost function is currently unrivaled in mathematical simplicity and the breadth of experimental results for planar movements that can be reproduced. The two-thirds power law was also the point of departure for examining what internal metrics the CNS uses to represent movement. In particular, it was shown that the two-thirds power law is compatible with movement at constant affine velocity. This observation led to a mathematical framework based on the use of affine differential geometry that was used both to describe and analyze complicated 2D and 3D drawing and scribbling hand trajectories.

We then proceeded to the analysis of the inverse kinematics problem for 3D arm movements. The case of movement in three dimensions is considerably more complex than those in the plane. This is because a planar movement described by $x$ and $y$ coordinates largely fixes the joint angles at the shoulder and elbow. However, for movement in three dimensions, all seven degrees of freedom available to the arm are used. The hand's position and orientation do not contain enough information to fix all the arm's parameters, implying a degrees-of-freedom problem. Despite this added complexity, we analyzed 3D arm movements from the perspective of Donders' and Listing's laws, which were first formulated in the context of the eye, and we examined whether similar constraints operate also for the human arm. Mathematical tools derived from Lie algebra were then used to model 3D arm movements and both monocular and binocular eye movements. While several studies have analyzed aspects of arm movement in three dimensions (Gielen et al., 1997; Soechting et al., 1995; Liebermann, 1999; Liebermann et al., 1999), as yet no comprehensive theory captures all these aspects of motion. We believe that such a theory, although likely to be relatively complex, represents an important theoretical aim for the fields of both motor control and robotics.

## Acknowledgments

The research described in the chapter was supported in part by the Moross Laboratory, the Israeli Ministry of Science, and the Minerva Foundation.

## References

Abend, W., Bizzi, E., and Morasso, P. (1982) Human arm trajectory formation. *Brain* 105: 331–348.

Atkeson, C.G., Hale, J., Kawato, M., Kotosaka, S., Pollick, F., Riley, M., Schaal, S., Shibata, S., Tevatia, G., and Ude, A. (2000) Using humanoid robots to study human behavior. *IEEE Intelligent Systems* 15: 46–56.

Atkeson, C.G., and Hollerbach, G.M. (1985) Kinematic features of unrestrained vertical arm movements. *J Neurosci* 5: 2318–2330.

Bernstein, N. (1967) *The coordination and regulation of movements.* Oxford: Pergamon Press.

Bizzi, E., and Mussa-Ivaldi, F.A. (1995) Toward a neurobiology of coordinate transformations. In Gazzaniga, M.S. (Ed.), *The cognitive neurosciences,* pp. 495–506, Cambridge, MA: MIT Press.

Bizzi, E., Mussa-Ivaldi, F.A., and Giszter, S. (1991) Computations underlying the execution of movement: A biological perspective. *Science* 253: 287–291.

Calabi, E., Olver, P.J., and Tannenbaum, A. (1996) Affine geometry, curve flows, and invariant numerical approximations. *Adv Math* 124: 154–196.

Desmurget, M., Jordan, M., Prablanc, C., and Jeannerod, M. (1997) Constrained and unconstrained movements involve different control strategies. *J Neurophysiol* 77: 1644–1650.

Donders, F.C. (1848) Beitrag zur Lehre von den Bewegungen des menschliches Auges. In *Holländische Beiträge zu den Anatomischen und Physiologischen Wissenschafter,* vol. 1, pp. 104–145. Amsterdam: Düsseldorf: August Bötticher'sche Buchhandlung.

Flash, T., and Hogan, N. (1985) The coordination of arm movements: An experimentally confirmed mathematical model. *J Neurosci* 5: 1688–1703.

Flash, T., and Hogan, N. (1995) Optimization principles in motor control. In Arbib, M. (Ed.), *Handbook of brain theory and neural networks,* pp. 682–685. Cambridge, MA: MIT Press.

Georgopoulos, A.P. (1986) On reaching. *Annu Rev Neurosci* 9: 147–170.

Georgopoulos, A.P., and Ashe, J. (2000) One motor cortex, two different views. *Nature Neurosci* 3: 963–965.

Georgopoulos A.P., Kalaska J.F., Caminiti R., and Massey J.T. (1982) On the relations between the direction of two-dimensional arm movements and cell discharge in primate motor cortex. *J Neurosci* 2: 1527–1537.

Gielen, C., Vrijenhoek, E.J., Flash, T., and Neggers, S. (1997) Arm position constraints during pointing and reaching in 3-D space. *J Neurophysiol* 78: 660–673.

Guggenheimer, H.W. (1977) *Differential geometry.* New York: Dover.

Haggard, P., and Richardson, J. (1996) Spatial patterns in the control of human arm movement. *J Exp Psychol Hum Percept Perform* 22: 42–62.

Handzel, A.A., and Flash, T. (1997) The coordinates of the binocular motor system. *Soc Neurosci Abstr.*

Handzel, A.A., and Flash, T. (1999) Geometric methods in the study of human motor control. *Cogn Stud* 6: 1–13.

Harris, C.M. (1998) On the optimal control of behaviour: A stochastic perspective. *J Neurosci Meth* 83: 73–88.

Harris, C.M., and Wolpert, D.M. (1998) Signal-dependent noise determines motor planning. *Nature* 394: 780–784.

Hollerbach, J.M., and Flash, T. (1982) Dynamic interactions between limb segments during planar arm movements. *Biol Cyber* 44: 67–77.

Hollerbach, J.M. (1982) Computers, brains, and the control of movement. *Trends Neurosci,* 5: 184–192.

Lacquaniti, F., Terzuolo, C., and Viviani, P. (1983) The law relating the kinematics and figural aspects of drawing movements. *Acta Psychol* 54: 115–130.

Liebermann, D.G. (1999) Intrinsic joint kinematic strategies for planning, reaching and pointing movements towards 3-dimensional targets. Ph.D. thesis, Department of Computer Science and Applied Mathematics, Weizmann Institute of Science, Rehovot, Israel.

Liebermann, D.G., Flash, T., and Gielen, C.C.A.M. (1999) The flat Listing's plane constraint applied to intrinsic joint kinematics planning and its effects on end-point path prediction. In *Proceedings, International Society of Biomechanics, XVIIth congress,* p. 357, Calgary, Canada, August 8–13.

Moran, D.W., and Schwartz, A.B. (2000) One motor cortex, two different views. *Nature Neurosci* 3: 963.

Morasso, P. (1981) Spatial control of arm movements. *Exp Brain Res* 42: 223–227.

Pollick, F.E., Flash, T., Giblin, P.J., and Shapiro, G. (1997) Three dimensional movements at constant affine velocity. *Soc Neurosci Abstr.*

Pollick, F.E., and Sapiro, G. (1997) Constant affine velocity predicts the 1/3 power law of planar motion reception and generation. *Vision Res* 37: 347–353.

Richardson, M.J.E., and Flash, T. (2002) Comparing smooth arm movements with the two-thirds power law and the related segmented-control hypothesis. *J Neurosci,* 15: 8201–8211.

Richardson, M.J.E., and Flash, T. (2000) The relation between kinematics and geometry as predicted by the planning of globally smooth human hand trajectories. *Soc Neurosci Abstr* 26: 1719.

Rossetti, Y., Stelmach, G.E., Desmurget, M., Prablanc, C., and Jeannerod, M. (1994) The effect of viewing the static hand prior to movement onset on pointing kinematics and variability. *Exp Brain Res* 101: 323–330.

Schaal, S. (1999) Is imitation learning the route to humanoid robots? *Trends Cogn Sci* 3: 233–242.

Schwartz, A.B. (1993) Motor cortical activity during drawing movements: Population response during sinusoid tracing. *J Neurophysiol* 70: 28–36.

Schwartz, A.B., and Moran, D.W. (1999) Motor cortical activity during drawing movements: Population representation during lemniscate tracing. *J Neurophysiol* 82: 2705–2718.

Scott, S.H. (2000) Reply to "one motor cortex, two different views." *Nature Neurosci* 3: 964–965.

Scott, S.H., Gribble, P.L., Graham K.M., and Cabel, W. (2001) Dissociation between hand motion and population vectors from neural activity in motor cortex. *Nature* 413: 161–165.

Soechting, J., Buneo, C., Hermann, U., and Flanders, M. (1995) Moving effortlessly in three dimensions: Does Donders law apply to arm movement? *J Neurosci* 15: 6271–6280.

Soechting, J.F., and Lacquaniti, F. (1981) Invariant characteristics of a pointing movement in man. *J Neurosci* 1: 710–720.

Soechting, J.F., and Terzuolo, C.A. (1987) Organization of arm movements: Motion is segmented. *Neuroscience* 23: 39–51.

Todorov, E. (2002) Cosine tuning minimizes motor errors. *Neural Computation* 14(6): 1233–1260

Todorov, E. (2000) Direct cortical control of muscle activation in voluntary arm movement: A model. *Nature Neurosci* 3(4): 391–398..

Todorov, E., and Jordan, M.I. (1998) Smoothness maximization along a predefined path accurately predicts the speed profiles of complex arm movements. *J Neurophysiol* 80: 696–714.

Uno, Y., Kawato, M., and Suzuki, R. (1989) Formation and control of optimal trajectories in human multijoint arm movements: Minimum torque-change model. *Biol Cyber* 61: 89–101.

Viviani, P., and Flash, T. (1995) Minimum-jerk, two-thirds power law, and isochrony: Converging approaches to movement planning. *J Exp Psychol* 21: 32–53.

Viviani, P., and Schneider, R. (1999) A developmental-study of the relationship between geometry and kinematics in drawing movements. *J Exp Psychol Hum Percept Perform* 17: 198–218.

Viviani, P., and Terzuolo, C. (1982) Trajectory determines movement dynamics. *Neuroscience* 7: 431–437.

Westheimer, G. (1957) Kinematics of the eye. *J Optical Soc Am* 47: 967–974.

Zhang, K., and Sejnowski, T.J. (1999) A theory of geometric constraints on neural activity for natural three-dimensional movements. *J Neurosci* 19: 3122–3145.

# 3

# Development
# of Turning and Reaching

*Patricia Bate and Esther Thelen*
Indiana University

Postural control is integral to goal-directed movement. Indeed, movement is so tightly embedded in postural set that the two are rightly considered as an ensemble, a whole-body synergy geared for effective action. In this chapter, we examine how the postural and transport components of reaching change over development. We illustrate, using our own work and that of others, how reaching skill emerges in the context of developmental changes in upright stability in sitting. Furthermore, we report a new study describing a postural context for reaching: turning toward an object.

In Western cultures, reaching develops over the period when infants are mostly lying down, reclining against support, and, later, sitting independently. Reaches in the sitting position require extensive postural control to prevent falling while the arm transports the hand to the object. The specific postural demands of seated reaching include positioning the center of mass over the base of support, preserving the upright configuration of the trunk segments, moving eyes and head smoothly to point at the target, and countering reactive forces originating in the arm movements.

The embedding of reaching in posture can be framed as an issue of the management of the degrees of freedom of body segments. Bernstein (1984) conceived the degrees of freedom of an action as those variables whose values are free to vary. He additionally proposed that ensembles of neuromuscular and skeletal components (called *coordinative structures* by Turvey et al., 1978) are put together to manage the degrees of freedom associated with each particular task. At a kinematic level the degrees of freedom can be viewed as the dimensions in Cartesian space through which each segment is free to move. For example, an infant seated on a moving platform could constitute a coordinative structure with one degree of freedom that reflects the trunk and head tipping forward and back around a horizontal axis through the hip joints. In contrast, a structure assembled to allow an infant to reach for an object at the side might include several degrees of freedom at different levels of the spine to allow rotation around a vertical axis and additional degrees of freedom in the arm and forearm to reach for the object and in the nonreaching arm for support or balance.

The degrees of freedom available in the joints are usually more than the six necessary to specify the position and orientation of an object in space. It is well-known that people can do the same task using different joint configurations. For example, adults can compensate for trunk movements during reaching by changing the angles of arm segments. Ma and Feldman (1995) and Adamovich et al. (2001) showed that when seated adults reach to an object placed within arm's length, the arm joint angles minimize the effects of trunk movement on hand trajectory. Also, if the object is placed beyond arm's length so that trunk movement must contribute to transportation of the hand, effects of unpredicted restriction of trunk movement are partially compensated by changes in arm joint kinematics (Kaminski et al., 1995; Moore et al., 1992; Rossi et al., 2002; Tyler and Hasan, 1995).

While many configurations are possible within each task, adults show preferred modes of combining movements. For example, there are many combinations of wrist, elbow, and shoulder angles that position the hand at an object (Klein and Huang, 1983), yet the relative timing between segments is invariant in certain tasks. The relative timing of the shoulder and elbow movement is consistent over changes in object size and distance in discrete pointing tasks (e.g., Soechting, 1984; Soechting and Lacquaniti, 1981). The transport and grasp components of reaching for an object show a constant relationship across distance and object size (e.g., Hoff and Arbib, 1991; Jeannerod, 1981), and the relative timing between wrist forward projection and forearm rotation is constant in reaching to rotate a bar (Kelso et al., 1994). It seems that for each task, we organize into one or more preferred coordination patterns because they are more stable, more efficient, or more comfortable (Kugler and Turvey, 1987). These preferred patterns of coordination might vary with task-specific factors, such as the position of the object, the nature of the external support, and effects of gravity. In standing adults, the muscle activations controlling the degrees of freedom for reaching vary with the velocity, predictability, and inertial load of the arm and the degree of external support (Aruin and Latash, 1995; Bouisset et al., 2000; Cordo and Nashner, 1982; Hay and Redon, 2001; Horak et al., 1984; Le Bozec et al., 2001; Van der Fits et al., 1998). Seated adults also assemble context-specific patterns of postural support for fast pointing movements. The order of activation of muscles for maintaining the sitting posture during fast pointing to a target in front is cranial to caudal: The ipsilateral back extensors are recruited first, followed in order by pelvis, thigh, and ankle muscles (Teyssedre et al., 2000). However, this order changes to caudal to cranial when mass is added to the arm. Moreover, the lower trunk and thigh muscle activity depends on whether the adult is standing, sitting, reclining, or supine (Van der Fits et al., 1998). Patterns of postural activity are also contingent upon which arm is raised (Teyssedre et al., 2000).

# Posture and Reaching in Infants

The primary task of infants, like that of adults, is to coordinate the degrees of freedom in posture and reaching to fit the particular task. But unlike adults, infants have developmental issues as well: Not all components of the posture and reaching system are equally available for any particular task. Here we tell a developmental story that shows how infants assemble their task-specific coordination within the changing background of other neuromuscular developments. In particular, infants solve task issues within a background of developing postural control that proceeds in a general head-to-tail direction. As infants gain control of successive segments—head, neck, shoulders, and trunk—they incorporate those postural sets into their reaching. We show that these changing postural constraints influence both infants' reaching to the front and the more complex action of turning and reaching to the side.

## *Postural Requirements for Early Reaching*

Infants are first able to successfully reach and grab objects when they are about 4 months old, although there is considerable individual variability. Reaching is a visually elicited task, so infants must be able to localize objects in space before them, have some motivation to grasp an object (usually to bring it to the mouth for exploration), and begin to match the "feel" of the arms moving in space to the location of the desired object. There is good evidence that infants' vision is sufficient for seeing a graspable object in three-dimensional space. By 3 or 4 months, they have had considerable experience in grasping and mouthing objects, fingers, and clothing, and they have been moving their arms continually and exploring the consequences of such movements. What seems to be needed is control of the arm—generating task-appropriate forces and trajectories—and the postural control that enables arm control.

### Control of Head and Shoulder Muscles

The first postural requirement for reaching is stability of the head. Head control is crucially needed to orient and stabilize the gaze and, thus, the target object. This is especially important because infants are born without even the ability to lift their heads against gravity and, for several months after birth, may rest their heads in an asymmetric posture. The asymmetric tonic neck reflex often seems obligatory and resistant even to contralateral visual stimuli. Clearly, without stable head control, stable localization is not possible.

Indeed, good head control is a prerequisite for the onset of reaching. In their longitudinal study of four infants, Spencer et al. (2000) found that all the babies developed consistent midline head position while supine before the onset of reaching. Three of the babies showed midline head posture just at the week of reaching onset, and the fourth, several weeks in advance of reaching. Thus, being able to balance the head appeared to be necessary, but not sufficient, for reaching onset.

Reaching by definition requires lifting the arm and, for many tasks, maintaining the arm in an extended position away from the body and perhaps without external support. Thus, muscles of shoulders and neck must be strong enough to lift the limb. Because of the gravity vector, holding the arms straight and extended while the body is supine is especially effortful. (Try reading when lying flat on your back.) Indeed, supporting a young infant vertically promotes reaching, probably because of the gravity issue. Infants in the Spencer et al. (2000) study reached a week or more earlier when supported vertically than when tested supine. Similarly, Savelsburgh and Van der Kamp (1994) found that 12- to 19-week-old infants reached with more mature frequency and duration when upright than when their chairs were tilted back. Also, upright-seated infants were more likely to reach unilaterally, while supine infants used both hands to reach (Rochat and Goubet, 1995).

The critical involvement of the muscles of neck and shoulder in reach onset emerged in Spencer and Thelen's (1998) longitudinal study of electromyographic (EMG) patterns before and after reach onset in four infants. Consistent with an important role for proximal muscles in reaching, Van der Fits et al. (1999) described frequent, variable activity in the neck muscles during forward reaches of 4-month-olds. Spencer and Thelen (1998) discovered dramatic changes in activation patterns associated with the onset of reaching. They developed a method to determine what proportion of time each of the four monitored muscles (biceps, triceps, deltoid, and trapezius) and all possible combinations of those muscles were active during all reaching and nonreaching movements. They found that prereaching movements were largely generated by activation in the upper-arm muscles, the biceps and triceps, which serve to flex and extend the elbow. In contrast, the proportion of time of deltoid and trapezius muscle activation significantly increased in the weeks following reaching onset. Further analysis revealed, however, that muscle pattern differences were not simply a function of a change in posture and movements of the arms between the prereaching and postreaching periods but were an actual shift in the muscles used. Even when prereaching infants reached to full extension, they used different muscles than older infants.

Newborn infants' limbs are in a primarily flexed posture, and the environment in utero provides little challenge to shoulder and neck antigravity muscles. Thus, it may take several months of moving in a gravitational environment for these muscles to become strong enough to support the extended limb.

**Emerging Control of Trunk**

In adults, reaching is preceded by anticipatory postural adjustments in trunk muscles to compensate for the reactive forces generated by the moving limb. At 4 months of age, when infants first reach for objects, however, they cannot sit independently and are always placed with various degrees of trunk support in infant seats, in cribs, or on parents' laps. There is initially little involvement of trunk muscles. For example, when Woollacott et al. (1987) and Hadders-Algra et al. (1996a) tested postural responses in infants seated on a moving platform, they found that 3.5- and 4-month-old infants produced electrical activity in neck muscles directionally appropriate to backward translation. Not until 5 to 6 months did infants show appropriate responses in both neck and trunk. However, trunk support for reaching may emerge earlier than reactions to platform perturbations. Van der Fits et al. (1999) found that, during forward reaches, trunk muscle activity was direction specific from 4 months.

In the months following the onset of reaching, infants gain considerable extensor strength in the back and explore lifting their shoulders away from the support surface when seated. Indeed, in the study described by Spencer et al. (2000), infants were lifting head and shoulders away from the seat soon after reaching onset. As infants gain more control of their heads, shoulders, and trunks, caregivers provide more opportunities to test these postural synergies by removing head supports, holding infants upright by the hips rather than the chest and head, and allowing babies to reach for objects with increasing involvement of the trunk.

## *Good Reaching Depends on Good Sitting*

There is considerable evidence linking improvements in reaching with infants' progress toward stable independent sitting. For instance, all four infants studied by Thelen and Spencer (1998) and Spencer et al. (2000) generated stable reaches in chair-supported sitting only after they had achieved 3 s or more of independent sitting on a mat. Fontaine and Le Bonniec (1988) grouped 96 infants into four levels of sitting ability. The infants were supported at the pelvis while seated on the experimenter's knees and presented with objects. Infants with better sitting ability were more successful, and sitting ability predicted quality and success of reaches better than age. Rochat et al. (1999) also found a connection between independent sitting ability and reaching. When infants were strapped into a chair, those who were able to balance independently while sitting reached toward far objects more often than infants who were not able to sit independently. Rochat et al. (1999) noted that the support would probably have allowed them to reach the object if they leaned on the straps, but infants did not use this strategy; only those who could balance independently in sitting reached frequently for far objects.

What can be special about the experience of sitting outside the confines of an adult's grasp or an infant chair? Infant seats provide external scaffolding but also permit the infant to move head and shoulders away from the support. By leaning forward into a more vertical position than that supported by the backward-tilted chair, infants have some opportunity to explore movements of the upper trunk. However it is less likely that infants will be able to move the trunk sufficiently far from the chair to gain experience in balancing the pelvis on the thighs. Thus, infants who are supported in infant chairs are likely to have experience of upper-trunk control but not the ability to lean the trunk forward by flexion at the hip, as is required in reaching toward far objects (Kaminski et al., 1995). The first demand for control of the entire trunk may occur when an infant is first released in sitting without support.

When released in sitting, young infants flop forward until their trunk is in a near horizontal position over the legs. The mechanism by which they develop the ability to maintain themselves propped on their hands, and then more upright, is control of the lower trunk. Harbourne et al. (1993) showed that the trunk leans less far forward as infants develop synergies between lumbar extensors and the hip and knee flexors or extensors. Van der Fits et al. (1999) showed that in children of 8 months the cephalocaudal order of postural recruitment during reaching in supported sitting changes to initial activity in the lumbar extensors when the child is placed in independent, long sitting, suggesting that control of lower-trunk degrees of freedom is a critical component of reaching from an independent position.

## Integration of Stability and Transport Roles of the Trunk

The coordination pattern used for reaching for near objects is different from that used for reaching for distant objects. In reaching for an object that lies within arm's length, postural functions are performed primarily by the trunk and legs, and transport functions by the arms. The arm transports the hand, while the trunk maintains the center of mass over the base of support and counters perturbations to trunk stability resulting from the reach. However, when an object is more than an arm's length distant, the trunk shares the transport function by leaning forward during reaching (Kaminski et al., 1995; Moore et al., 1992; Tyler and Hasan, 1995). Control of degrees of freedom at the hip joint and lower trunk enables the trunk to carry the arms closer to the object while maintaining stability.

This integration of stability and transport roles is apparently so difficult that 6-month-old infants who reach enthusiastically for a toy tend not to reach when trunk leaning is required (Clifton et al., 1991; Yonas and Hartman, 1993). However, if nonsitting infants are provided with external stability, they use their trunk for transport. Rochat and Goubet (1995; experiment 1) measured the distance of the hand and the head from a ball approaching along the sagittal plane. They found that infants unable to sit alone did not move their heads forward; that is, these infants did not recruit degrees of freedom at the hip or spinal joints. However, when provided with a high level of support from an inflated cushion pressing laterally on the pelvis, nonsitters leaned forward as they reached (Rochat and Goubet, 1995; experiment 2).

In summary, to reach into the space around them, infants formulate coordination patterns specific to the position of the target object. Control of degrees of freedom at the upper trunk, shoulder, lower trunk, and pelvis permits stable reaches in sitting and allows release of the trunk to meet transport requirements when the object is distant. Active control of the lumbar spine and pelvic tilt is learned in independent sitting, hence the close relationship in time between acquisition of independent sitting and emergence of smooth, straight reaching.

## Task-Appropriate Synergies Within Cephalocaudal Control

Infants' increasing control in erect positions follows a general head-to-tail progression, and as we have seen, the ability to reach at all, and then to reach well, is intimately tied to their postural set. Head control is needed to stabilize looking, head and shoulder strength is needed to lift the arms, and trunk control is needed to anticipate lifting the arm and to stabilize the arm and trunk. The ability to rotate around the hip joint is necessary to extend the trunk to reach for objects beyond arm's length.

Within this general progression, however, we have some evidence of task-specific recruitment of synergies. Infants assemble different coordination patterns depending on their level of support. For instance, Thelen et al. (1993) reported that elbow extension contributed extensively to midline reaches. In contrast, infants of similar ages described by Berthier et al. (1999) restricted their elbow movements by co-contraction of flexors and extensors. The difference was their level of support. Thelen et al. (1993) restrained infants at the chest in a chair. The infants were prevented from leaning forward and so recruited elbow degrees of freedom. Berthier et al.'s (1999) infants were seated on their parents' laps. They used forward movements of their trunks and may have stiffened their elbows to reduce threats to balance while leaning forward.

The level of support and relation to gravity also influence whether infants used one or two hands to reach. Rochat (1992) and Rochat and Goubet (1995) elicited reaches to displays mounted in front of infants supported to different degrees in various relationships to gravity. They showed that across all postures, nonsitting infants more frequently yoked their arms into a bilateral reach pattern than the independent sitters. These nonsitting infants, who primarily used bimanual reaching while supine, reached unilaterally when placed in supported sitting.

## Turning to Reach

In every study of infant reaching and its postural context, infants are presented objects directly in front of them. This makes sense because it is common for caregivers to deal with babies face on and to make objects available to them in their visual field. However, as infants become more independent and sit alone, they do not confine their reaching to only those objects directly in their gaze. Seated infants reach all around them for toys, but we do not know how they meet the complex transport and stability requirements of this task or how this ability develops.

To turn and reach for a toy at the side, infants must construct coordination patterns quite different from those required for forward reaching. The synergy entails transport by the trunk as the rotating spine and head carry the eyes and arm toward the object. The trunk also maintains stability as the infant turns and balances to reach. In our study, we asked how infants assemble synergies for this specific task of turning to reach, within the general developmental constraints of postural control.

## Methods

In this attempt to capture the changing coordination patterns of infant turning, we report on a single infant from age 16 weeks to 35 weeks. We modeled the spine with three degrees of freedom, allowing rotation of the head, trunk, and pelvis in horizontal planes. We envisaged that the coordinative structures of the turns would be expressed in the amplitude and timing relationships of movements in each of these kinematic dimensions.

To document movement in each degree of freedom, we fixed reflective markers to the head, upper trunk (spines of scapulae), and sacrum, sampled the positions of these markers, and calculated kinematic indices. To identify coordination patterns in turning, we examined relationships between these variables and plotted developmental trajectories.

### *Data Collection*

We recorded each weekly session with three video cameras and a force platform. (The force-platform data are not presented here.) The infant (Peter) was seated on the force platform with his mother in front and a researcher behind. He wore tights, a closely fitted hat, and reflective markers (figure 3.1).

We manually triggered each trial to start when Peter was sitting independently and looking to the front. A few seconds after the beginning of a trial, a researcher moved a toy into a specific position on a virtual line circling Peter at approximately his shoulder height and arm length. When the toy was in position, the researcher shook it to elicit a sound; this shaking continued to the end of the recording period at 10 s.

If Peter reached for the toy, the researcher moved it slightly away along a radial line from shoulder joint to toy so that he did not contact it during the trial, although we encouraged him to grasp and play with the toy between trials when it seemed necessary to maintain his interest. We continued data collection until two trials had been collected at each position or the infant became fussy; we ended most sessions for the second reason.

The full design tested six toy positions: to the left and right sides in line with the acromial processes of the shoulders (90° to the sagittal plane where 0° is the projection of the sagittal plane directly in front of the body), behind and in front in the sagittal plane, and to the left and right at 45° to the line of the acromial

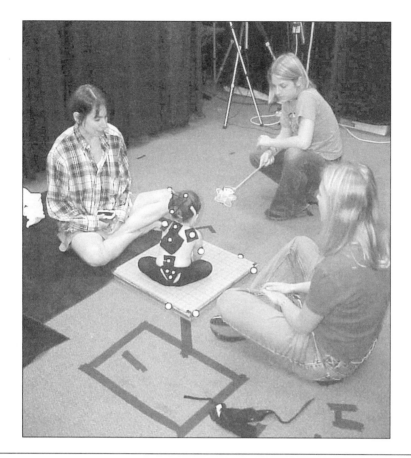

**Figure 3.1**    Infant seated on a force platform, wearing reflective markers, and turning to a toy presented at the position 90° to the right.

Photo courtesy of S. Tolen.

processes (135° to the sagittal plane). Peter's tolerance was low initially, so we limited trials to the 90° positions only; we introduced the other positions as Peter's endurance increased. Here we report the first turn to each 90° and 135° position. Turns to the 90° position began at 17 weeks, and turns to the 135° positions were first tested at 23 weeks.

## Data Reduction

We classified arm and body movements by behavioral coding and analyzed segmental kinematics. We digitized videotaped data at 60 Hz and constructed 3D coordinates using the Peak system; we smoothed the position data using a low-pass Butterworth filter (Jackson, 1979). Where possible, we selected the first trial at each toy position

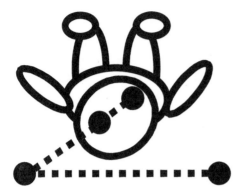

**Figure 3.2** Lines between two markers on the head and two on the force platform were used to calculate the horizontal angular amplitude of the head.

for analysis. We replaced trials containing procedural errors, technical errors, or marker occlusions with later trials of the same toy position.

### Classification of Postural Functions of the Arms

We developed a mutually exclusive and exhaustive coding scheme to classify postural functions of the arms. Using this scheme, we recorded the onset times for four sitting behaviors: supported by the researcher or parent and independent with two, one, or no hands on the force platform.

### Classification of Reaches

We used an event-based coding scheme to identify reaches. We recorded a reach onset if one hand (or two) moved toward the toy while the head was turned toward the toy or if the head turned toward the toy during this hand movement, and we marked the end of a reach if the hand touched the force platform or the body or if the head turned away from the toy. We allocated each reach to one of three mutually exclusive and exhaustive categories: use of the arm ipsilateral or contralateral to the toy, use of both arms, or no reach.

### Kinematic Analysis of Segment Movements During Turns

We identified the onset and offset time of each turn by behavioral coding, using criteria that directed the observer to identify rotations of the head, trunk, or pelvis around a vertical axis (figure 3.2). We used these times to locate the turn on the kinematic record, and we then used a graphical interface (MATLAB) to identify the onset and offset times of each segment at the time of the nearest-velocity zero crossing of the correct sign. Occasionally, if the kinematic record and reexamination of the videotape suggested a more appropriate time, we shifted to an earlier or later zero crossing.

## Results

The postural synergies used for sitting and the kinematics of turning and reaching are presented in the following sections.

## Postural Synergies for Sitting

We discerned three postural synergies in Peter's attempts to maintain the sitting position. In one pattern Peter leaned his trunk far forward while he prevented collapse onto the extended legs by propping on both hands. In another synergy his trunk was more vertical, and his hands rested on his legs or were held in the air as if they were balancing poles. In the third synergy his arms worked asymmetrically; Peter leaned on one hand while he held the other in the air.

Three developmental periods were characterized by different uses of the hands. During weeks 16 to 21, Peter predominantly supported himself by propping on two hands ("propping"). During weeks 22 to 30, Peter spent most time with both his hands resting on his legs or in the air ("balancing"). From week 31, Peter's sitting posture was characterized by versatility in the role of the arms ("mixed"): All three patterns were present in approximately the same extent (figure 3.3).

Within these postural control synergies, how did Peter manage to turn to reach for the toy? We found a stable element in the turns, but within this stability, the structure of the turns changed coincidentally with changes in postural strategies.

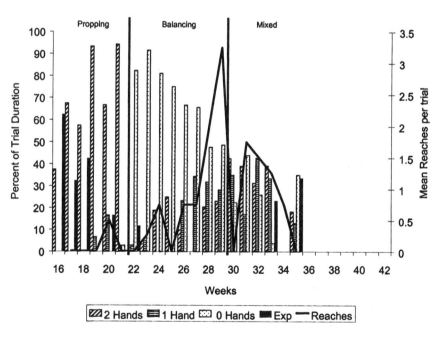

**Figure 3.3**    Proportional trial durations for 3 postural synergies, using no, one, or two hands, showing the three developmental periods: propping, balancing, and mixed. The solid black bars indicate where experimenters supported Peter to keep him from toppling or restrained him if he attempted to crawl away.

## *Head-Trunk-Pelvis Turns*

We first examined turns to the 90° toy position. We found that the turning movements of all segments were in the direction of the toy. The relative contribution of
the head to the amplitudes of these turns was consistent throughout development:
The head turned farther than the trunk or the pelvis in nearly all turns. We termed
this turning pattern the head-trunk-pelvis (HTP) turn; kinematic data for an exemplar
HTP turn are presented in figure 3.4. The relative amplitudes of trunk and pelvis
rotation in these HTP turns became more consistent over development. The head
turned farther than the trunk and the trunk turned farther than the pelvis in 3 of 7
turns during the propping period, 8 of 14 turns in the balancing period, and 3 of 3
turns in the mixed period.

Although the distributions of turning amplitudes between the segments were
similar for the propping and balancing periods, mean amplitudes suggested that when
Peter used his arms as props, he turned less in the head and trunk. In general, head
and trunk movements were smaller for turns that occurred when the arms were
yoked into the sitting structure as props than for those generated from postures in
which the arms were balancing (figure 3.5). Table 3.1 reports the mean relative
amplitude of each segment for turns during the propping, balancing, and mixed
periods (see the definition of swivel turns on page 68). The freeing of the proximal
segments in the balancing period was also apparent in the differences between turns.
The head and trunk amplitudes varied more during the balancing period.

Although the relative amplitudes of the head and trunk rotations were more
variable during the balancing period, the relative onset times of these segments

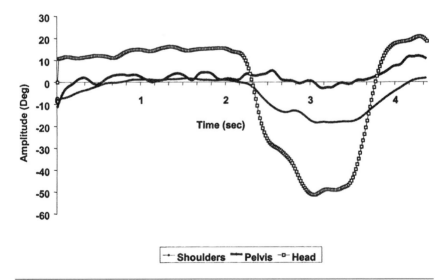

**Figure 3.4**   Exemplar HTP turn. Horizontal angular displacements of the head, trunk, and
pelvis are plotted against time.

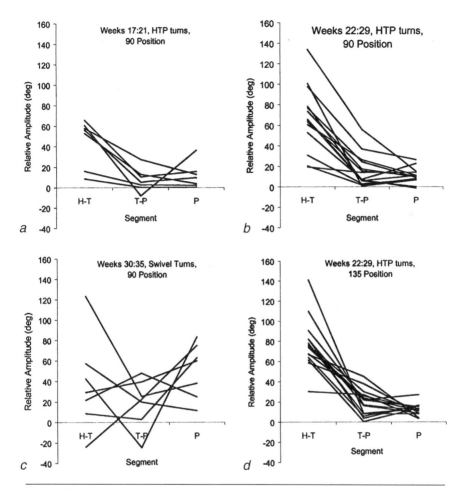

**Figure 3.5**    Segment turn amplitudes. *(a)* HTP turns to the 90° toy position during the propping period. *(b)* HTP turns to the 90° position during the balancing period. *(c)* Swivel turns to the 90° position during the mixed period. *(d)* HTP turns to the 135° position during the balancing period. (H= head, T = trunk, P = pelvis.)

became more consistent. The mean lag of the pelvis was longer than that of the trunk (table 3.2). However, when we looked for this pattern in individual turns, we found that it was more common during the arm-balancing period. While the arms were propping, the head started before the trunk in 5 of 7 turns, and the trunk before the pelvis in 3 of 7 turns; both these orders were present in only one turn. However, during the balancing period the head started before the trunk in 12 of 14 turns, and the trunk before the pelvis in 9 of 14 turns; both these orders were present in 7 of 14 turns. The order of onset of segment movement was becoming more consistently cephalocaudal.

**Table 3.1   Mean Relative Amplitudes of Segment Turns**

| | Head–trunk | | Trunk–pelvis | | Pelvis | |
|---|---|---|---|---|---|---|
| | 90° | 135° | 90° | 135° | 90° | 135° |
| Weeks 17–21, HTP | 42.7 (28.7) *n* = 7 | † | 7.5 (11.3) | † | 11.7 (12.3) | † |
| Weeks 22–29, HTP | 60.2 (41.1) *n* = 14 | 77.2 (24.8) *n* = 15 | 15.8 (15.8) | 19.7 (12.8) | 10.8 (7.5) | 11.4 (23.6) |
| Weeks 30–35, swivel | 29.3 (147.5) *n* = 7 | 46.3 (106.2) *n* = 3* | 22.5 (72.5) | 26.8 (11.2) | 50.8 (26.6) | 24.9 (32.0) |
| Weeks 30–35, HTP | 47.8 (7.6) *n* = 3* | 44.9 (13.9) *n* = 2* | 20.4 (12.2) | 23.7 (9.4) | 17.3 (19.6) | 28.9 (20.9) |

Mean relative amplitudes calculated by subtracting the horizontal angular amplitude of the head from that of the trunk (head–trunk) and that of the trunk from that of the pelvis (trunk–pelvis). Standard deviations are in parentheses.

†Toy position 135° not tested.

*These values are medians and ranges.

## *Emergence of Swivel Turns*

After Peter had achieved some mastery of sitting and turning, he began to more flexibly use his arms for sitting stability, and he demonstrated a second turning style. Peter turned by placing his hands down on the floor and pushing with his arms, translating the pelvis backward and rotating the pubic bone toward the toy (figure 3.6). The turn ended with his face, chest, and pelvis facing the toy front on. We named these turns, characterized by leaning on the hands while sliding the pelvis, swivel turns. Of the 10 turns during weeks 30 to 35, 7 were of this type. While some turns incorporated large head movements or small pelvis movements, mean head amplitude was less and pelvis amplitude greater than for the HTP turns (table 3.1); the pelvis moved farther than the head or trunk in 5 of the 7 swivel turns (figure 3.5c).

The swivel turns reflected the cephalocaudal order of segmental recruitment that developed in the HTP turns. The mean lag of the trunk was less than that of the pelvis (table 3.2). In 6 of the 7 swivel turns the head moved before the trunk, and in 3 of the 7 the trunk moved before the pelvis; both these orders were present in 3 of the 7 turns.

**Table 3.2 Mean Durations for Head, Trunk, and Pelvis Segments and Onset Lags of Trunk and Pelvis Relative to Head**

| | Head | | Trunk | | Pelvis | |
|---|---|---|---|---|---|---|
| | 90° | 135° | 90° | 135° | 90° | 135° |
| **_Duration (ms)_** | | | | | | |
| Weeks 17–21, HTP | 1652 (955) n = 7 | † | 1507 (773) | † | 1226 (911) | † |
| Weeks 22–29, HTP | 1568 (702) n = 14 | 2023 (601) n = 15 | 1769 (813) | 1830 (642) | 1487 (888) | 1680 (825) |
| Weeks 30–35, swivel | 3570 (4990) n = 7* | 3320 (2830) n = 3* | 2930 (5200) | 2920 (288) | 3100 (4820) | 2830 (2470) |
| Weeks 30–35, HTP | 1110 (890) n = 3* | 1805 (1105) n = 2* | 1220 (660) | 1652 (806) | 1320 (600) | 1050 (800) |
| **_Lag (ms)_** | | | | | | |
| Weeks 17–21, HTP | | | 83 (282) n = 7 | † | 207 (244) | † |
| Weeks 22–29, HTP | | | 77 (285) n = 14 | 139 (205) n = 15 | 241 (214) | 198 (342) |
| Weeks 30–35, swivel | | | 150 (163) n = 14 | 33 (450) n = 3 | 250 (417) | 233 (427) |
| Weeks 30–35, HTP | | | 33 (67) n = 3* | 150 (0) n = 2* | 133 (217) | 500 (0) |

Standard deviations are in parentheses.

†Toy position 135° not tested.

*These values are medians and ranges.

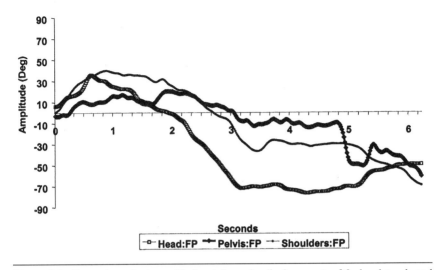

**Figure 3.6**  Exemplar swivel turn. Horizontal angular displacements of the head, trunk, and pelvis are plotted against time. A swivel is visible late in the turn in the pelvis trace.

## *Turns to 135°*

As part of our investigation of the development of turning, we sought to determine how Peter would assemble synergies for a larger turn. During weeks 22 to 35, we added a condition to the study in which we presented toys at 135° to the sagittal plane. We will first discuss the turns performed while the arms were balancing (weeks 22 to 29).

Peter turned farther when the toy was positioned at 135°. Examining the movement of the head relative to the external environment, we found that the mean head amplitude to the 90° toy position was 92° (SD = 52°), and to the 135° position it was 109° (SD = 25°).

The synergies Peter assembled for the larger turns were similar to those for the 90° toy position. The turns to the 135° position preserved the relative ranking of the segment amplitudes: In all turns the relative amplitude of the head was greater than that of the trunk, and in 10 of the 15 turns the relative amplitude of the trunk was greater than amplitude of the pelvis. Both these relationships were present in 10 of the 15 turns.

Despite the common structure of the turns to 90° and 135°, we noted a relative lack of mobility at the pelvis segment in the larger turns. Mean amplitudes suggested that while Peter displaced head and trunk segments farther to achieve the greater range, he did not move his pelvis farther than for the 90° position (table 3.1). The distribution of the amplitudes across the individual turns showed that more turns with large amplitudes of head and trunk were present in the 135° position (figure 3.5). It seemed that while the head and trunk contributed to both stability and transport functions, the pelvis was not free to contribute extensively to transport.

The onset order of segments was also similar for the turns to the two positions. The order that became consolidated over this period for the 90° turns also dominated the 135° turns: Head movement preceded trunk movement in 12 of 15 turns, and trunk preceded pelvis in 10 of 15 turns. A consistent sequence of head, then trunk, and then pelvis was present in 7 of 15 turns. Consistent with this, mean lags showed that the trunk followed the head and the pelvis followed the trunk (table 3.2). We concluded that the kinematic structure of the turns to 135° was that of the HTP category, characterized by relative segmental amplitudes and onset orders.

From weeks 30 to 35, Peter used the swivel pattern three times and the HTP pattern twice in turns to 135°. All five turns demonstrated a cephalocaudal order of initiation of segments.

## Reaches

Peter's reaching was integrated with the postural roles of the arms. He reached only twice during the propping period, when weight bearing through the arms was a component of sitting stability. However when he released his arms into the balancing role, he reached more than once per trial. The number of reaches was highest in the last weeks of the balance period and the first weeks of the mixed period (figure 3.3).

Peter's reaches also reflected his turning style. He changed the arm used for reaching concomitantly with the onset of swivel turns. While most reaches were performed with the arm ipsilateral to the toy, from week 30 Peter sometimes reached with the contralateral arm (figure 3.7). These contralateral reaches ($n = 4$) all followed swivel turns. The 7 swivel turns in weeks 30 to 35 were associated with either ipsilateral ($n = 4$) or contralateral ($n = 3$) reaches or both ($n = 1$).

# Discussion

Although we report data from only one infant, our study illustrates the sharing of transport and postural functions between body segments in the development of turning and reaching. Traditionally, the trunk has been viewed as providing stability for the reach. While this is no doubt true, we suggest a more complex developmental story: The trunk supports the transport function of the arms, and the arms also support the transport function of the trunk. The shifting roles of these segments over development illustrate how the infant "softly assembled" the turning structure. He used his available capacities to turn and reach, and as these abilities changed, so did the assembled synergies.

## An Account of the Development of Seated Turning

We found that the transport role of the spine was organized in a cephalocaudal direction: In the HTP turns of the first two periods, the head contributed greater

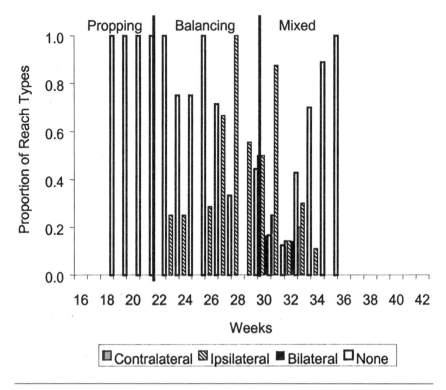

**Figure 3.7**    Average number of reaches of each type per trial, for the 90° toy position.

amplitude than the trunk or pelvis. Pelvis and trunk amplitude increased later with the introduction of swivel turns. This order is consistent with the order of progression of postural stability described by Woollacott et al. (1987) and Hadders-Algra et al. (1996a) for responses to external perturbations and with other evidence that head stability develops before stability of other segments (e.g., Hopkins et al., 1990).

All together, these findings suggest a possible account for the integration of transport and stability requirements of seated turning during development. If both the stability capacities and the transport capacities necessary for turning develop in a cephalocaudal direction, then in order for the infant not to fall over during turning, the degrees of freedom at any segment can be recruited for transport only after more caudal segments have developed ability to maintain postural stability. Turns in which the head is the only moving segment would become possible when stability could be provided by the trunk and pelvis, turns that include both the head and trunk would emerge only when the pelvis was stable, and turns involving all three segments would require stabilization by the legs.

The present data show that this account requires extension to include not only transport but also postural roles for the arms. In our study of a single infant, we found that the arms filled multiple roles through the development of seated turning.

They took on two postural roles during early development: Initially they acted as props, and later their position in the air or on the thighs suggested that they were used as balancing poles to counter shifts in center of mass and as generators of tactile information for balance. Later in development one or both of the hands came back to the floor to carry weight and to serve as a fulcrum for transport of the pelvis. In these ways the coordinative structures assembled for turning included stabilizing and transport functions by the arms. It is clear that an account of seated turning must include the arms in addition to axial segments.

We propose that the trend toward early limitation of the range of the trunk and head in turning is a consequence of the postural stability strategy. When trunk and pelvis control was poor, axial movement was limited to the head; turning at the trunk and pelvis was minimal. The muscles of the shoulder girdle fixed the arms in the propping position in relation to the support surface and the trunk. This fixation permitted transmission of body weight through the hands, widened the base of support, and prevented forward collapse of the trunk and pelvis. Through the shoulder muscle attachments at the skull and spinous processes, this strategy also limited the available range of rotation at the head and spine, which in turn limited reactive forces resulting from head and trunk movements. Later in development, when control of the trunk had improved, the arms moved away from the chest wall in balancing strategies. While the arms were still constrained to act symmetrically, they were not fixed between trunk and floor and thus did not limit head movement. The arms counterbalanced reactive forces, and the trunk degrees of freedom became available to transport head and arms toward the toy.

The amplitudes and timings of spinal segment movements converged on a stable pattern. The emergent picture was one in which all three segments contributed amplitude: the head most and the pelvis least. The segments moved for similar durations; the head started moving first, and the pelvis last.

Convergence on this stable turning pattern emerged in the context of developmental changes in many system components. The postural role of the arms, body mass, strength, and skill all changed during the period of the study. While we cannot tease apart the interrelated contributions of these factors, the consistency in the relationships between spinal segments in the presence of these changes suggests that the HTP turning style represents a preferred coordinative structure for axial degrees of freedom (Kugler and Turvey, 1987). Furthermore, the adoption of relatively large amplitudes of the pelvis after week 30 suggests that the initial pattern may have been the only form of coordination of spinal segments for turning that was available to Peter at his early levels of postural stability. Each time we presented a toy, Peter assembled from his available components a synergy that generated the best possible solution to the problem of turning to reach. This solution was stable until certain changes in the components permitted emergence of a new structure and a new turning style.

The return of the hands to a weight-bearing role during sitting and turning was a dramatic sequel to the 9-week period during which Peter mostly held his hands in the air. This change in the postural role of the arms from pillars to pivots is characteristic of the recursive nature of patterns of motor development (Gesell, 1946; Corbetta and Thelen, 1996). It may have been triggered by several factors. The record of motor milestones showed that Peter started using his arms for locomotion at the same time that use of the arms for postural maintenance became more versatile. He started belly crawling, which provides experience in the propulsive and weight-bearing functions of the arms, in the week before he first swivel-turned. Also, the video record of the data collection sessions showed that Peter engaged in activities that appeared preparatory for weight bearing by the arms over several weeks prior to week 30: He frequently engaged in rhythmically hitting the force platform with both hands and repeatedly rocked his weight forward onto his hands to the extent that his pelvis lifted. Practice in weight bearing and propulsion may have contributed to the emergence of the swivel turns.

While rocking and belly crawling may be essential precursors to the performance of swivel turns, they do not explain why the swivel turns emerged or why they were repeated. From week 30 to 35 we identified 10 turns to toys at the side, of which 3 were of the HTP type and 7 swivel type. We argue that because swivel turns were more frequent than HTP turns, they must have presented some advantage. Perhaps the endpoint of a swivel turn constituted a better position from which to look at or reach for the toy.

In searching for criteria under which the swivel-turn end position may have been preferable to that of an HTP turn, we considered the possibility that it was more comfortable. It has been demonstrated that people prefer to finish movements near the midrange of most joints (Rosenbaum, 1995; Cruse et al., 1993), yet many HTP turns ended with the head and trunk rotated through a considerable range. To test the possibility that the end positions of HTP turns were uncomfortable, we constructed a crude index reflecting the relative extents of segment contributions. We assumed that a turn would be more comfortable if the maximal amplitudes of segment contributions were similar than if they were disparate. We found that the swivel turns were organized such that the ratios of head-to-trunk and trunk-to-pelvis amplitudes were much smaller than for HTP turns (table 3.3). We concluded that Peter might have switched to swivel turns because the end positions were more comfortable. This explanation is consistent with Bernstein's proposal that preferred patterns are adopted because they are more comfortable (Kugler and Turvey, 1987).

In addition to the possibility that the swivel turns were more comfortable, some aspect of reaching, or of the relationship between reaches and turns, may have precipitated the change in turning style. The exclusive association of contralateral reaches with swivel turns led us to consider the possibility that at 30 weeks Peter began to prefer a particular hand for reaching and that this preference drove the emergence of swivel turns. Handedness has been demonstrated to fluctuate over the first year (Corbetta and Thelen, 1999). If a preference for using a particular hand emerged in week 30, then this preference may have driven swiveling of the pelvis into a position from which the preferred arm could easily reach. This explanation predicts that reaches with the arm contralateral to the toy would be more prevalent on one side than the other. However, examination of the data showed contralateral

**Table 3.3 Ratios of Mean Horizontal Angular Amplitudes of Head–Trunk and Trunk–Pelvis Segments**

| | Weeks 17–29 | | Weeks 30–35 | | | |
| | All turns | | HTP turns | | Swivel turns | |
| | 135° | 90° | 135° | 90° | 135° | 90° |
|---|---|---|---|---|---|---|
| Head–trunk | 3.8 | 3.4 | 2.3 | 1.9 | 1.4 | 2.2 |
| Trunk–pelvis | 1.9 | 2.5 | 2.3 | 1.8 | 1.1 | 2.1 |

reaches were equally prevalent with each hand, so we discarded the explanation that handedness contributed to the emergence of swivel turns.

We further examined the differential associations of the reaching hand with the two turn types in relation to an earlier finding that infants rarely reach into the extremes of the reach space (Spencer and Thelen, 1998). One possible explanation for this behavior is that structures assembled for reaching maintain a linear relationship between shoulder and elbow dynamic muscle torques (Gottlieb, Song, Hong, Almeida, and Corcos, 1996; Gottlieb, Song, Hong, and Corcos, 1996; Gottlieb et al., 1997; Zaal et al., 1999). In the present study, HTP turns ended with the trunk only partially turned toward the toy, so contralateral reaches to the toy would necessarily end in an extreme position at the far side of the anterior work space. Such reaches may violate the proposed linear synergy constraint. Whatever the reason for infants' failures to reach into extremes of the reach space, the present data were consistent with Spencer and Thelen's (1998) observations. Almost all reaches following HTP turns were performed with the ipsilateral arm. In contrast, swivel turns ended with the chest facing the toy, so reaches that ended close to the midline would be equally frequent with each arm, as was seen in our data set.

There is another reason why the partially rotated end position following HTP turns may have proved an unsatisfactory position from which to reach. From this position movement of the ipsilateral hand toward the toy would extend the arm outside the base of support, which was only the width of the pelvis, bringing the center of mass of the body close to the safety margin for balance. It is possible that this reach entailed undesirable levels of risk of balance loss or of attention, energy, or strength to maintain balance. In contrast, at the end of a swivel turn, Peter's body was positioned so that the toy was in the center of the anterior work space. Reaching from this position projects the mass of the arm over the long axis of the base of support provided by the extended legs, so balance was less threatened. Perhaps swivel turns' highly stable base for reaching led to the adoption of this coordination pattern.

Swivel turns may have provided a more satisfactory base for reaching. The arms' postural role in sitting and belly crawling prepared them for a propulsive role in turning by providing opportunities for weight bearing, propulsion, and strengthening. When

Peter was placed in a sitting position during week 30, his arms, newly released from exclusive duty in sitting as balancing poles or props, were suddenly available to push. Swivel turns were evoked by the simultaneous occurrence of the toy at the side and factors such as increased ability to push through the arms, instability, discomfort associated with ipsilateral reaching from a semiturned position, and constraints against reaches into extreme positions. The swivel turns ended with the body facing the toy, so reaches with the ipsilateral and contralateral arms were equally comfortable or equally consistent with the linear synergy, and these reaches became equally probable.

Moreover, some characteristics of the swivel turns suggest that they use more energy than HTP turns. They produced larger amplitudes than the HTP turns; amplitudes of the trunk and pelvis movements were more than twice as large. Indeed, in some turns the pelvis and trunk amplitudes approached or exceeded those of the head. The movements of the trunk were slow, and lags between segments were long; these turns moved the entire body mass to a new position on the force platform. The higher energy cost associated with this turning style may not have been an important factor, or it may have been countered by the benefits discussed previously.

The reaches reflected the postural roles of the arms. Consistent with previous reports of reaching success and quality being contingent on control of the sitting posture (e.g. Rochat, 1992; Rochat and Goubet, 1995; Spencer et al., 2000; Thelen and Spencer, 1998), we found that the number of reaches increased when the postural role of the arms changed from propping to balancing. We contend that the abilities to control the pelvis and spinal extension in sitting are critical in determining the release of the arms from their weight-bearing role and the associated emergence of reaching.

Peter's experiences in postural functions immediately prior to the escalation of reach frequency suggest that the inability to counter reaction forces limits reaching in the early weeks. For much of the 6 weeks immediately preceding the steep increase in number of reaches, Peter maintained independent sitting with his hands in the air. This position probably provided him the opportunity to learn to counter torques generated by arm movements and so may have prepared him to counter the reactive forces associated with reaching. The age at which Peter achieved belly crawling constituted a second indicator of the importance of postural stability to the generation of reaches. In previous weeks Peter probably spent a lot of time in the pivot prone position in preparation for belly crawling, which emerged at 29 weeks. We proposed earlier that belly crawling promotes the propulsive use of the arms. Now we suggest that, in addition, learning to belly crawl develops the strength and coordination necessary to achieve an extended position of the trunk against gravity. This ability to extend the spine while stabilizing the pelvis in an anteriorly tipped position appears to be essential for successful reaching (Harbourne et al., 1993; Van der Fits et al., 1999) and, together with practice countering arm reaction forces in sitting, probably permitted the steep increase in reach frequency seen at 28 weeks.

If postural stability were a major contributor to the increase in reaching, why did Peter's reach frequency decline over weeks 31 to 35? Since his postural control was good, we can only conclude that he had become bored with the testing paradigm, and locomotion-related goals were more salient than our toys. Indeed, he crawled away from the experiment as soon as he was able, at week 36.

We expect that the development of turning behaviors in other infants would be different to the extent that important aspects of their structural contexts and experiences vary. In particular, we have identified one factor that limits the generalizability of the data. Although our findings are consistent with previous reports that reaches are unilateral during development of independent sitting ability (Rochat, 1992; Rochat and Goubet, 1995; Rose and Berthenthal, 1998) and most of Peter's motor milestones were achieved at ages similar to those reported in the literature, the repeated measurements may have had a training effect. Comparing our data with reports in the literature, we found that Peter sat earlier than commonly reported in Western-reared infants. Peter balanced himself with his hands in the air for longer than 10 s at week 22, but McGraw (1945) and Touwen (1976) found 32 to 36 weeks to be the usual age of emergence of independent sitting, Spencer et al. (2000) found the age at which four infants were able to sit alone for more than 3 s was between 24 and 27 weeks, Van der Fits et al. (1998) found that none of 10 infants could sit independently for 10 s at 24 weeks although 6 of the 10 sat for less than 10 s, and Hopkins and Ronnquist (2002) found that none of six infants ages 22 to 26 weeks could sit independently for longer than 5 s. There have been previous reports that practice improves postural stability in infants. Hadders-Algra et al. (1996b) found that practice in reaching caused more mature responses to platform perturbations in seated infants, and Sveistrup and Woollacott (1997) found that practice with 300 perturbations over a week shifted muscle response selection toward more mature patterns in newly standing infants. We noted that by the beginning of week 22 we had propped Peter on his hands and replaced him many times while we recorded 48 trials over 81 min since his first test at 16 weeks. It is possible that participation in the study improved Peter's ability to sit independently. We are replicating this study in several more infants, and comparison of their data with reported times of acquisition of motor skills may provide more evidence of a training effect.

It is possible that the swivel turns also may have emerged as a result of participation in the study. To collect the data we repeatedly elicited turns while Peter sat on a smooth surface wearing spandex tights. Consistent with a dynamic systems interpretation of development, it may be that the progressive freeing of the pelvis and emergence of the pelvis sliding strategy in week 30 resulted from the interactive effects of all these factors. These swivel turns may have been specific to this environment and Peter's experience and may not be seen, or may emerge later, in infants wearing bulky diapers or seated on carpet.

## Conclusions

Our study revealed the softly assembled nature of the action of turning to reach. We showed how the head, trunk, and pelvis developed transport functions in the context of changes in postural functions of the arms. Release of degrees of freedom for turning developed top down as the arms were released from their weight-bearing role and the head and trunk increasingly contributed to the transport component of turning.

We found that the postural and transport functions also dovetailed in the relationship between reaches and turns. Early in development the infant reached exclusively with the arm ipsilateral to the toy. However, he ultimately transported his pelvis while pivoting on his arms, creating a new work space for reaching. Reach frequency and reach type changed concurrently with the synergy assembled for turning, and Peter's preference for a front-on position to the toy as a base for reaches with the contralateral arm extended previous reports that postural support determines reach strategy (Thelen et al., 1993; Berthier et al., 1999; Van der Fits et al., 1999).

## Acknowledgments

We appreciate the extensive contributions of undergraduate students during the data collection and processing phases of this study: in particular Sarah Tolen and Sarah Levinson, who appear in Figure 3.1. We are also indebted to Dexter Gromley for managerial and technical contributions, Jing Feng for assistance with software development and psychology staff and graduate students for other support. Most importantly, we thank Peter and his mother who attended lengthy sessions regularly, over many months, in order to share Peter's development. Supported by NIH NICHD HD 22830 to E.T.

## References

Adamovich, S.V., Archambault, P.S., Ghafouri, M., Levin, M.L., Poizner, H., and Feldman, A.G. (2001) Hand trajectory invariance in reaching movements involving the trunk. *Exp Brain Res* 138: 288-303.

Aruin, A., and Latash, M. (1995) Directional specificity of postural muscles in feed-forward postural reactions during fast voluntary arm movements. *Exp Brain Res* 102: 323-332.

Bernstein, N. (1984) The problem of the interrelation of coordination and localization. In Whiting, H.T.A. (Ed.), *Human motor actions: Bernstein reassessed.* Advances in Psychology, vol. 17, pp. 77-120, Amsterdam: North-Holland.

Berthier, N.E., Clifton, R., McCall, D.D., and Robin, D.J. (1999) Proximo-distal structure of early reaching in human infants. *Exp Brain Res* 127: 259-269.

Bouisset, S., Richardson, J., and Zattara, M. (2000) Do anticipatory postural adjustments occurring in different segments of the postural chain follow the same organizational rule for different task movement velocities, independently of the inertial load value? *Exp Brain Res* 132: 79-86.

Clifton, R.K., Perris, E.E., and Bullinger, A. (1991) Infants' perception of auditory space. *Dev Psychobiol* 27: 187-197.

Corbetta, D., and Thelen, E. (1999) Lateral biases and fluctuations in infant's spontaneous arm movements and reaching. *Dev Psychobiology* 34: 237-255.

Corbetta, D., and Thelen, E. (1996) The developmental origins of bimanual coordination. *J Exp Psychol Hum Percept Perform* 22: 502-522.

Cordo, P.J., and Nashner, L.M. (1982) Properties of postural adjustments associated with rapid arm movements. *J Neurophysiol* 47: 287-302.

Cruse, H., Bruwer, M., and Dean, J. (1993) Control of three and four joint arm movement: strategies for a manipulator with redundant degrees of freedom. *J Motor Behavior* 25: 131-139.

Fontaine, R., and Le Bonniec, G.P. (1988) Postural evolution and integration of the prehension gesture in children aged 4 to 10 months. *Br J Dev Psychol* 6: 223-233.

Gesell, A. (1946) The ontogenesis of infant behavior. In Carmichael, L. (Ed.), *Manual of child psychology*, pp. 295-331. New York: Wiley.

Gottlieb, G.L., Song, S., Almeida, G.L., Hong, D., and Corcos, D. (1997) Directional control of planar arm movement. *J Neurophysiol* 78: 2985-2998.

Gottlieb, G.L., Song, S., Hong, D., Almeida, G.L., and Corcos, D. (1996) Coordinating movement at two joints: A principle of linear covariance. *J Neurophysiol* 75: 1760-1763.

Gottlieb, G.L., Song, S., Hong, D., and Corcos, D. (1996) Coordinating two degrees of freedom during human arm movement: Load and speed invariance of relative joint torques. *J Neurophysiol* 75: 3196-3206.

Hadders-Algra, M., Brogren, E., and Forssberg, H. (1996a) Ontogeny of postural adjustments during sitting in infancy: Variation, selection and modulation. *J Physiol* 493.1: 273-288.

Hadders-Algra, M., Brogren, E., and Forssberg, H. (1996b) Training affects the development of postural adjustments in sitting infants. *J Physiol* 493.1: 289-298.

Harbourne, R.T., Guiliani, C., and Mac Neela, J. (1993) A kinematic and electromyographic analysis of the development of sitting posture in infants. *Dev Psychobiol* 26: 51-64.

Hay, L., and Redon, C. (2001) Development of postural adaptation to arm raising. *Exp Brain Res* 139: 224-232.

Hoff, B., and Arbib, M. (1991) A model of the effects of speed, accuracy and perturbation on visually guided reaching. In Caminiti, R., Johnson, P.B., and Bernod, R. (Eds.), *Control of arm movement in space.* Experimental Brain Research Series, suppl. 22, pp. 258-306. Berlin: Springer.

Hopkins, B., Lems, Y.L., Van Wulfften Palthe, T., Hoeksma, J., Kardaun, O., and Butterworth, G. (1990) Development of head position preference during early infancy: A longitudinal study in the daily life situation. *Dev Psychobiol* 23: 39-53.

Hopkins, B., and Ronnquist, L. (2002) Facilitating postural control: Effects on reaching behavior of 6-month-old infants. *Dev Psychobiol* 40: 168-182.

Horak, F., Esselman, E., Anderson, M., and Lynch, M. (1984) The effects of movement velocity, mass displacement and task certainty on associated postural adjustments made by normal and hemiplegic subjects. *J Neurol Neurosurg* 47: 1020-1028.

Jackson, K.M. (1979) Fitting of mathematical functions to biomechanical data. *IEEE Trans Biomed Eng* 26: 122-124.

Jeannerod, M. (1981) Intersegmental coordination during reaching at natural visual objects. In Long, J., and Baddeley, A. (Eds.), *Attention and performance,* pp. 153-169. Hillsdale, NJ: Erlbaum.

Kaminski, T., Bock, C., and Gentile, A. (1995) The coordination between trunk and arm motion during pointing movements. *Exp Brain Res* 106: 457-466.

Kelso, J.A.S., Buchanan, J.J., and Murata, T. (1994) Multifunctionality and switching in the coordination dynamics of reaching and grasping. *Human Movement Science* 13:63-94.

Klein, C.A., and Huang, C.H. (1983) Review of pseudo-inverse control for use with kinematically redundant manipulators. *IEEE Trans Syst Man Cybern* 13: 245-250.

Kugler, P.N., and Turvey, M.T. (1987) *Information, natural law and the self-assembly of movement.* Mahwah, NJ: Erlbaum.

Le Bozec, S., Lesne, J., and Bouisset, S. (2001) A sequence of postural muscle excitations precedes and accompanies isometric ramp efforts performed while sitting in human subjects. *Neurosci Lett* 303: 72-76.

Ma, S., and Feldman, A.G. (1995) Two functionally different synergies during arm reaching movements involving the trunk. *J Neurophysiol* 73: 2120-2122.

McGraw, M.B. (1945) *The neuromuscular maturation of the human infant.* London: Mac Keith Press.

Moore, S., Brunt, D., Nesbitt, M., and Juarez, T. (1992) Investigation of evidence for anticipatory postural adjustments in seated subjects who performed a reaching task. *Phys Ther* 72: 335-343.

Rochat, P. (1992) Self sitting and reaching in 5 to 8 month old infants: The impact of posture and its development on early eye-hand coordination. *J Mot Behav* 24: 210-220.

Rochat, P., and Goubet, N. (1995) Development of sitting and reaching in 5- to 6-month-old infants. *Infant Behav Dev* 18: 53-68.

Rochat, P., Goubet, N., and Senders, S.J. (1999) To reach or not to reach? Perception of body effectivities by young infants. *Infant Child Dev* 8: 129-148.

Rose, J.L., and Berthenthal, B.L. (1998) A longitudinal study of the development of the visual control of posture. In Berthenthal, B., and Von Hofsten, C.L. (Eds.), *Eye, head, and trunk control: The foundation for manual development.* Neuroscience and Biobehavioral Reviews, 22(4): 515-520.

Rosenbaum, D.A., Loukopoulos, L.D., Meulenbrock, R.G., Vaughn, J., and Engelbrecht, S.E. (1995) Planning reaches by evaluating stored postures. *Psychological Review* 102:28-67.

Rossi, E., Mitnitski, A., and Feldman, A.G. (2002) Sequential control signals determine arm and trunk contributions to hand transport during reaching in humans. *J Physiol* 538.2: 659-671.

Savelsburgh, G.J., and Van der Kamp, J. (1994) The effect of body orientation to gravity on early infant reaching. *J Exp Child Psychol* 58: 510-528.

Soechting, J.F. (1984) Effect of target size on spatial and temporal characteristics of a pointing movement in man. *Exp Brain Res* 54: 121-132.

Soechting, J.F., and Lacquaniti, F. (1981) Invariant characteristics of a pointing movement in man. *J Neurosci* 1: 710-720.

Spencer, J., and Thelen, E. (1998) Spatially specific changes in infants' muscle co-activity as they learn to reach. *Infancy* 1: 275-302.

Spencer, J., Vereijken, B., Diedrich, F.J., and Thelen, E. (2000) Posture and the emergence of manual skills. *Dev Sci* 3: 216-233.

Sveistrup, H., and Woollacott, M.H. (1997) Practice modifies the developing automatic postural response. *Exp Brain Res* 114: 33-43

Teyssedre, C., Lino, F., Zattara, M., and Bouisset, S. (2000) Anticipatory EMG patterns associated with preferred and non-preferred arm pointing movements. *Exp Brain Res* 134: 435-440.

Thelen, E., Corbetta, D., Kamm, D., Spencer, J.P., Schneider, K., and Zernicke, R.F. (1993) The transition to reaching: Matching intention and intrinsic dynamics. *Child Dev* 64: 1058-1098.

Thelen, E., and Spencer, J. (1998) Postural control during reaching in young infants: A dynamic systems approach. *Neurosci Biobehav* 22: 507-514.

Touwen, B.C.L. (1976) *Neurological development in infancy.* Clinics in Developmental Medicine no. 59. London: Heineman.

Turvey, M.T., Shaw, R.A., and Mace, W. (1978) Issues in the theory of action: Degrees of freedom, coordinative structures and coalitions. In Requin, J.E. (Ed.), *Attention and performance VI,* pp. 557-595. Hillsdale, NJ: Erlbaum.

Tyler, A., and Hasan, Z. (1995) Qualitative discrepancies between trunk muscle activity and dynamic postural requirements at the initiation of reaching movements performed while sitting. *Exp Brain Res* 107: 87-95.

Van der Fits, I.B., Klip, A.W., Van Eykern, L.A., and Hadders-Algra, M. (1998) Postural adjustments accompanying fast pointing movements in standing, sitting and lying adults. *Exp Brain Res* 120: 202-216.

Van der Fits, I.B., Otten, E., Klip, A.W., Van Eykern, L.A., and Hadders-Algra, M. (1999) The development of postural adjustments during reaching in 6 to 18 month old infants: Evidence for two transitions. *Exp Brain Res* 126: 517-528.

Woollacott, M., Debu, B., and Mowat, M. (1987) Neuromuscular control of posture in the infant and child: Is vision dominant? *J Mot Behav* 19: 167-186.

Yonas, A., and Hartman, B. (1993) Perceiving the affordance of contact in 4- and 5-month-old infants. *Child Dev* 64: 298-308.

Zaal, F.T., Daigle, K., Gottlieb, G.L., and Thelen, E. (1999) An unlearned principle for coordinating natural movements. *J Neurophysiol* 82:255-259.

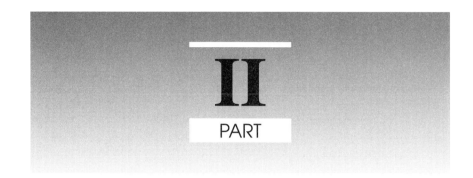

# New Approaches
# to Motor Variability

# 4

# Dynamical Systems Approaches to Understanding the Generation of Movement by the Nervous System

*Gregor Schöner*
Ruhr-Universität Bochum

To generate a movement, the nervous system must specify task-relevant movement parameters, generate a movement plan in time, and control the effector system. There is evidence that all of these processes are continuously linked to ongoing sensory information. This suggests that control-theoretic (dynamical) stability is an important property of the movement system at all levels, including the level of movement planning. The dynamic field representation of movement parameters provides movement plans with dynamic properties. A dynamic field model of movement preparation addresses how prior information, the recent motor history, and current perceptual information are integrated into a movement plan that evolves continuously in time and is graded in its metric contents. Such movement plans are characterized as stable states of the dynamic field. Conversely, instabilities in the dynamic field account for how decisions about movement plans are made when sensory information is insufficient to fully specify an upcoming movement. Through the concept of population coding, the dynamic field concept is linked to the cortical neurophysiology of movement planning.

Psychophysicists studying sensation and perception have had great success at isolating individual feature representations, levels of perception, and specific subsystems, primarily through careful control of the information contained in the stimulus. Students of motor behavior, by contrast, have found it much more difficult to limit their experimental manipulations to any specific level of motor control. Movement is always an active behavior that is not determined exclusively by a stimulus. Minimally, performing a motor act involves representing relevant spatial information about movement goals, planning and initiating the motor act, generating the time courses of control variables, and real-time control of the movement. These different components of action are closely interconnected (figure 4.1). When a limb is mechanically perturbed or loaded, for instance, this manipulation affects not only the peripheral motor control system but also the timing system (coordination) and even the spatial planning of the action (motor equivalent solutions). Varying the timing constraints of a movement always affects control (as changed speeds and accelerations provide changed control problems) and often alters the spatial characteristics of the resulting trajectories too (through space-time invariances, for example). Conversely, varying the spatial constraints affects both timing and control problems.

In light of the highly integrated nature of these systems that generate movement, one might wonder how different levels of motor control can be distinguished at all. One line of attack is through the abstract notion of stability. In the most radical stance, the different levels can actually be defined in terms of the kind of variables that they keep stable (Schöner, 1994).

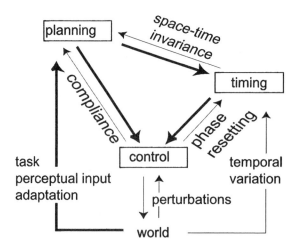

**Figure 4.1** Levels of planning, timing, and control are needed to generate movement. The flow of information is typically assumed to go from planning to timing and control (thick arrows). Many other directions of flow (thin arrows) may occur, however, leading to a web of interconnected processes.

# Stability

The stationary state of a system is *stable* if it persists in the face of external or random perturbations. This abstract notion is familiar to all of us from control theory, which in the context of motor control describes how particular states of the mechanical degrees of freedom of the motor apparatus can be stabilized and assigned specific values. Biomechanically, stability might arise just from the physics of effector systems (e.g., by damping due to the viscous properties of muscles). More generally, feedback control can steer systems into desired states.

Mathematically, the concept of stability is formalized (as *asymptotic stability*) within the framework of the theory of dynamical systems (Braun, 1994). This abstract concept is relevant to state variables other than effector positions, velocities, or accelerations. For instance, the relative timing between different effectors can be characterized by stable states such that a perturbation of the timing of one limb engages a process leading to the recovery of the target relative timing (for a review of theoretical issues about timing, see Schöner, 2002). The fact that relative timing must have stability properties becomes obvious when that stability is lost, as in instabilities of coordination (Schöner and Kelso, 1988).

Movement parameters such as the direction in space of the end-effector path, the movement extent, or the movement time characterize a motor act as a whole. Because such parameters typically have well-defined values from the start of the movement, the specification of these parameters can be viewed as a form of planning. Movement plans, however, can be updated any time during movement preparation and execution (e.g., Goodale, Pélisson, and Prablanc, 1986; van Sonderen, van der Gon, and Gielen, 1988, 1989; Prablanc and Martin, 1992). Moreover, movement plans can evolve continuously in time in graded fashion (e.g., Ghez et al., 1997). In the experiments that support these statements, movement plans were perturbed at only a single moment in time. In real life the sensory information that specifies actions varies all the time. The ongoing linkage of motor plans to such time-varying information conceptually requires that motor plans have stability properties as well.

In theoretical terms, stability at the level of the control of effector systems is addressed by all models of motor control. In equilibrium-point theory, for instance, viscosity ensures that postural states are stable (for a review see Latash, 1993). In neural network models of control, stability is generated from recurrence (e.g., Kawato, 1990), although the muscular system contributes as well. Stability at the level of timing arises from the coupling of stable limit cycle oscillators (conceived abstractly as in Haken, Kelso, and Bunz, 1985, or neuronally as in Grossberg, Pribe, and Cohen, 1997; see Schöner, 2002, for a review). How can stability be conceived at the level of the planning of motor acts? Neural network models of motor planning typically have not addressed this issue directly, although some models contain stability properties implicitly (for instance, by using graded representations of movements, e.g., Hinton, 1984).

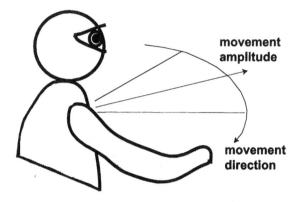

**movement amplitude**

**movement direction**

**Figure 4.2** The space of possible goal-directed movements can be spanned by continuous movement parameters such as movement direction or movement amplitude.

## Dynamic Field Theory

Dynamic field theory was developed with the goal of making the stability of movement plans explicit (Kopecz and Schöner, 1995; Erlhagen and Schöner, 2002). Movement planning is conceived of as the process of generating values for all relevant movement parameters. Movement parameters are continuous in nature (e.g., movement direction and amplitude; see figure 4.2 ) or can be embedded in a continuous description (e.g., degree of involvement of a limb in a movement). These parameters can thus be thought of as spanning a metric space of possible movements. Any particular motor act is a point in that space.

### Activation Fields

To represent information about planned motor acts, we invoke the concept of activation (e.g., Williams, 1986). Large levels of activation indicate the presence of information; low levels, its absence. Graded information (such as expecting a particular probability of the need to perform a particular movement) can be represented by intermediate levels of activation. Every possible movement is thus characterized by an activation variable. This leads to a high-dimensional field of activation: Along each dimension of the space of possible movements, a continuous number of activation variables represent information about planned movements.

In typical experiments, the different movements that a participant is asked to perform vary along one or a small number of dimensions. We therefore simplify the concept by describing the high-dimensional field merely along one particular dimension (say, along the parameter "movement direction," as illustrated in figure 4.3). A peak of activation then represents a particular planned movement in the direction represented at the site of the field where the peak is localized (figure 4.3a).

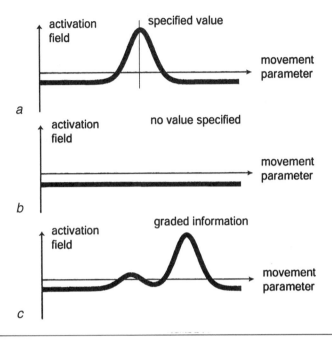

**Figure 4.3**   A field of activation is defined over a movement parameter and represents information about that movement parameter.

The absence of information is represented by a homogeneous pattern of activation (figure 4.3b). Varying amounts of information can be represented by graded patterns of activation (figure 4.3c). We assume that any single motor act is represented by a peak of activation that has a nonzero width rather than by an arbitrarily sharp activation spike. This implies that when the single movement parameter value that is specified by the location of the maximum of the field is activated, movement parameter values nearby representing similar movements are coactivated. This assumption can be justified empirically based on results from the timed movement initiation paradigm (Ghez et al., 1997; see further discussion later in this chapter) and based on mapping activation fields onto cortical distributions of population activation (Erlhagen et al., 1999).

## Field Dynamics

Input drives the activation patterns of the field. Sensory signals specifying movement targets, for instance, are conceived of as sources of input to the field. Such inputs might come from imperative signals preceding the initiation of a motor act, but also from prior information about possible movement targets obtained, for example, from the perceptual layout of work space, from explicit prior sensory information (precues), or from the recent movement history.

Studies in the timed movement initiation paradigm have varied the time between the imperative signal and the initiation of the motor act (by controlling the latter through a sequence of metronome signals). Using this technique, Ghez and colleagues (reviews in Ghez, Hening, and Favilla, 1990; Ghez et al., 1997) have observed that histograms of the movement field parameter values that describe the performed movements evolve continuously, with an increasing stimulus-response interval from an initial "default" distribution to a distribution centered on the specified value. At intermediate stimulus-response intervals, the transient distributions can be centered over parameter values that are never specified in the task.

We assume that the activation field evolves continuously in time as described by a dynamical system of field activation. Here is a mathematical formulation for an activation field, $u(\phi, t)$, representing the direction $\phi$ of a planned movement:

$$\tau\dot{u}(\phi,t) = -u(\phi,t) + h + s_{spec}(\phi,t) + s_{pre}(\phi,t) \tag{4.1}$$

where $\tau$ is the time scale over which activation patterns evolve, $h < 0$ is the resting level of the field in the absence of input, $s_{spec}$ is input from sensory information that encodes an imperative signal to make a particular movement, and $s_{pre}$ is input representing prior information about possible movements. Input is meaningful when it is localized along the field dimension, so that an activation peak arises at a particular location representing the movement parameter value "computed" from the inputs (figure 4.4). In such an input-driven description, the field essentially sums and low-pass filters different inputs. Many neural network models address this aspect, with a concern of understanding the various transformations needed to extract information about movement parameter values from various sources of sensory information. The formulation given above takes these transformations for granted.

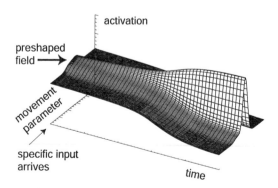

**Figure 4.4**   An activation field representing a movement parameter evolves in time under the influence of inputs and interaction. The field is initially preshaped around a range of possible values through input representing the task layout. The imperative signal provides input specifying the upcoming movement. The activation peak that arises is stabilized and sharpened by competitive interaction.

## Decision Making and Interaction

The preparation of an upcoming movement involves more than "computation" of the appropriate movement parameter values from sensory input, however. In daily life, initiating a motor act obviously requires selecting a particular movement goal out of a typically extensive range of perceived possible movement targets. That a part of such decision processes is performed relatively closely to the processes of movement preparation discussed here is clear from laboratory experiments in which the imperative signal does not uniquely specify a single movement parameter value or contains distracting information. Such paradigms have been extensively used in the domain of visually driven saccadic eye movements (recent review in Glimcher, 2001) and recently also in the domain of goal-directed reaching movements (recent review in Tipper, Howard, and Houghton, 2000). Figure 4.5 illustrates an exemplary early study by Ottes, van Gisbergen, and Eggermont (1985). From an initial fixation point, a saccadic eye movement is elicited by presenting two visual targets. Per instruction, the color indicates which of the two targets the saccade must be directed to. Saccades with short latencies, however, are frequently directed to an averaged retinal position between the two possible targets when the two targets are close to each other (figure 4.5a) or to either of the two targets when the targets are farther apart (figure 4.5b).

To account for the capacity of the saccadic eye movement system to generate averaged responses for metrically close targets and make a decision for metrically distant targets, Kopecz and Schöner (1995) postulated that a dynamic field representing the planned saccadic endpoint evolves under the influence of not only input information but also interactions within the activation field. Neighboring field sites were assumed to be mutually facilitatory, while field sites representing metrically distant saccadic endpoints were assumed to be mutually inhibitory, introducing effective competition between activation peaks when these are at a sufficient distance from each other. These interactions make the field dynamics nonlinear because only activated field sites are allowed to participate in the interaction. This is character-

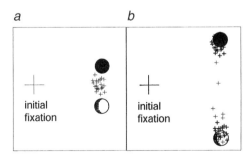

**Figure 4.5**    Saccadic eye movements directed toward one of two visual targets. See text for explanation.

From Ottes, van Gisbergen, and Eggermont (1985).

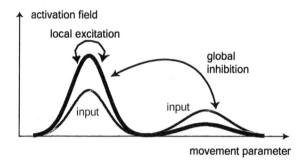

**Figure 4.6**   Locally excitatory and globally inhibitory interaction enable the dynamic field to make decisions. When two field locations receive input (gray line), an activation peak positioned over one of the activated sites may inhibit growth of a peak at the other site while stabilizing its own activation. The sigmoid nonlinearity causes the suppressed activation levels at the alternative site to be insufficient to destabilize the peak.

ized by a sigmoid nonlinearity $\sigma(u)$ that mediates the interaction strength $w(\phi - \phi')$ between two field sites, $\phi$ and $\phi'$:

$$\tau\dot{u}(\phi,t) = -u(\phi,t) + h + s_{spec}(\phi,t) + s_{pre}(\phi,t) + \int d\phi' w(\phi - \phi')\sigma(u(\phi')) \quad (4.2)$$

How the sigmoid nonlinearity $\sigma(u)$ and the interaction kernel $w(\phi - \phi')$ lead to nonlinear interaction was analyzed mathematically by Amari (1977) and is illustrated in figure 4.6.

The resulting field dynamics generate a stable peak at an averaged location when two inputs specify metrically close saccadic endpoints (figure 4.7a). This averaging mode is mediated by the facilitatory short-range interaction. When the two inputs specify metrically distant saccadic endpoints (figure 4.7b), the dynamic field becomes bistable. An activation pattern with a strong peak located over one input site may be stabilized, but an alternative pattern with a strong peak located over the other input site is also stable. Which of the two patterns arises depends on any prior activation patterns in the field or on chance (mediated through stochastic inputs to the field). In a thought experiment in which the metric distance between the two saccadic targets is gradually increased, the field dynamics go through an instability in which the averaging solution becomes unstable and gives way to the two stable solutions centered over the two inputs. This conceptually illustrates how stability is an essential ingredient of the model.

## Preshape

In daily life, movements are never planned starting from a tabula rasa. There is always a perceptual and motor context out of which the new motor act arises. This is true most of the time in the laboratory as well, where previous movements, the perceptual layout of the work space, instructions, or explicit prior information all

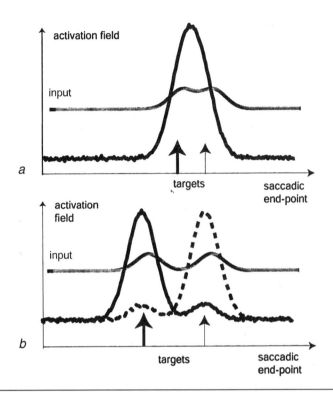

**Figure 4.7**   A dynamic field simulation of decision making in visually driven saccades. The dynamic field is bistable in *b;* the two activation patterns (solid and dashed black lines) shown are both possible.

From Kopecz and Schöner (1995).

prestructure the representation of possible movements. Such factors are one source of input to the dynamic field. Because such inputs can arise earlier than the imperative signal specifying a particular movement, they preshape the field, preactivating parameter values that characterize the expected movements.

Many classic effects in movement preparation can be understood in terms of such preshaping. For instance, it can be observed that with an increasing number of choices or decreasing probability of the choices, the time from stimulus to response increases (the Hick-Hyman law; Hick, 1952; Hyman, 1953). This observation can be accounted for by assuming that the more probable choices are more strongly preactivated, providing them with a head start in the growth of activation that is required to initiate the movement. Figure 4.8 illustrates this effect for a two-choice task. The two sites representing the two possible movements are preactivated to varying degrees, expressing different probabilities. Activation in the field reaches equivalent levels earlier when the more probable choice is specified. When the two choices differ more strongly in probability (figure 4.8, b and e compared with a and d), this time advantage is larger.

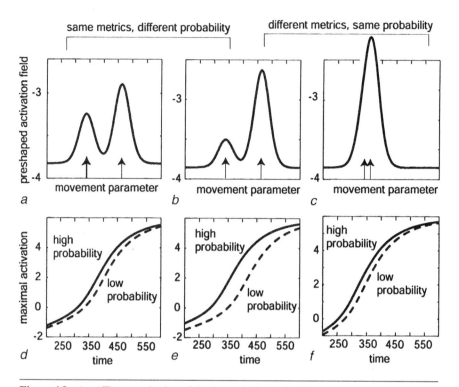

**Figure 4.8** *(a-c)* The preactivation of the dynamic field when in a two choice task the probabilities or the choice metrics are varied. *(d-f)* The temporal evolution of the maximal level of activation in the field is shown for the case that the more probable (solid line) or the less probable choice (dashed line) is specified.

In the field, however, not only the amount of activation but also the metric structure in the space of possible movements matters. The center and right columns of the figure (figure 4.8, b and e compared with c and f) compare situations with identical ratio of probabilities; the two choices are movements that are close to each other in parameter space (figure 4.8, c and f) or not (figure 4.8, b and e). The reaction time advantage of the probable choice is reduced when the choices consist of similar movements, because the two activation peaks overlap and facilitatory interaction helps activate the field when the less probable choice is specified.

McDowell and colleagues (2002) tested this prediction. Participants made pointing movements to one of two targets (figure 4.9). In the wide condition, the targets required an upward movement in one case and a movement in a direction 120° away from the up direction in the other case. In the narrow condition, the same vertical movement represented one choice, and the alternative was a movement in a direction 20° from the up direction. The vertical movement common across both conditions was the rare choice, occurring in 20% of the trials; the other movement was the frequent condition, occurring in 80% of the trials. (The actual experiment contained additional and control conditions.)

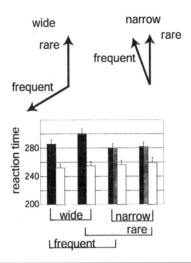

**Figure 4.9** Pointing movements to one of two targets separated by either a wide or narrow angle. At the bottom, the dark bars indicate reaction times for the pointing task, while the white bars represent reaction times from a control task in which the same response (lifting a finger from a home button) was made to all stimuli. See text for details.

From McDowell et al. (2000).

When the two choices involved dissimilar movement directions (120° apart, wide), a longer reaction time was observed for the rare choice, a replication of the classic Hyman effect. When the two choices involved similar movement directions (20° apart, narrow), this effect was no longer observed. The identical movement with identical probability as in the wide condition was initiated at the same latency as the frequent movement in the narrow condition. This is the effect predicted by dynamic field theory: The rare movement now gets a boost from its neighbor. The effect is the opposite of what one might expect were one to conceive of the process of movement initiation as involving a categorical decision between two choices. Such decisions are known to take longer, the more metrically similar the choices are (e.g., Johnson, 1939).

# Conclusions

The framework of dynamic field theory extends the concept of stability from motor control to the representation of information about movements. This makes it possible to account for the graded and continuous evolution of movement representations and provides the conceptual basis for understanding how motor plans can be continuously linked to sensory input. The nonlinear nature of the field dynamics leads to instabilities, from which new qualities of movement preparation emerge. We illustrated how the selection of one movement target from two possible targets can be understood in terms of nonlinear interactions. The transition to averaging for narrowly spaced targets delineates two qualitatively different modes of movement representation, which emerge from the same underlying field dynamics. Ghez and colleagues (1997) similarly observed two different modes in the early phase of movement preparation using the timed movement initiation paradigm: In a discrete mode a decision is made to move to one of multiple targets, whereas in a continuous mode a weighted average of possible movement targets determines which movement is made. These modes emerge quite analogously as two dynamic regimes from the field dynamics, again controlled by the metric distance between the possible movements (Erlhagen and Schöner, 2002).

Parametric activation fields have direct neurophysiological plausibility through a link to the concept of population code. Abstractly speaking, the population code concept of Georgopoulos and colleagues (1984) could be interpreted as a projection from cortical space into the space spanned by the movement parameter "direction": The cortical neurons broadly tuned to movement direction are labeled in terms of their preferred movement directions rather than in terms of their cortical location. A distribution of population activation constructed from this projection can then be considered an estimate of an underlying activation field (Erlhagen et al., 1999). Bastian and colleagues (1998) observed the temporal evolution of distributions of population activation obtained from neurons in the motor and premotor cortex of macaque monkeys, who performed a center-outward pointing task. When prior information about upcoming movement targets was manipulated, the preactivation of the appropriate region of the activation field was observed, providing direct evidence in favor of the postulated preshaping of input.

The simplest cognitive properties of movement representations such as decision making and short-term memory emerge from the dynamic field through instabilities. Broader insights from this observation may lead to a new look at cognitive processes with a renewed emphasis on their direct link to the motor and sensory surfaces (see discussion in Thelen et al., 2001).

# References

Amari, S. 1977. Dynamics of pattern formation in lateral-inhibition type neural fields. *Biological Cybernetics* 27: 77-87.

Bastian, A., A. Riehle, W. Erlhagen, and G. Schöner. 1998. Prior information preshapes the population representation of movement direction in motor cortex. *Neuroreports* 9: 315-319.

Braun, M. 1994. *Differential equations and their applications.* 4th edition. Springer Verlag, New York.

Erlhagen, W., A. Bastian, D. Jancke, A. Riehle, and G. Schöner. 1999. The distribution of neuronal population activation (DPA) as a tool to study interaction and integration in cortical representations. *Journal of Neuroscience Methods* 94: 53-66.

Erlhagen, W., and G. Schöner. 2002. Dynamic field theory of movement preparation. *Psychological Review,* July. 109: 545-572.

Georgopoulos, A.P., J.F. Kalaska, M.D. Crutcher, R. Caminiti, and J.T. Massey. 1984. The representation of movement direction in the motor cortex: Single cell and population studies. In G.M. Edelman, W.E. Gall, and W.M. Cowan, editors, *Dynamic aspects of neocortical function,* pp. 501-524. John Wiley, New York.

Ghez, C., M. Favilla, M.F. Ghilardi, J. Gordon, R. Bermejo, and S. Pullman. 1997. Discrete and continuous planning of hand movements and isometric force trajectories. *Experimental Brain Research* 115: 217-233.

Ghez, C., W. Hening, and M. Favilla. 1990. Parallel interacting channels in the initiation and specification of motor response features. In M. Jeannerod, editor, *Attention and performance XIII*, pp. 265-293. Erlbaum, Hillsdale, NJ.

Glimcher, P.W. 2001. Making choices: The neurophysiology of visual-saccadic decision making. *Trends in Neurosciences* 24 (11): 654-659.

Goodale, M.A., D. Pélisson, and C. Prablanc. 1986. Large adjustments in visually guided reaching do not depend on vision of the hand or perception of target displacement. *Nature* 320: 748-750.

Grossberg, S., C. Pribe, and M.A. Cohen. 1997. Neural control of interlimb oscillations. I. Human bimanual coordination. *Biological Cybernetics* 77: 131-140.

Haken, H., J.A.S. Kelso, and H. Bunz. 1985. A theoretical model of phase transitions in human hand movements. *Biological Cybernetics* 51: 347-356.

Hick, W.E. 1952. On the rate of gain of information. *Quarterly Journal of Experimental Psychology* 4: 11-26.

Hinton, G.E. 1984. Parallel computations for controlling an arm. *Journal of Motor Behavior* 16: 171-194.

Hyman, R. 1953. Stimulus information as a determinant of reaction time. *Journal of Experimental Psychology* 45: 188-196.

Johnson, D.M. 1939. Confidence and speed in the two-category judgment. *Archives of Psychology* 241: 1-52.

Kawato, M. 1990. Computational schemas and neural network models of multijoint arm trajectory. In W.T. Miller, III, R.S. Sutton, and P.J. Werbos, editors, *Neural networks for control*, pp. 197-228. MIT Press, Cambridge, MA.

Kopecz, K., and G. Schöner. 1995. Saccadic motor planning by integrating visual information and pre-information on neural, dynamic fields. *Biological Cybernetics* 73: 49-60.

Latash, M. 1993. *Control of human movement.* Human Kinetics, Champaign, IL.

McDowell, K., J.J. Jeka, G. Schöner, and B.D. Hatfield. 2002. Behavioural and electrocortical evidence of an interaction between probability and task metrics in movement preparation. *Experimental Brain Research.* 144: 303-313.

Ottes, F.P., J.A.M. van Gisbergen, and J.J. Eggermont. 1985. Latency dependence of colour-based target vs. nontarget discrimination by the saccadic system. *Vision Research* 25: 849-862.

Prablanc, C., and O. Martin. 1992. Autonomous control during hand reaching at undetected two-dimensional target displacements. *Journal of Neurophysiology* 67: 455-469.

Schöner, G. 1994. From interlimb coordination to trajectory formation: Common dynamical principles. In S. Swinnen, H. Heuer, J. Massion, and P. Casaer, editors, *Interlimb coordination: Neural, dynamical, and cognitive constraints*, pp. 339-368. Academic Press, San Diego.

Schöner, G. 2002. Timing, clocks, and dynamical systems. *Brain and Cognition* 48: 31-51.

Schöner, G., and J.A.S. Kelso. 1988. Dynamic pattern generation in behavioral and neural systems. *Science* 239: 1513-1520.

Thelen, E., G. Schöner, C. Scheier, and L. Smith. 2001. The dynamics of embodiment: A field theory of infant perseverative reaching. *Brain and Behavioral Sciences* 24: 1-33.

Tipper, S.P., L.A. Howard, and G. Houghton. 2000. Behavioral consequences of selection from neural population codes. In S. Monsell and J. Driver, editors, *Attention and performance XVIII: Control of cognitive processes*, pp. 223-245. MIT Press, Cambridge, MA.

van Sonderen, J.F., J.J. Denier van der Gon, and C.C.A.M. Gielen. 1988. Conditions determining early modifications of motor programmes in response to changes in target location. *Experimental Brain Research* 71: 320-328.

van Sonderen, J.F., J.J. Denier van der Gon, and C.C.A.M. Gielen. 1989. Motor programmes for goal-directed movements are continuously adjusted according to changes in target location. *Experimental Brain Research* 78: 139-146.

Williams, R.J. 1986. The logic of activation functions. In D.E. Rumelhart, J.L. McClelland, and the PDP research group, editors, *Parallel distributed processing,* volume 1, pp. 423-424. MIT Press, Cambridge, MA.

# 5

# Coordination of Multielement Motor Systems Based on Motor Abundance

*Mark L. Latash*
Pennsylvania State University

*Frederic Danion*
Université de la Méditerranée

*John F. Scholz*
University of Delaware

*Gregor Schöner*
Ruhr-Universität Bochum

In the tradition of Gelfand and Tsetlin, we revisit the principle of minimal interaction and focus on one of its consequences: error correction among elements of a structural unit. We introduce an uncontrolled manifold (UCM) hypothesis, together with a toolbox that allows the analysis of different performance variables with respect to their possible selective stabilization by the controller during natural motor tasks. We review evidence supporting the UCM hypothesis, including studies of whole-body movements, multijoint limb movements, two-limb movements, and multifinger force production tasks. The reviewed material suggests that the UCM hypothesis offers a fruitful framework for analysis of multielement motor systems. Challenges facing the UCM hypothesis are discussed, together with promising future directions of its development.

## The Problem of Motor Redundancy

A long time ago, Bernstein (1935, 1947) noticed that the anatomical design of human limbs allowed numerous kinematic solutions to most everyday motor problems. He used the example of the human arm, with its seven major axes of joint rotation, to illustrate that a typical task (e.g., to touch an object with the tip of the index finger) leads to a problem that has no unique solution. Such problems are equivalent to solving a system of equations when the number of equations is smaller than the number of unknowns. This example has turned into a proverbial illustration for one of the most notorious problems in the area of movement studies, the problem of motor redundancy.

At each level of analysis of the system for the production of voluntary movements, many more elements contribute to performance than are absolutely necessary to solve a motor task. For example, the trajectory of the endpoint of a limb does not define a unique pattern of joint rotations (cf. the problem of inverse kinematics, Mussa-Ivaldi et al., 1989) or a unique pattern of joint torques (cf. the problem of inverse dynamics, Atkeson, 1989). Similarly, the value of a joint torque does not define a unique combination of activation levels of muscles crossing the joint, and a level of muscle activation does not define a unique pattern of motor unit recruitment, and so on (cf. Latash, 1996). In other words, a motor task formulated at a certain level of analysis does not prescribe a single particular pattern at a lower, multielement level, so the controller (the central nervous system) always seems to be confronted with a problem of choice: How to select a particular way of solving each particular problem? Problems of this type belong to an ill-posed class that have been termed *problems of motor redundancy* or *Bernstein's problems* (Turvey, 1990). Bernstein himself (1947, 1967) viewed the problem of the elimination of redundant degrees of freedom as the central issue of motor control.

Bernstein was somewhat vague in his writings on this issue, and it is unclear whether he seriously implied an elimination of biomechanical degrees of freedom (DFs) using his examples. One should be absolutely clear that, for a natural movement, the only way to eliminate a biomechanical DF is to perform a major surgery. The efficacy of a particular mechanical DF can be modulated, explored, limited, and so on, but one can never eliminate a DF. However, elimination of biomechanical DFs is rather commonly invoked in contemporary studies of human motor behavior (e.g., Newell, 1991; Piek, 1995; Vereijken et al., 1992). In many studies, the presence or the lack of visible motion of a joint has been viewed as a sign of a biomechanical DF being either recruited or eliminated. Along somewhat similar lines and following Bernstein's (1996) traditions, studies of motor learning commonly use notions of freezing and releasing DFs at different stages of skill acquisition (Piek, 1995; Vereijken et al., 1992) with an implicit assumption that it is easier to control an object with fewer biomechanical DFs (cf. Fentress, 1976).

There have been many attempts to address the problem of motor redundancy in its original formulation. These have involved, in particular, application of optimization methods based on certain mechanical, engineering, psychological, or complex cost functions (for reviews see Latash, 1993; Rosenbaum et al., 1995; Seif-Naraghi and Winters, 1990). However, in this chapter, we suggest that the problem itself has been inadequately formulated and needs to be reconsidered.

## Motor Variability Suggests That the Problem of Motor Redundancy Is Ill Posed

The inadequacy of the original formulation of the problem of motor redundancy has been implicit in many studies of natural voluntary movements, particularly those that have focused on the issue of motor variability. Motor variability is arguably the most reproducible phenomenon in the realm of motor behavior: Several attempts at the same task always lead to somewhat different patterns of performance, including kinematics, kinetics, patterns of neural firing, muscle activation, and so on. This feature of human movements did not escape Bernstein's attention. Bernstein (1947) used the expression "repetition without repetition" when he described consecutive attempts at solving a motor task. He implied that each repetition of a motor act involves unique, nonrepetitive neural and motor patterns. This phenomenon was a major argument used by Bernstein against the then-prevalent Pavlov's theory of conditioned reflexes that considered effects of motor practice as "beating a path" through the central nervous system (CNS).

During the last half century, motor variability has become an object of study in its own right, with review papers and monographs dedicated to this topic (e.g., Newell and Corcos, 1993). At present, most motor control researchers view variability not as a nuisance that forces experimenters to record many trials of each motor task, but rather as a window into the central organization of the system that produces voluntary movements.

In the 1920s, Bernstein performed a study of the kinematics of hitting movements, specifically, professional blacksmiths' striking the chisel with the hammer. His subjects were perfectly trained. They had performed the same movement hundreds of times a day for years. For this analysis, Bernstein (1927) used a very sophisticated method to record movement kinematics: kimocyclography, an ancestor of contemporary optoelectronic systems. The method used a photographic camera with slow-moving film and a high-speed shutter (Popova and Mogilyanskaya, 1934). This camera recorded displacements of light bulbs placed on the moving objects. By the end of the 1920s, Bernstein could record at a speed of over 500 snapshots per second (Bernstein and Popova, 1929). In the precomputer age, data processing created the bottleneck. It was not unusual to spend months measuring and analyzing the kinematics of a single trial. Using this system, Bernstein (1927, 1967) noticed that the variability of the trajectory of the tip of the hammer over a series of strikes by a blacksmith was smaller than the variability of the trajectories of the individual joints of the arm holding the hammer. Since the brain apparently could not send signals directly to the hammer, Bernstein concluded that the joints were not acting independently but were correcting each other's errors. This observation suggested that the CNS does not try to find a unique solution for the problem of kinematic redundancy by eliminating redundant DFs but rather uses the apparently redundant set of joints to ensure more accurate (less variable) performance of the task. Of course, Bernstein's was a qualitative observation because variability in the space of joints is not directly comparable to variability in end-effector space.

This observation by Bernstein was followed some 50 years later by a series of studies showing that during multielement movements, elements show *error compensation,* that is, changes in their activity when a spontaneous or externally produced perturbation occurs in the course of a well-learned movement (Abbs and Gracco, 1984; Berkinblit et al., 1986; Li et al., 1998). The phenomenon of error compensation is hardly compatible with the original formulation of the problem of motor redundancy. It implies that no unique solution is being computed by the CNS, but rather whole families of solutions are facilitated, leading to the same desired functional outcome (cf. the notion of motor equivalence reviewed in Berkinblit et al., 1986).

## Synergies and Structural Units

By the end of the 19th century, the great British neurologist Hughlings Jackson (1889) formulated a theory of multiple cortical representations of the motor apparatus. In particular, he wrote, "The central nervous system knows nothing about muscles, it only knows movements" (p. 358). Hughlings Jackson probably implied that the brain controls movements not in a "marionette fashion," that is, computing and sending signals to each effector (cf. Turvey and Carello, 1996), but by uniting effectors (muscles) into groups that we would now probably address as synergies. A synergy is arguably the most frequently used and least precisely described notion in the area of movement studies. Most readers of this chapter are probably familiar with this notion, so before going any further, we would like the reader to try to formulate a definition for a synergy that distinguishes a synergy from a nonsynergy or introduces a measure of the "strength" of a synergy.

To start an analysis of a biological system at a selected level of description, one needs to define an element, the smallest sensible structure, that can be used at the chosen level of analysis. For example, the motor unit can be viewed as an element of an intact muscle, and a muscle with its central neuronal apparatus can be viewed as an element of a multijoint limb. Gelfand and Tsetlin (1966) formulated a principle of nonindividualized control, according to which elements of a

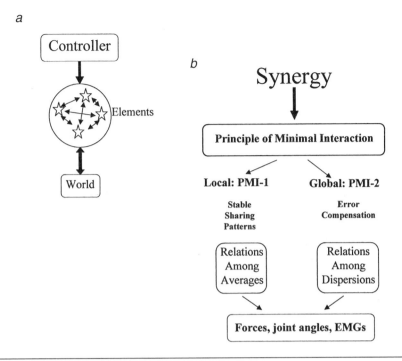

**Figure 5.1**  *(a)* The general structure of a synergy, consisting of a controller and a set of elements interacting with the environment. *(b)* Synergies obey the principle of minimal interaction (PMI), which has two components: PMI-1 tends to preserve a sharing pattern among the elements, while PMI-2 tends to minimize deviations of the functional output of the synergy from a required value.

complex system are not controlled individually but united into task-specific or intention-specific structural units (cf. Hughlings Jackson, 1889, and the notion of action units in Greene, 1972). Structural units are organized by the controller in a flexible, task-specific way for purposes, which can be termed *synergies* (figure 5.1). External behavior generated by a structural unit is defined by its purpose (i.e., by the synergy) and by current external conditions. In contemporary literature, the term *synergy* is more commonly used as a synonym of *structural unit*. This definition has two components that are necessary to consider a system a synergy: task specificity and the presence of a controller.

Elements of a structural unit (of a synergy) are also structural units (synergies): For example, a multimuscle synergy has muscles as its elements, while each muscle is a synergy of motor units. A multijoint kinematic synergy can be composed of a few multijoint subsynergies (cf. Alexandrov et al., 1998).

Gelfand and Tsetlin (1966) also suggested a principle of minimal interaction (PMI), which states that the interaction among elements at a lower level of a hierarchy is organized in such a way that the external input to each of the elements in minimized. The originally somewhat vague formulation was developed later (Gelfand and Latash, 1998; Lestienne et al., chapter 1 in this volume), and the principle of minimal interaction was reformulated at two levels:

- PMI-1 (at the level of interaction among elements, local): The effect of a change in the magnitude of a common functional output on the relative contribution of an element to that common functional output is minimized by changes in the output of all elements.

- PMI-2 (at the level of interaction between individual elements and the higher level of the hierarchy, global): The effect of a change in the output of an element on the common, functionally defined outcome of the structural unit is minimized by changes in the output of other elements.

In other words, elements within a synergy interact in such a way that each of them tries to function in its preferred mode while simultaneously keeping the functional output at a desired level so that no intervention from the higher level of the hierarchy is required, even when one or more of the elements change their contributions.

For example, imagine that you are the conductor of a choir and you need the choir to produce a certain level of sound. One strategy would be to tell each singer how loudly he or she is supposed to sing. This strategy will solve the problem, but the solution will be unstable: If one singer makes a mistake or quits singing altogether, the task will not be performed properly since other singers will continue to sing at their instructed levels. An alternative would be to make use of the fact that the singers have ears: Let the singers hear the required sound level, and then tell them to sing more loudly if sound level is too soft and to sing more softly if it is too loud. This instruction unites the singers in a task-specific way into a synergy. They will produce the required level of sound, although with a certain variability, and the solution will be stable, even if one singer suddenly decides to stop singing.

Figure 5.1 illustrates the introduced definition of synergy and the principle of minimal interaction. The local PMI (PMI-1) defines a particular preferred relationship among the elements' average outputs. Such relationships have been described for a variety of tasks, including vertical posture, locomotion, reaching, and finger force production (Desmurget et al., 1995; Macpherson et al., 1986; Pelz et al., 2001; Santello and Soechting, 2000; Smith et al., 1985; Wang and Stelmach, 1998). If we assume, for simplicity, that the elements are contributing in an additive way to a common functional output, PMI-1 favors positive correlations among outputs of individual elements such that the *sharing pattern* (cf. Li et al., 1998) is preserved. Principal component analysis (PCA) is one commonly used method to identify such sharing patterns over the time when an action is realized or over a range of task parameters.

The global PMI (PMI-2) has also been addressed as the principle of error compensation (Latash, Li, and Zatsiorsky, 1998). In general, if the elements are contributing in an additive way to a common functional output, PMI-2 favors negative correlations among outputs of individual elements to minimize the effects of a spontaneous change in the output of an element (an error) on the common functional output.

As illustrated in figure 5.1, PMI-1 and PMI-2 seem to be in competition since they tend to promote opposite changes in the outputs of elements of a synergy. Imagine that a person is asked to press with two effectors (for example, hands) and produce a ramp pattern of total force increasing from zero to some high level of force. Imagine also that the person is right-handed and, on average, produces 55% of the total force with the right hand. If individual force changes over such a ramp are analyzed, a strong positive correlation between the forces will be found (see PMI-1 in figure 5.1 and Li et al., 1998). Imagine that the person is now asked to perform this task many times. In half way through one trial, the right hand produces a spontaneous error (its force is too high). What would be the deviation of the force of the left hand from its average preferred value? PMI-1 predicts that it will be proportionally *higher,* so that its share stays at 45%, while PMI-2 predicts that it will be *lower* to keep the total force closer to its required instantaneous level. An experiment is required to see which prediction is true.

Let us now consider another example. A person takes a fork and presses the four prongs on four force sensors. The total force changes to produce a ramp similar to the one in the previous example. If the person presses down without rotating the fork around its longitudinal axis, there will be a strong positive correlation between the forces produced by individual prongs, so PMI-1 will be satisfied. However, in no situation will PMI-2 be satisfied: If in one trial, a prong produces an error, all other prongs will produce errors in the same direction such that the error in the total force will not be reduced but amplified!

According to our definition, the fork is not a synergy, since there is no controller that can modify relationships among the outputs of its elements (prongs) in a task-specific way. No natural, inanimate object can represent a synergy since such objects do not have controllers that can ensure their flexibility and task specificity. A different definition could be introduced that considers all objects that comply with PMI-1 as synergies. However, this would mean that any inanimate object becomes a synergy: For example, a stone on the ground can be viewed as a synergy of its parts, which produce pressure on the ground in proportion to the weight of an object placed on the stone. This is absurd. Therefore, PMI-1 and its consequences (stable sharing patterns among elements) are insufficient to declare a system a synergy. In contrast, PMI-2 is applicable to synergies but not to inanimate objects.

In a biological system, both PMI-1 and PMI-2 are applicable to synergies, in particular, to motor synergies. However, as mentioned earlier, these two forms of the principle of minimal interaction can come into conflict. Hence, analysis of both averages and dispersions is required to discover the purposes of a synergy and its intrinsic design. Until recently, analysis of averages has dominated motor control studies, and stable relationships among outputs of elements (joint angles, muscle activation levels, joint torques, finger forces, etc.) have commonly been declared synergies (Gottlieb et al., 1996; Henry et al., 1998; Keshner et al., 1988; Saltiel et al., 2001; Vernazza-Martin et al., 1999). As the fork example shows, however, such conclusions may be premature. For example, a covariation among joint trajectories or joint torques may be due to inertial coupling or the presence of biarticular muscles, not to a particular organization of control. In this chapter, we focus on the other side of synergies reflected in the relationships among dispersions in the outputs of individual elements. This analysis is more related to PMI-2 and thus is more sensitive to a crucial feature of synergies: error compensation.

Gelfand and Tsetlin (1966) formulated a set of axioms for the organization of structural units and a principle of minimal interaction: "An element of a structural unit tries to minimize the total input it receives from the controller, the environment, and other elements of the structural unit." Later, Gelfand and Latash (1998) reformulated this principle: A structural unit (a synergy) is always organized in a task-specific way so that if an element introduces an error into the common functional output, other elements change their contributions to minimize the original error, and no corrective action is required of the controller. We suggest using the term *synergy* only for systems that function according to this principle and demonstrate error compensation among their elements. Let us emphasize that this definition makes synergies always task specific: A multielement system can be a synergy with respect to a particular task and a nonsynergy with respect to other tasks.

One of the original axioms suggested by Gelfand and Tsetlin in 1966 has been further developed into a principle of abundance (Gelfand and Latash, 1998; Latash, 2000). This principle states that, within a multielement synergy, all the elements (DFs) form an abundant (rather than redundant) set and always participate in all the tasks, ensuring both the stability and the flexibility of the performance. Thus, the principle of abundance renders the problem of motor redundancy irrelevant: No DFs are ever eliminated or frozen. The idea of motor abundance allows the introduction of elements of exactness into one of the most commonly (ab)used terms in the area of movement studies, synergy.

# The Uncontrolled Manifold Hypothesis

Within the Uncontrolled Manifold (UCM) hypothesis, control is associated with selective stabilization of particular performance variables corresponding to particular directions within the state space of the system. In a sense, it can be viewed as a particular optimization approach in which an optimized (selectively stabilized) function is selected each time in a task-specific manner. The UCM hypothesis assumes that, for a given task, the controller (the CNS) selects a variable or set of variables whose value or values it tries to stabilize at each moment in time. The value of such a variable corresponds to a subspace in the state space of the elements within which the value does not change (a null space). When elements of the system change their outputs within this subspace, the selected value of the selected variable remains unchanged. If changes in the elements' output take the system out of the subspace, however, the value of the variable changes. This may be associated with an error in the system's performance. Such a subspace has been termed the *uncontrolled manifold.* After forming a UCM, the controller focuses on directions within the state space that do not belong to the UCM and selectively restricts the variability of elements along these "essential" directions, but not along directions within the UCM. This means that the controller allows the elements to show high variability as long as it does not affect the desired value of the variable.

Consider the following example: A person is asked to press with two hands to produce a total force of 50 N. Let this person perform the task 100 times, and plot the values of individual hand forces on the force-force plane (the state space of the system). The data points form a cloud (in figure 5.2, the ovals indicate the data distribution shapes). Let us consider two possibilities. First, the cloud may be circular (figure 5.2a). This means that if one hand by chance produced a higher than usual force, the other hand produced with equal probability higher than usual or lower than usual forces. In other words, if one hand introduced an error into the common output, the probability is equal that the other hand would amplify or reduce the error. By definition, this is not a synergy. Let us consider the alternative illustrated

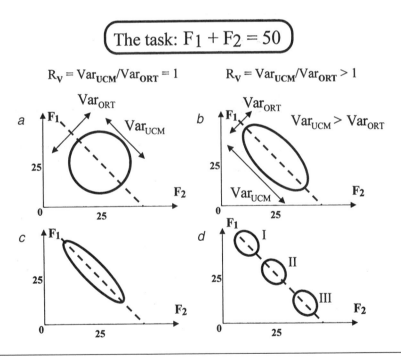

**Figure 5.2** Ellipses show possible distributions of data points across many trials of the task in which the subject is asked to produce the total force of 50 N by pressing with two hands. Dashed lines show uncontrolled manifolds (UCMs) for the task $F_1 + F_2 = 50$. Relationships between components of variance parallel and orthogonal to the UCM can be described by their ratio $R_V$. *(a)* This is not a synergy; $R_V = 1$. *(b)* This is a synergy; $R_V > 1$. Practice leading to better performance (smaller variance orthogonal to the UCM) can result in *(c)* a stronger synergy or *(d)* a weaker synergy.

in figure 5.2b. The cloud of points is elongated along a line corresponding to the equation $F_1 + F_2 = 50$ (the dashed line in figure 5.2). In this case, if by chance one hand produced a larger force, the other hand would more likely produce a lower force to keep the sum closer to the required value. The two elements are at least partly compensating for each other's errors. This is a synergy, and the dashed line is the UCM.

To analyze such clouds of data points quantitatively, a particular measure of variability can be used, the variance. Variance is particularly useful because, if several elements contribute to a common output with certain errors and these errors are uncorrelated, the variance of the output is equal to the sum of the variances of the elements. This property of variance allows us to compare it across subspaces with different dimensions. Let us introduce two measures of variance for the data clouds illustrated in figure 5.2. One of them is the projection of the variance on the UCM ($Var_{UCM}$), and the other is the projection of the variance on the orthogonal to the UCM direction ($Var_{ORT}$). Let us normalize both $Var_{UCM}$ and $Var_{ORT}$ by the number of dimensions (DFs) within the UCM and within the orthogonal subspace. (In figure 5.2, no normalization is required since the dimensions of UCM and orthogonal subspace are both unity.) If $Var_{UCM}$ is significantly higher than $Var_{ORT}$ after the normalization, as in figure 5.2b, the system functions according to the UCM hypothesis, that is, it establishes a link between errors in the outputs of the elements. If there is no difference between $Var_{UCM}$ and $Var_{ORT}$, the system controls the elements independently. This may be quantified using the ratio $R_V = Var_{UCM}/Var_{ORT}$. If $R_V > 1$, the system functions according to the UCM hypothesis with respect to the selected criterion, and it is therefore a synergy.

Note that, by definition, a UCM always reflects a control hypothesis, that is, a hypothesis about the value of a performance variable, which the system is assumed to stabilize. In the example in figure 5.2, the control hypothesis is that the system tried to stabilize the total force at 50 N. Other control hypotheses may be considered, for example, that the total force is stabilized at a different value or that another function (e.g., the difference) in the two forces is stabilized at a certain value. For a control hypothesis $R_V > 1$, the hypothesized performance variable is selectively stabilized. If $R_V = 1$, the organization of control is indifferent to the selected performance variable. If $R_V < 1$, the organization of control is such that the selected performance variable is destabilized; that is, if an element introduces an error into the common output, changes in the outputs of other elements are more likely to amplify the error. This may mean, in particular, that the system stabilizes a different variable so that the analyzed variable is destabilized. We consider such examples later in the chapter.

If a multielement system is organized so that it uses the UCM method of control, only certain relationships between variance components can be predicted, not their absolute magnitudes. Thus, this particular mode of control can lead to good or bad performance and is compatible with better, equal, or worse performance as compared with performances obtained by controlling each element of the system independently (as by a nonsynergy).

Imagine that, as a result of practice, a system improved its performance with respect to a particular criterion, for example, it became less variable with respect to a required value of a performance variable. Such an improvement in performance theoretically can be associated with an increased or a decreased $R_V$ computed with respect to the selected variable (figure 5.2, c and d). In both cases, the component of variance orthogonal to the UCM ($Var_{ORT}$) should decrease, implying less-variable production of the common output, that is, better performance. In figure 5.2c, this is associated with no change in $Var_{UCM}$, leading to an increase in $R_V$. In figure 5.2d, $Var_{UCM}$ decreased more than $Var_{ORT}$, leading to a drop in $R_V$. Figure 5.2d also illustrates the relative independence of the two formulations of the principle of minimal interaction, PMI-1 and PMI-2: The same degree of error compensation (the same $R_V$ values) can be associated with different sharing patterns, as in the data distributions I, II, and III.

A multielement system can selectively stabilize several performance variables at the same time. This is true as long as the number of elements is at least as high as the number of task constraints plus the number of stabilized variables.

## Generalizing the UCM Hypothesis

Figure 5.2 illustrated the simplest case, in which two elements contributed to a common output. To use the UCM approach to analyze the functioning of a multi-element system, we need a Jacobian ($\mathbf{J}$) of the system, that is, a set of coefficients that describe how infinitesimally small changes in the outputs of individual elements are reflected in the magnitude of a selected performance variable. This is formalized as a matrix of partial derivatives of the selected variable with respect to outputs of the elements. In some cases, the $\mathbf{J}$ matrix can be computed based on the geometric properties of the system. For example, when we are interested in how individual joint rotations are organized to produce a particular motion of the endpoint of a multijoint limb, coefficients for a Jacobian can be computed as trigonometric functions with coefficients reflecting the relative configuration and size of the segments (Zatsiorsky, 1999). In other situations, however, getting an estimate of the $\mathbf{J}$ matrix itself becomes a major problem. Such problems can be particularly hard to solve for a system whose apparent output elements may not be independently controlled.

Consider the situation when a person tries to produce force by pressing with the tip of a finger. Other fingers of the hand also show involuntary force production. This phenomenon is called *enslaving* (Hager-Ross and Schieber, 1999; Kilbreath and Gandevia, 1994; Zatsiorsky et al. 1998, 2000). It is due both to peripheral connections among the fingers, such as shared muscles and interdigit tendinous connections (Kilbreath and Gandevia, 1994; Leijsne et al., 1993), and to neural factors such as overlapping cortical representations for individual fingers (Roullier, 1996). Enslaving is not specific to particular tasks and can be seen in virtually all motor activities involving the hand. Such built-in dependencies among the fingers imply that the CNS cannot control the force output of a finger independently of the force outputs of other fingers.

Let us introduce another set of hypothetical variables that the CNS manipulates independently when it tries to coordinate the fingers of a hand. Such variables can be associated with patterns of force changes when a person tries to produce force with only one finger (cf. Zatsiorsky et al., 1998). These hypothetical variables have been termed *modes* (Latash et al., 2001; Scholz et al., 2002). Figure 5.3 illustrates the notion of modes. Each mode contributes to force production by each finger of the hand, and individual modes can be independently involved to different degrees by the CNS. An attenuation of the combined effects of several force modes acting simultaneously leads to the phenomenon of force deficit, that is, a lower force generated by a finger when it acts together with other fingers than in a single-finger task.

Most contemporary scientists would probably agree that muscles are not controlled independently by the CNS (see the earlier cited quotation by Hughlings Jackson, 1889). The notion of multimuscle synergies is commonly invoked in studies of different motor activities (e.g., Chong and Franklin, 2001; De Serres and Milner, 1991; Henry et al., 1998; Macpherson, 1988; Saltiel et al., 2001; Tresch et al., 1999). If one wants to perform a formal analysis of a multimuscle synergy using the framework of the UCM hypothesis, a relationship between small changes in the activity of individual

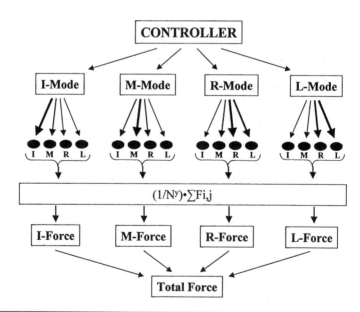

**Figure 5.3**    In four-finger force production tasks, the controller manipulates four independent variables, termed *modes*. A single mode is recruited when the subject tries to press with only one finger. Each mode contributes to force production by each finger (enslaving). The outputs of modes are summed up and attenuated with a coefficient that reflects the total number of recruited modes, $N$ (force deficit), yielding the actual finger force patterns.

muscles and a common functional output variable (an EMG Jacobian) is necessary. To obtain the coefficients composing such a matrix, an experimenter cannot simply tell a subject "Now change the activity of only your left brachioradialis," because this is a nonsensical instruction. Multimuscle modes therefore need to be discovered by more subtle means. Such means are currently being developed.

## Kinematic Studies Using the UCM Hypothesis

Several studies so far have used the UCM hypothesis to analyze motor systems and tasks of different complexity. Table 5.1 presents a summary of these studies. It specifies the tasks, methods of analysis, and control hypotheses that were tested in particular studies. Control hypotheses refer to particular time courses of perfor-

**Table 5.1 Main Results of Studies Using the UCM Framework**

| Study | Task | Analysis | Hypotheses* | Results |
|-------|------|----------|-------------|---------|
| Scholz and Schöner, 1999 | Sit-to-stand | Planar kinematic | H1—center of mass (CM) path H2—head position | $R_v > 1$ for horizontal and vertical CM path (H1); $R_v > 1$ for H2, horizontal path only. |
| Scholz et al., 2001; Reisman et al., 2002 | Sit-to-stand | Planar kinematic, kinetic | H1—CM path H2—head path H3—linear momentum of CM | $R_v > 1$ for H1, H2, and H3 for horizontal but not vertical path; $R_v >> 1$ for H1 for horizontal path, when task is more challenging. |
| Domkin et al., 2002; Laczko et al., 2001 | Bimanual pointing | Planar kinematic | H1—target trajectory H2—pointer trajectory H3—vectorial distance between pointer and target | All hypotheses confirmed. H3 showed higher $R_v$. Practice led to better performance and smaller $R_v$. |

*continued*

**Table 5.1**   *(continued)*

| Study | Task | Analysis | Hypotheses* | Results |
|-------|------|----------|-------------|---------|
| Scholz et al., 2000 | Quick-draw shooting | 3D kinematic | H1—pistol orientation H2—pistol position H3—CM position | H1 confirmed over the whole movement; H2 and H3 confirmed only during early phase. |
| Scholz et al., 2002 | Four-finger cyclic force production | Kinetic | H1—total force H2—total moment | H1 confirmed only at high forces; H2 confirmed over the whole cycle. |
| Latash et al., 2001 | Marginally redundant, two- and three-finger cyclic force production | Kinetic, stable and unstable conditions | H1—total force H2—total moment | H1 confirmed only at high forces; H2 confirmed over much of the cycle. Moment was stabilized at the expense of force destabilization. |

*Analyses were performed with respect to particular control hypotheses: The hypotheses specify variables whose time profiles were assumed to be selectively stabilized by the CNS. More details are in the text.

mance variables that the CNS was assumed to stabilize during particular tasks. The last column of the table summarizes the main findings of the studies regarding the tested control hypotheses. The studied tasks included whole-body motion, joint coordination during a bimanual task, joint coordination during a single-limb task, and finger coordination in multifinger force production tasks.

Scholz and his colleagues (Reisman, Scholz, and Schöner, 2002; Scholz et al., 2001; Scholz and Schöner, 1999) performed a kinematic analysis of the sit-to-stand task. This particular task was selected because it is a common, everyday action that involves the coordination of rotation at several major joints and has apparent constraints, such as keeping the projection of the center of mass (CM) within the area of support. Another intuitive consideration is that during such an action unexpected changes in the head position should be avoided, particularly to maintain the constancy of visual perception. Based on these considerations, Scholz and colleagues formulated and tested the following control hypotheses:

- H1-StS: Rotations of major leg and trunk joints are coordinated to stabilize the average trajectory of the CM and the linear momentum of the CM.

- H2-StS: Joint rotations are coordinated to stabilize the instantaneous position of the head in space. Exact results depend on the experimental condition.

There was a large difference between the two variance components computed with respect to the UCMs underlying control of the horizontal path of the CM and its linear momentum ($R_V > 1$) and, to a lesser extent, the horizontal path of the head. When the task was made more challenging by decreasing the support area under the feet, $R_V$ increased due to a selective increase in $Var_{UCM}$ (Scholz et al., 2001). This selective increase in $Var_{UCM}$ may reflect an additional advantage of a UCM control strategy other than error compensation. That is, reducing control action by freeing directions in joint space from control may reduce unnecessary perturbations that occur due to the mechanical coupling of joints (Scholz et al., 2000). In contrast to the results for horizontal motion, the value of $R_V$ for control of the vertical path of the CM differed across conditions and was approximately unity for more challenging task conditions.

In experiments by Domkin et al. (2002; also see Laczko et al., 2001), subjects performed a two-arm "fast and accurate" pointing task in which one arm moved the target while the other arm moved the pointer. By instruction, the motion was nearly planar. As a result, three joints (shoulder, elbow, and wrist) in each arm formed redundant sets. The authors asked a number of questions regarding the joint coordination both within each limb and between the two limbs. The following control hypotheses were tested using the UCM approach:

- H1-P: Joint rotations in the left arm are coordinated to stabilize the average trajectory of the target.

- H2-P: Joint rotations in the right arm are coordinated to stabilize the average trajectory of the pointer.

- H3-P: Joint rotations of both arms are coordinated to stabilize the vectorial distance between the pointer and the target.

Series of pointing movements were analyzed both before and after a three-day practice. All three hypotheses were supported both before and after the practice in the sense that $R_V$ was larger than unity for each of them. However, $R_V$ for H3-P was significantly higher than for H1-P or H2-P. This result suggests that the joints of the two arms were indeed united in a bimanual synergy rather than a simple superposition of two unimanual synergies.

After practice, the subjects improved their performance and showed smaller indices of variability in the final position of the pointer with respect to the center of the target. The UCM analysis, however, led to somewhat unexpected results. Both $Var_{UCM}$ and $Var_{ORT}$ decreased with practice for all three hypotheses, H1-P, H2-P, and H3-P. However, $Var_{UCM}$ decreased more, leading to smaller $R_V$ values after practice (similar to the case illustrated in figure 5.2d). Thus, the subjects decreased their variability more within the UCM, that is, in directions that did not affect their performance. We might speculate that the task was so simple that there was not much room for decreasing $Var_{ORT}$. Other factors, outside the explicit task, could play a role in making the movements more stereotypical, for example optimizing postural stability. Finally, the uncontrolled manifold analysis by Domkin et al. (2002) looked at separate "snapshots" of UCMs along the trajectory. Note, however, that the smooth path of the end effector required that such a sequence of different UCMs form a continuum. It is conceivable that joint angles lying in certain regions of one UCM may be more suited than other joint angle combinations within the same UCM for a transition to the next UCM. Thus, subjects might have learned to limit the range of joint combinations within a given UCM to improve efficiency in transitions from one UCM to another. More studies are required to answer these questions.

While the studies by Scholz and his colleagues (2001; Scholz and Schöner, 1999) and by Domkin et al. (2002; also see Laczko et al., 2001) were essentially planar, Scholz et al. (2000) analyzed unrestricted movement of human arm in three-dimensional space during quick-draw pistol shooting. The task was selected because accurate shooting depends on two angles (pitch and yaw) describing the orientation of the pistol with respect to the target at the time the trigger is pressed, but not on the third angle (roll) and not on the position of the pistol along the line of shooting (figure 5.4). Scholz and his colleagues tested three hypotheses related to the coordination of the seven major joint rotations of the arm:

- H1-Sh: Instantaneous orientation of the pistol barrel with respect to the direction from the back-sight to the target is selectively stabilized.
- H2-Sh: Instantaneous position of the pistol is selectively stabilized.
- H3-Sh: Instantaneous location of the center of mass of the arm-plus-pistol system is stabilized.

Hypothesis H1-Sh looks trivial since, if the barrel is not oriented along the direction to the target, the target is not going to be hit. However, this is correct only at the moment the trigger is pressed, not along the whole trajectory of the movement. When the angle between the barrel and direction to the target is differ-

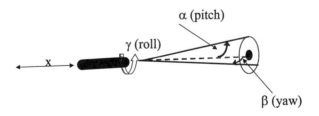

**Figure 5.4** Two angles characterizing the orientation of the barrel of the pistol in space, pitch and yaw, are crucial for accurate shooting. The third angle (roll) and the actual location of the pistol on the line of shooting (*x*) do not matter.

ent from zero, hypothesis H1-Sh is not trivial: Why should one stabilize this angle when the pistol is pointing away from the target? Moreover, it is conceivable that the pistol's orientation with respect to the target could be controlled by choosing a unique combination of joint motions through application of cost constraints (cf. Rosenbaum et al., 1995) such that no UCM effect is expected. Hypothesis H2-Sh implies simply that each subject tried to reproduce a preferred trajectory of the pistol in space. Hypothesis H3-Sh may be justified if we consider the mechanical effects of a fast arm movement on more proximal body parts. Such a movement creates a postural perturbation at more proximal joints. A common mechanism to stabilize posture against such self-generated perturbations is by anticipatory postural adjustments (APAs; Belenkiy et al., 1967; Cordo and Nashner, 1982; Massion, 1992). APAs have been shown to play an important role during shooting (Belenkiy et al., 1967). However, the APAs are generated by the CNS prior to actual perturbations, based on their estimated mechanical effects (Bouisset and Zattara, 1987). If the perturbation is predictable in time, the controller may be able to anticipate it and minimize its effects on shooting performance. Since mechanical coupling effects are related to the kinematics of the distal segments, stabilization of the trajectory of the center of mass can be viewed as a means of making this perturbation more predictable so that the efficacy of the APAs is higher.

In the study by Scholz et al. (2000), hypothesis H1-Sh was confirmed over the whole duration of the pistol trajectory ($R_V > 1$). In other words, rotations of the seven major joints were coordinated to stabilize the instantaneous orientation of the pistol with respect to the target, even when the pistol was directed away from the target. Hypotheses H2-Sh and H3-Sh were supported ($R_V > 1$) during the initial phase of the trajectory but not at its most crucial later phase, which determined whether the target was hit. With respect to H2-Sh, it is conceivable that this result was due to the fact that the subjects started each movement from a rather clumsy posture (selected to ensure significant joint rotations in all major joints). As a result, they might have been forced along a particular trajectory leading to more comfortable joint configurations. Selective stabilization of the CM trajectory early in the movement might be related to the typical acceleration profile seen during the movements. The movements were very fast (movement time on the order of 300 ms) with an asymmetrical velocity profile. There was an early, large acceleration peak, while deceleration was typically longer and showed smaller absolute magnitudes. Such a kinematic profile suggests larger coupling forces early in the movement; these forces could have led to the selective stabilization of the CM trajectory to ensure better efficacy of the APA mechanism.

# Multifinger Force Production Studies Using the UCM Hypothesis

Multifinger force production is a very attractive object for studies of multielement systems. Synergies within such a system are very "human"; they are well practiced throughout life in a variety of complex coordination tasks such as drinking from a glass, eating with a spoon, or writing with a pen. It is relatively easy to measure outputs of the individual elements (forces of individual fingers) and to present tasks to subjects. Earlier studies showed signs of finger interaction during such tasks that suggested the action of an error compensation mechanism among the fingers of a hand. In particular, Li et al. (1998) studied ramp force production by four fingers acting in parallel. This study showed that the variance of the total force at high force levels was smaller than the sum of the variances of individual finger forces. This finding suggests that there is a degree of error compensation among the fingers that tends to stabilize total force. In a study by Latash, Li, and Zatsiorsky (1998) subjects were asked to produce a constant force with three fingers of a hand and then to tap a few times with one of the fingers. During the first tap, the tapping finger obviously lost contact with the surface and stopped contributing to the total force. The other, nontapping fingers showed an out-of-phase increase in their forces such that over 90% of the lost force was compensated for.

There are complicating factors, however. In particular, as mentioned earlier, individual fingers are not controlled independently by the CNS. Hence, a direct UCM analysis of finger forces could be expected to lead to spurious "UCMs" as a result of the built-in relationships among the forces (enslaving; Li et al., 1998). To avoid this problem, analysis needs to be performed using a different set of variables that are presumably manipulated independently by the CNS. Earlier we mentioned this problem and also a solution: switching from a set of finger forces to a set of variables (modes) that describe force changes when a subject tries to produce force with only one finger. This approach was used in two studies discussed in the following paragraphs.

In these studies, the subjects were paced by a metronome and asked to draw a sinelike wave on a screen such that its extrema touched two horizontal lines. In one study (Scholz et al., 2002), all four fingers of the right hand were acting in parallel. In a modification of the procedure, the middle and ring fingers were taped together and placed on one force transducer. This manipulation was based on the expected importance of the total moment generated by the fingers with respect to the longitudinal axis of the forearm and the hand (cf. the principle of minimization of secondary moments; Zatsiorsky et al., 1998, 2000). Coupling the two central fingers and placing them on one transducer was expected to emphasize the coordination of the index and little fingers in the moment production.

Another study used two (index and middle) or three (index, middle, and ring) fingers (Latash et al., 2001). In this study, the subjects produced force profiles in stable and unstable conditions. The unstable conditions were created by placing the frame with the force sensors on a narrow supporting surface located midway between the two lateral fingers. Both studies tested two control hypotheses:

- H1-F: Individual finger forces are coordinated to stabilize the average total force profile.

- H2-F: Individual finger forces are coordinated to stabilize the average profile of total moment generated by all involved fingers with respect to the midpoint between the two lateral fingers.

As mentioned earlier, in these two studies, patterns of individual finger forces were recomputed as force-mode patterns; then, force-mode patterns were analyzed with respect to the two control hypotheses. The results of the two studies had much in common (figure 5.5). The force-control hypothesis (H1-F) was confirmed only within a narrow phase range of the force cycle, close to the peak total force. The moment-control hypothesis (H2-F) was confirmed over most of the cycle.

When only two fingers participate in such a task, force-control and moment-control requirements become incompatible. Figure 5.5 illustrates that selective force stabilization requires a negative correlation between the forces of the two fingers (gray ellipse), while selective moment stabilization requires a positive correlation between the two forces (black ellipse). Thus, force stabilization necessarily means moment destabilization, while moment stabilization necessarily means force destabilization. In other words, the subjects were forced to choose which of the two variables to stabilize at the expense of destabilizing the other. Let us emphasize that the subjects were explicitly asked to reproduce a pattern of total force and got force feedback on the monitor, but there was no explicit feedback on total moment. In unstable conditions, moment stabilization was implicit; however, basically identical results were seen in stable conditions when the moment did not need to be stabilized at all.

In three- and four-finger tasks, however, the system is rich enough to stabilize both force and moment at the same time. However, for three-finger tasks, the results were similar to those for two-finger tasks; that is, total force was destabilized over most of the force cycle. Actually, the only change was that the third finger was used to stabilize moment over the whole cycle, not to stabilize force better! Only when all four fingers were used were the subjects able to avoid apparent force destabilization. However, they still stabilized force only within a relatively narrow phase range close to high magnitudes of total force, whereas moment was stabilized over the whole cycle.

These seemingly unexpected findings are likely to reflect the neural coordination of fingers (i.e., multifinger synergies) elaborated by the CNS based on a lifetime of everyday tasks. Most everyday tasks, such as drinking from a glass, writing with a pen, or working with a screwdriver, impose much stronger constraints on permissible errors in total moment than in total force. In such tasks, grip force should be only sufficiently large to prevent the object from slipping out of the hand. It should also be less than a magnitude that could potentially crush the object. These are relatively weak constraints. The moment, however, needs to be controlled much more precisely to write legibly and to avoid spilling the contents of the glass (see figure 5.6).

Let us focus attention on another finding in the cited studies of multifinger force production (Latash et al., 2001; Scholz et al., 2002). The UCM analysis of the

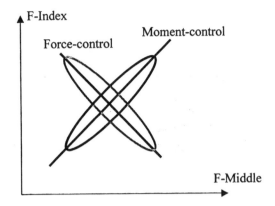

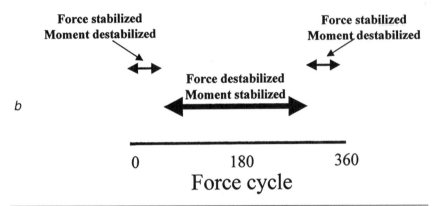

**Figure 5.5** *(a)* The requirements of total force and total moment stabilization are in conflict when only two fingers participate in the task. *(b)* Experiments with oscillatory force production with the index and middle fingers showed moment stabilization and force destabilization over most of the force cycle.

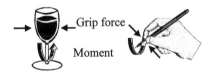

**Figure 5.6** In a variety of everyday motor tasks, such as taking a sip from the glass or writing with the pen, a time pattern of the total moment generated by the fingers needs to be controlled much more precisely than the total grip force.

two components of total variance for the moment-control hypothesis consistently showed that $Var_{UCM}$ had an "inverted Mexican hat" shape, with peaks at 1/4 and 3/4 of the force cycle, that is, at phases when force changes were most rapid while force magnitudes had intermediate values. By contrast, $Var_{ORT}$ showed a smooth change within the force cycle, more or less in proportion to the actual force level. According to the model suggested by Gutman and Gottlieb (1992), such patterns are likely to reflect the different relative roles of the magnitude and timing errors in the two variance components. In particular, the apparent relation of $Var_{UCM}$ to the rate of change of force suggests that the timing errors played an important role. The apparent lack of relation of $Var_{ORT}$ to the rate of force change suggests that the timing errors were small. Since the variance of the total force was, by definition, affected only by $Var_{ORT}$, we can conclude that the timing errors in individual finger forces were preferentially compensated for by the interaction that led to the observed moment stabilization.

## Advantages and Promises of the UCM Hypothesis

The UCM hypothesis suggests a particular realization of the principle of abundance (Gelfand and Latash, 1998) and a toolbox that can be used to ask the CNS questions about particular variables, which may or may not be selectively stabilized in motor actions. The hypothesis is therefore deeply rooted in the traditions of motor control research that originated from the seminal work by Gelfand and Tsetlin (1961; 1966). This work has inspired many researchers in the area of motor control (Kugler et al., 1990; Saltzman and Kelso, 1987; Turvey, 1990). However, to our knowledge, the UCM hypothesis is the first attempt to introduce exactness and quantification into the notion of error compensation as a salient feature of motor synergies. We would like to conclude that the attempt has been successful, based on the reviewed experimental material. Besides providing an opportunity to quantify error compensation, this approach has already led to unexpected findings that suggest particular neural strategies of motor coordination. We believe, in particular, that the approach promises direct application to the area of disordered movements and motor rehabilitation, when the injured CNS is likely to show adaptive strategies leading to atypical motor coordination (Latash and Anson, 1996). The UCM method promises to help researchers understand the purposes of such adaptive strategies by enabling them to test control hypotheses about different characteristics of performance that may be selectively stabilized in patients but not in healthy persons.

Although the computational aspect of the UCM hypothesis looks similar to the well-known technique of principal component analysis (PCA), there are at least two significant differences. First, PCA is "objective"; it allows the computation of the magnitudes and directions of the main axes of a multidimensional ellipsoid describing a data distribution. It does not give information on possible relationships of the main axes to particular functionally important performance variables. In contrast, the UCM toolbox always analyzes data sets with respect to a control hypothesis, that is, a hypothesis about a certain potentially important performance variable. Second, PCA is performed dimension by dimension, while the UCM toolbox allows comparison of the variances between multidimensional subspaces with different dimensionalities.

The hypothesis is based on an assumption that all available DFs within a synergy are always used to solve motor tasks. Obviously, if a synergy is inadequate for a particular motor task, it cannot be used to solve it. In that case, it can be expected to break down and be taken apart into elements, which are then used to create a new synergy. Let us consider what can happen during such a transition period, acquiring a new motor skill.

Practice during motor rehabilitation or mastering a new skill has commonly been described as including steps of "freezing" and "releasing" DFs (Newell, 1991; Vereijken et al., 1992). Following Bernstein's (1996) traditions, freezing DFs has been considered the means of simplifying control of a multielement system when appropriate synergies do not exist yet. This reasoning is not obvious, however. First, preventing a joint rotation during a fast movement of a multijoint kinematic chain does not mean easier control. Because of mechanical coupling, control signals to muscles crossing a joint need to be controlled very precisely to avoid joint flapping (Dounskaia et al., 1998; Latash et al., 1995). However, a drop in the excursion of particular joints, sometimes accompanied by excessive muscle co-contraction at the joints, has been commonly described at early stages of motor skill acquisition (Bernstein, 1947, 1996; Piek, 1995). What could be the reason for these phenomena if we look at them not as the means of eliminating redundancy but as occurring within an abundant system?

Imagine that the CNS needs to control a multielement system to stabilize a particular performance variable $X(t)$. Note that elements within such a multielement system can themselves be synergies (structural units). If a multielement synergy with respect to $X$ does not exist, a new motor skill needs to be learned, that is, a new synergy $S_X$ needs to be developed. During practice, however, the elements have to be controlled independently to produce a required trajectory of $X(t)$ within a permissible error margin. Each element is characterized by its typical contribution to $X$ and also by its typical inherent error. The more elements used to produce $X(t)$, the larger the expected error since there is no error compensation among the elements ($S_X$ does not exist yet). Hence, an optimal strategy could be to use a minimal set of elements to produce $X(t)$ while keeping changes in the outputs of the rest of the elements at a minimum. In such a case, the principle of abundance is violated since no synergy exists. But this strategy reduces typical errors in the outputs of the "expelled" elements since output errors typically increase with the magnitude of the output (e.g., Newell et al., 1984). After $S_X$ is created, error compensation among its elements makes it advantageous to involve more elements (to release DFs). Jaric and Latash (1999) showed that in an arm-pointing task the spatial error in the final position of the pointer tip could be smaller or larger than the spatial error of the final position of a distal point on the forearm. In the former case, wrist motion amplitude was larger, suggesting that the wrist was incorporated into the multijoint synergy and partly compensated for errors created by more proximal joints. In the latter case, the wrist motion was smaller, and it only added to the overall error; the wrist can be viewed as "frozen" or expelled from the synergy.

The last example shows that the UCM approach can be used to test quantitatively whether an alleged element of a multielement synergy actually contributes to stabilization of a particular performance variable. If considering the contribution of this element leads to better error compensation (higher $R_V$ values) with respect to the selected variable, the element indeed takes part in the synergy. Otherwise, the element can be viewed as alien to the synergy.

We would also like to mention an approach suggested recently by Todorov (2001) based on the idea of optimal control of a multielement system in the presence of a certain irreducible level of noise. Simulations performed by Todorov showed data distributions very similar to those illustrated in figure 5.2b, implying that error compensation between two elements contributed to a common output.

## Challenges Facing the UCM Hypothesis

The UCM hypothesis is presently in its infancy. All the studies performed to date can be criticized for involving major simplifications. These studies failed to address certain issues crucial for understanding the physiological mechanisms underlying the coordination of abundant systems. However, these same shortcomings of the early studies can be viewed as a source of excitement. They show not only that the UCM approach is inherently rich and able to offer answers to current interesting questions, but, more important, that it invites new questions to be formulated and explored.

Let us only touch on the following major challenges facing the UCM hypothesis:

1. To quantify the two components of variance with respect to a control hypothesis, all the cited studies analyzed selected times in the course of a motor act over several trials. Effectively, these studies analyzed data distributions with respect to instantaneous UCMs at certain snapshots of a movement trajectory. Apparently, UCMs need to evolve over the course of a movement, even if the same performance variable is stabilized over the whole movement duration. This is because the variable is likely to be stabilized at different values corresponding to different subspaces within the state space of the system. Reconstructing and quantifying the time evolution of variance components with respect to an evolving UCM is a challenge to be met.

2. To stabilize a particular performance variable, elements of a synergy (certainly including their central control structures) need to monitor either changes in the performance variable or changes in the outputs of other elements. Information on changes in the performance variable is more relevant to stabilizing it. However, using feedback loops that involve peripheral receptors is likely to involve time

delays that may destabilize performance or make such information obsolete (during very fast movements). On the other hand, intrinsic feedback loops within the CNS can be used to ensure that changes in the output of an element induce corrective changes in the outputs of other elements with minimal time delays. Such intrinsic loops may work with very short time delays; however, their efficacy may not be perfect since corrections will be based on an estimate of the effects of an original error on an essential performance variable rather than on actual changes in the variable. It is conceivable that both peripheral and central feedback loops can be used in task-specific ways to ensure proper functioning of a synergy.

3. Related to the previous point is the issue of the sources of sensory information that is used to ensure error compensation among elements of a synergy. Most likely, most synergies can function using information of different modalities. A movement performed under haptic control is more likely to use information from cutaneous receptors and proprioceptors. A movement performed under visual control is more likely to use visual information to stabilize the same performance variable. For example, synergetic behavior has been described for two persons who were involved in a mutually coordinated motor activity while observing each other's actions (Schmidt et al., 1990). It is also easy to imagine interpersonal coordination happening through an exchange of haptic information, for example, when two or more persons are manipulating a large object, such as carrying a piano upstairs.

4. With the exception of the finger force production studies, the cited experiments used outputs of apparent elements to test the UCM hypothesis. In particular, kinematic studies considered rotations at individual joints as independent variables manipulated by the CNS. It is well known, however, that joints of the human body are coupled so that a small change in the motion of one joint hypothetically can lead to changes in the motion of all other joints. The coupling is partly due to purely passive mechanical effects and partly to the presence of biarticular muscles that provide adjustable, springlike links between adjacent joints (van Ingen Schenau, 1989; Prilutsky, 2000; Zajac and Gordon, 1989). The presence of such links always implies a possibility of spurious UCM effects due to the design of the system rather than to its control. The finger force studies (Latash et al., 2001; Scholz et al., 2002) employed a different level of description using hypothetical central variables in order to circumvent this problem. However, to address the problem adequately, researchers need to answer the following question: What independently controlled variables are used by the CNS to produce voluntary movements?

It is theoretically possible to apply the general theoretical framework of the UCM hypothesis and the associated computational approaches to more physiological variables, such as muscle activation patterns and patterns of neural signals associated with motor tasks. There are methodological challenges to be met. However, the main problems may not be methodological but philosophical. Since Bernstein (remember "repetition without repetition"), there has been a growing understanding of a basic difference between central control variables and performance variables. The former are supposed to be primarily under control of the CNS, while the latter always reflect, to an equal degree, factors external to the organism, such as external force fields. In an ideal world, we would perform UCM analysis on central control variables. However, two factors prevent this from happening. First, there is no agreement in the motor control community on the nature of these variables (Stein, 1982; Feldman and Levin, 1995). (We think that the equilibrium-point hypothesis is the only one in the area that promises a feasible approach to this problem; see Latash, 1993, 2000.) Second, even if such an agreement is achieved, there will be one more obstacle: how to measure the time profiles of these control variables with sufficient reliability and accuracy to allow the variance analysis inherent to the UCM approach.

Despite all the difficulties and challenges at the present time, we do not see alternatives to the central organization of abundant motor systems. It offers at least a glimpse of hope in dealing with the main problem of motor control and biology in general: the lack of an adequate language (Gelfand, 1991). We think that *synergy* is a candidate for a keyword in such a language, and the UCM approach is the only one that permits analysis of synergies in an exact way.

## Conclusions

We conclude that studies of motor variability provide a window into how the central nervous system deals with the problem of motor redundancy. Such studies also allow researchers to test different hypotheses regarding a range of performance variables that may or may not be purposefully stabilized by the controller. So far, the framework of the UCM hypothesis has been applied to kinematic and kinetic studies of whole-body movements, multijoint limb movements, two-limb movements, and multifinger force production tasks. Since this chapter was written, promising results have been obtained in studies of clinical populations, including patients after stroke and persons with Down syndrome, and in the application of the UCM hypothesis to physiological variables such as patterns of muscle activation. We are only at the early stages of the development of this fascinating hypothesis and associated tools, which promise a breakthrough in both basic and applied motor control research.

## Acknowledgments

Supported in part by NIH grants HD-35857 and NS-35032 and by NSF grant IBN-0078127.

## References

Abbs, J.H., and Gracco, V.L. (1984) Control of complex motor gestures: Orofacial muscle responses to load perturbations of the lip during speech. *J Neurophysiol* 51: 705-723.

Alexandrov, A., Frolov, A., and Massion, J. (1998) Axial synergies during human upper trunk bending. *Exp Brain Res* 118: 210-220.

Atkeson, C.G. (1989) Learning arm kinematics and dynamics. *Annu Rev Neurosci* 12: 157-183.

Belenkiy, V.E., Gurfinkel, V.S., and Paltsev, E.I. (1967) On the elements of control of voluntary movements [in Russian]. *Biofizika* 12: 135-141.

Berkinblit, M.B., Feldman, A.G., and Fukson, O.I. (1986) Adaptability of innate motor patterns and motor control mechanisms. *Behav Brain Sci* 9: 585-638.

Bernstein, N.A. (1927) Kymozyclographion, ein neuer Apparat fur Bewegungsstudium. *Pflugers Arch gesamte Physiol Menschen Tiere* 217: 783-793.

Bernstein, N.A. (1935) The problem of interrelation between coordination and localization [in Russian]. *Arch Biol Sci* 38: 1-35.

Bernstein, N.A. (1947) *On the construction of movements* [in Russian]. Moscow: Medgiz.

Bernstein, N.A. (1967) *The co-ordination and regulation of movements.* Oxford: Pergamon Press.

Bernstein, N.A. (1996) On dexterity and its development. In Latash, M.L., and Turvey, M.T. (Eds.), *Dexterity and its development,* pp. 3-246. Mahwah, NJ: Erlbaum.

Bernstein, N.A., and Popova, T.S. (1929) Untersuchung uber die Biodynamik des Klavieranschlagers. Arbeitsphysiol. *Z Physiol Menschen Arbeit Sport* 1: 396-432.

Bouisset, S., and Zattara, M. (1987) Biomechanical study of the programming of anticipatory postural adjustments associated with voluntary movement. *J Biomech* 20: 735-742.

Chong, R.K., and Franklin, M.E. (2001) Initial evidence for the mixing and soft assembly of the ankle, suspensory, and hip muscle patterns. *Exp Brain Res* 136: 250-255.

Cordo, P.J., and Nashner, L.M. (1982) Properties of postural adjustments associated with rapid arm movements. *J Neurophysiol* 47: 287-302.

De Serres, S.J., and Milner, T.E. (1991) Wrist muscle activation patterns and stiffness associated with stable and unstable mechanical loads. *Exp Brain Res* 86: 451-458.

Desmurget, M., Prablanc, C., Rossetti, Y., Arzi, M., Paulignan, Y., Urquizar, C., and Mignot, J.C. (1995) Postural and synergic control for three-dimensional movements of reaching and grasping. *J Neurophysiol* 74: 905-910.

Domkin, D., Laczko, J., Jaric, S., Johansson, H., and Latash, M.L. (2002) Structure of joint variability in bimanual pointing tasks. *Exp Brain Res* 143: 11-23.

Dounskaia, N.V., Swinnen, S.P., Walter, C.B., Spaepen, A.J., and Verschueren, S.M. (1998) Hierarchical control of different elbow-wrist coordination patterns. *Exp Brain Res* 121: 239-254.

Feldman, A.G., and Levin, M.F. (1995) Positional frames of reference in motor control: Their origin and use. *Behav Brain Sci* 18: 723-806.

Fentress, J.C. (1976) Dynamic boundaries of patterned behavior: Interactions and self-organization. In Bateson, P.P.G., and Hindle, R.A. (Eds.), *Growing points in ethology,* pp. 135-170. Cambridge: Cambridge University Press.

Gelfand, I.M. (1991) Two archetypes in the psychology of man. *Nonlinear Sci Today* 1: 11-16.

Gelfand, I.M., and Latash, M.L. (1998) On the problem of adequate language in movement science. *Motor Control* 2: 306-313.

Gelfand, I.M., and Tsetlin, M.L. (1961) On certain methods of control of complex systems [in Russian]. *Adv Math Sci* 17: 103.

Gelfand, I.M., and Tsetlin, M.L. (1966) On mathematical modeling of the mechanisms of the central nervous system [in Russian]. In Gelfand, I.M., Gurfinkel, V.S., Fomin, S.V., and Tsetlin, M.L. (Eds.), *Models of the structural-functional organization of certain biological systems,* pp. 9-26. Moscow: Nauka. A translation is available in 1971 edition by MIT Press, Cambridge, MA.

Gottlieb, G.L., Song, Q., Hong, D.A., Almeida, G.L., and Corcos, D. (1996) Coordinating movement at two joints: A principle of linear covariance. *J Neurophysiol* 75: 1760-1764.

Greene, P.H. (1972) Problems of organization of motor systems. *Prog Theor Biol* 2: 303-338.

Gutman, S.R., and Gottlieb, G.L. (1992) Basic functions of variability of simple pre-planned movements. *Biol Cybern* 68: 63-73.

Hager-Ross, C.K., and Schieber, M.H. (1999) Independence of finger movements in humans. Progress in Motor Control II, p. 86, August 19-22, 1999, State College, PA.

Henry, S.M., Fung, J., and Horak, F.B. (1998) EMG responses to maintain stance during multidirectional surface translations. *J Neurophysiol* 80: 1939-1950.

Hughlings Jackson, J. (1889) On the comparative study of disease of the nervous system. *Br Med J* (August 17): 355-362.

Jaric, S., and Latash, M.L. (1999) Learning a pointing task with a kinematically redundant limb: Emerging synergies and patterns of final position variability. *Hum Mov Sci* 18: 819-838.

Keshner, E.A., Woollacott, M.H., and Debu, B. (1988) Neck, trunk and limb muscle responses during postural perturbations in humans. *Exp Brain Res* 71: 455-466.

Kilbreath, S.L., and Gandevia, S.C. (1994) Limited independent flexion of the thumb and fingers in human subjects. *J Physiol* 479: 487-497.

Kugler, P.N., Turvey, M.T., Schmidt, R.C., and Rosenblum, L.D. (1990) Investigating a nonconservative invariant of motion in coordinated rhythmic movements. *Ecol Psychol* 2: 151-189.

Laczko, J., Jaric, S., Domkin, D., Johansson, H., and Latash, M.L. (2001) Stabilization of kinematic variables in the control of bimanual pointing movements. Proceedings of the International Joint Conference on Neural Networks, July 14-19, 2001, Washington, DC.

Latash, M.L. (1993) *Control of human movement.* Champaign, IL: Human Kinetics.

Latash, M.L. (1996) How does our brain make its choices? In Latash, M.L., and Turvey, M.T. (Eds.), *Dexterity and its development,* pp. 277-304. Mahwah, NJ: Erlbaum.

Latash, M.L. (2000) There is no motor redundancy in human movements. There is motor abundance. *Motor Control* 4: 257-259.

Latash, M.L., and Anson, J.G. (1996) What are normal movements in atypical populations? *Behav Brain Sci* 19: 55-106.

Latash, M.L., Aruin, A.S., and Shapiro, M.B. (1995) The relation between posture and movement: A study of a simple synergy in a two-joint task. *Hum Mov Sci* 14: 79-107.

Latash, M.L., Li, Z.M., and Zatsiorsky, V.M. (1998) A principle of error compensation studied within a task of force production by a redundant set of fingers. *Exp Brain Res* 122: 131-138.

Latash, M.L., Scholz, J.F., Danion, F., and Schöner, G. (2001) Structure of motor variability in marginally redundant multi-finger force production tasks. *Exp Brain Res* 141: 153-165.

Leijsne, J.N., Snijiders, C.C.J., Bonte, J.E., Landsmeer, J.M., Kalker, J.J., Van Der Meulen, J.C., Sonneveld, G.J., and Hovius, S.E. (1993) The hand of the musician: The kinematics of the bidigital finger system with anatomical restrictions. *J Biomech* 26: 1169-1179.

Li, Z.M., Latash, M.L., and Zatsiorsky, V.M. (1998) Force sharing among fingers as a model of the redundancy problem. *Exp Brain Res* 119: 276-286.

Macpherson, J.M. (1988) Strategies that simplify the control of quadrupedal stance: II. Electromyographic activity. *J Neurophysiol* 60: 218-231.

Macpherson, J.M., Rushmer, D.S., and Dunbar, D.C. (1986) Postural responses in the cat to unexpected rotations of the supporting surface: Evidence for a centrally generated synergic organization. *Exp Brain Res* 62: 152-160.

Massion, J. (1992) Movement, posture and equilibrium: Interaction and coordination. *Prog Neurobiol* 38: 35-56.

Mussa-Ivaldi, F.A., Morasso, P., and Zaccaria, R. (1989) Kinematic networks: A distributed model for representing and regularizing motor redundancy. *Biol Cybern* 60: 1-16.

Newell, K.M. (1991) Motor skill acquisition. *Annu Rev Psychol* 42: 213-237.

Newell, K.M., Carlton, L.G., and Hancock, P.A. (1984) Kinetic analysis of response variability. *Psychol Bull* 96: 133-151.

Newell, K.M., and Corcos, D.M. (1993) *Variability in motor control.* Champaign, IL: Human Kinetics.

Pelz, J., Hayhoe, M., and Loeber, R. (2001) The coordination of eye, head, and hand movements in a natural task. *Exp Brain Res* 139: 266-277.

Piek, J.P. (1995) The contribution of spontaneous movements in the acquisition of motor coordination in infants. In Glencross, D.J., and Piek, J.P. (Eds.), *Motor control and sensory motor integration: Issues and directions,* pp. 199-230. Amsterdam: Elsevier.

Popova, T.S., and Mogilyanskaya, Z.V. (1934) *Technika isuchenija dvigenii: Prakticheskoe rukovodstvo po ciklogrammetrii* [Techniques for studies of movements: A practical manual on cyclographic methods]. Standartizacia i Razionalizaciaja, Moscow.

Prilutsky, B.I. (2000) Coordination of one- and two-joint muscles: Functional consequences and implications for motor control. *Motor Control* 4: 1-44.

Reisman, D.S., Scholz, J.P., and Schöner, G. (2002) Coordination underlying control of the whole-body momentum during sit-to-stand. *Gait Posture.* 15: 45-55.

Rosenbaum, D.A., Loukopoulos, L.D., Meulenbroek, R.G.M., Vaughan, J., and Engelbrecht, S.E. (1995) Planning reaches by evaluating stored postures. *Psychol Rev* 102: 28-67.

Roullier, E.M. (1996) Multiple hand representations in the motor cortical areas. In Wing, A.M., Haggard, P., and Flanagan, J.R. (Eds.), *Hand and brain: The neurophysiology and psychology of hand movements*, pp. 99-124. San Diego: Academic Press.

Saltiel, P., Wyler-Duda, K., D'Avella, A., Tresch, M.C., and Bizzi, E. (2001) Muscle synergies encoded within the spinal cord: Evidence from focal intraspinal NMDA iontophoresis in the frog. *J Neurophysiol* 85: 605-619.

Saltzman, E.L., and Kelso, J.A.S. (1987) Skilled actions: A task-dynamic approach. *Psychol Rev* 94: 84-106.

Santello, M., and Soechting, J.F. (2000) Force synergies for multifingered grasping. *Exp Brain Res* 133: 457-467.

Schmidt, R.C., Carello, C., and Turvey, M.T. (1990) Phase transitions and critical fluctuations in the visual coordination of rhythmic movements between people. *J Exp Psychol Hum Percept Perform* 16: 227-247.

Scholz, J.P., Danion, F., Latash, M.L., and Schöner, G. (2002) Understanding finger coordination through analysis of the structure of force variability. *Biol Cybern* 86: 29-39.

Scholz, J.P., Reisman, D., and Schöner, G. (2001) Effects of varying task constraints on solutions to joint control in sit-to-stand. *Exp Brain Res* 141: 485-500.

Scholz, J.P., and Schöner, G. (1999) The uncontrolled manifold concept: Identifying control variables for a functional task. *Exp Brain Res* 126: 289-306.

Scholz, J.P., Schöner, G., and Latash, M.L. (2000) Identifying the control structure of multijoint coordination during pistol shooting. *Exp Brain Res* 135: 382-404.

Seif-Naraghi, A.H., and Winters, J.M. (1990) Optimized strategies for scaling goal-directed dynamic limb movements. In Winters, J.M., and Woo, S.L.-Y. (Eds.), *Multiple muscle systems: Biomechanics and movement organization*, pp. 312-334. New York: Springer-Verlag.

Smith, J.L., Hoy, M.G., Koshland, G.F., Phillips, D.M., and Zernicke, R.F. (1985) Intralimb coordination of the paw-shake response: A novel mixed synergy. *J Neurophysiol* 54: 1271-1281.

Stein, R.B. (1982) What muscle variable(s) does the nervous system control in limb movements? *Behav Brain Sci* 5: 535-577.

Todorov, E. (2001) What can peripheral properties tell us about processing in motor cortex? Abstracts of the International Conference on Progress in Motor Control III, p. 10, University of Montreal, August 15-18, 2001, Montreal.

Tresch, M.C., Saltiel, P., and Bizzi, E. (1999) The construction of movement by the spinal cord. *Nat Neurosci* 2: 162-167.

Turvey, M.T. (1990) Coordination. *Am Psychol* 45: 938-953.

Turvey, M.T., and Carello, C. (1996) Dynamics of Bernstein's level of synergies. In Latash, M.L., and Turvey, M.T. (Eds.), *Dexterity and its development*, pp. 339-376. Mahwah, NJ: Erlbaum.

Van Ingen Schenau, G.J. (1989) From rotation to translation: Constraints on multi-joint movements and the unique action of bi-articular muscles. *Hum Mov Sci* 8: 301-337.

Vereijken, B., van Emmerick, R.E.A., Whiting, H.T.A., and Newell, K.M. (1992) Free(z)ing degrees of freedom in skill acquisition. *J Mot Behav* 24: 133-142.

Vernazza-Martin, S., Martin, N., and Massion, J. (1999) Kinematic synergies and equilibrium control during trunk movement under loaded and unloaded conditions. *Exp Brain Res* 128: 517-526.

Wang, J., and Stelmach, G.E. (1998) Coordination among the body segments during reach-to-grasp action involving the trunk. *Exp Brain Res* 123: 346-350.

Zajac, F.E., and Gordon, M.E. (1989) Determining muscle's force and action in multi-articular movements. *Exerc Sport Sci Rev* 17: 187-230.

Zatsiorsky, V.M. (1999) *Kinematics of human movement.* Champaign, IL: Human Kinetics.

Zatsiorsky, V.M., Li, Z.M., and Latash, M.L. (1998) Coordinated force production in multi-finger tasks: Finger interaction and neural network modeling. *Biol Cybern* 79: 139-150.

Zatsiorsky, V.M., Li, Z.M., and Latash, M.L. (2000) Enslaving effects in multi-finger force production. *Exp Brain Res* 131: 187-195.

# 6

# On the Role
# of the Primary Motor Cortex
# in Arm Movement Control

*Emanuel Todorov*
University of California, San Diego

The primary motor cortex (M1) plays a fundamental role in the control of voluntary arm movements, as evidenced by profound deficits following M1 lesions. Precisely what that role is has been the subject of lasting debate. This debate is fueled by the numerous correlations found between the activity of M1 neurons and various behavioral parameters.

The earliest experiments in awake, behaving monkeys (Evarts, 1968) showed that M1 firing is better correlated with isometric force than limb position. Given the dense projection from M1 to the spinal cord, sometimes directly to motoneurons, it is natural to interpret these early observations as evidence that M1 controls muscle force or activation (Evarts, 1981). It was later observed, however, that in multijoint movement tasks the majority of M1 neurons encode not the acceleration (which is proportional to force) but the direction (Georgopoulos et al., 1982) or velocity (Schwartz, 1994) of hand movement. In addition, the M1 directional tuning curves were quite broad, which, in the context of the single-joint studies that dominated the field at the time, seemed inconsistent with low-level muscle control. These observations, and the ability of the population vector (PV) to recover movement direction, led to the opposing view that M1 sends a much more abstract signal specifying a 3D vector in extrapersonal space.

To distinguish between the two alternatives, movement velocity and external load were varied separately in the same experiment (Kalaska et al., 1989). The results, however, supported both views: velocity- and load-related signals were both present and combined additively in the activity of the same neurons. Although the directional coding hypothesis can be extended to incorporate the observed tuning for load (Kalaska et al., 1989; Georgopoulos et al., 1992; Taira et al., 1996) as well as position (Georgopoulos et al., 1984; Kettner et al., 1988), it offers no explanation as to why all these parameters should be encoded simultaneously. Furthermore, many additional correlations have been observed that do not seem to fit in either view of M1 function (see Todorov, 2000a). We can use regression analysis to identify the multiple parameters correlated with the activity of each neuron (Ashe and Georgopoulos, 1994; Fu et al., 1995; Taira et al., 1996). The activity of any one neuron is, of course, correlated with some parameters better than others, but the presence of simultaneous correlations makes it impossible to determine what that neuron really encodes (Fetz, 1992).

Is it then possible to make any coherent statement regarding the role of M1 in arm movement control, at least to a first approximation? Is there *one* parameter of motor behavior that, if encoded in the M1 population, would explain most available results? I argue that of all the parameters previously considered, the only one that can provide the basis for a coherent model of M1 is muscle activation. This chapter summarizes a series of recent studies (Todorov, 2000a, 2002; Todorov et al., 2000) as well as unpublished work in which I have developed a model of direct cortical control of muscle activation.

## The Case for Muscle-Based Encoding

If one were to approach the M1 literature without a preexisting bias and search for the single idea that is most likely to lead to a simple yet successful quantitative model, which idea should one choose? I found the idea of muscle-based encoding to be the most promising candidate, for the following reasons:

- *Evidence for muscle control.* M1 neurons and muscles display similar patterns of directional variation in their onset times and activation magnitudes (Scott, 1997). The distributions of preferred directions of both M1 neurons and muscles are roughly uniform in the natural posture but become substantially elongated (along the same axis) when the arm is constrained to the horizontal plane (Scott and Kalaska, 1997; Scott et al., 2001). Increased muscle co-contraction is accompanied by increased M1 activity (Humphrey and Reed, 1983; see also the section "Muscle Co-contraction"). M1 and muscle activity are synchronized in certain frequency bands (Conway et al., 1995).

- *Evidence against directional coding.* Several studies have found systematic differences in M1 activity between experimental conditions with identical movement directions in extrapersonal space but different joint configurations (Caminiti et al., 1991; Scott and Kalaska, 1995; Sergio and Kalaska, 1998; Kakei et al., 1999). Such results clearly contradict the hypothesis of directional coding in extrapersonal space. The changes of M1 activity observed in most of these experiments are consistent with both muscle- and joint-based encoding, except for the wrist movement task used by Kakei et al. (1999), which quite convincingly ruled out a joint-based encoding (see also the section "Using the Redundancy of Population Codes"). Interestingly, neural activity in the ventral premotor cortex (PMv) was not affected by arm posture (Kakei et al., 2001), suggesting that the directional coding hypothesis is much more applicable to PMv than M1.

• *Direct projections.* Some M1 neurons (labeled corticomotoneuronal, or CM, neurons) project monosynaptically to motoneurons (Fetz and Cheney, 1980; Lemon et al., 1986). If the M1 population encoded just one parameter and that parameter was not closely related to muscle activation, motoneurons would not be able to "decode" the descending signal correctly, and this direct pathway would have no reason to exist. Note that although monosynaptic projections are a minority, there is an evolutionary trend for their percentage to increase: They are most prominent in the hand muscles of humans. Therefore, the existence of this pathway is not an accident that can be ignored.

• *Proprioceptive feedback.* Most M1 neurons are affected at short latencies by proprioceptive feedback, so that imposed movement in the preferred direction suppresses the activity of the neuron in a stretch-reflex-like manner (Evarts, 1981). The existence of this pathway indicates that the M1 output is compatible with such feedback; that is, adding the two signals at the level of individual neurons produces a meaningful quantity. It is hard to imagine how the combination of abstract directional signals encoded in extrapersonal space, and proprioceptive feedback encoded in a muscle- or joint-related frame of reference, could be useful or even interpretable.

• *Evolutionary considerations.* One would expect the general function of the spinal cord in primates, to the extent that it is used, to be related to functions that it performed long before any supraspinal systems existed. The supraspinal systems most likely evolved to enhance those functions by modulating the state of the spinal interneuronal networks in a way that helped them solve whatever problems they were already trying to solve (Loeb, 1999). The interpretation of abstract motor commands was not among these problems. A descending signal that modulates the state of the spinal networks should be compatible with the representation they use, and that representation is likely to be closely related to the pattern of muscle activation.

• *Computational considerations.* While the motor system is clearly hierarchical, the division of labor implicit in the directional coding hypothesis is unlikely. According to that hypothesis, the vast supraspinal system is dedicated to the rather trivial calculation of a 3D vector, while all the difficult control problems (e.g., coordinating redundant nonlinear actuators, dealing with complex interaction forces, ensuring stability in the presence of delays and uncertainty) are left to the ancient spinal circuitry.

# Model Overview

As explained previously, there are plenty of reasons to adopt a muscle-based model of M1. The question is, How can such a model account for the correlations with various behavioral parameters that seem unrelated to muscle activation? The main contribution of our work is in answering that question. Here I outline the features of the model and explain intuitively how they help account for the many disparate results.

## *M1 Output*

The model focuses exclusively on M1 neurons projecting to the spinal cord. Interneurons and output neurons projecting to other areas are not modeled, since most of the arguments in the previous section do not apply to them. The activity of such neurons can be systematically different, and so by focusing on the M1 output, the model avoids some of the response diversity that a more complete model would have to explain.

## *M1-to-Behavior Mapping*

We are interested only in the instantaneous activity of the M1 output neurons and its causal relationship to instantaneous motor behavior at some later point in time. All predictions regarding M1 are derived by inverting that causal relationship (see figure 6.1a). Motor planning, sensorimotor transformations, and transcortical feedback corrections are all enclosed in the black box labeled "Brain" in figure 6.1a and do not concern us here. The "brain" receives online feedback; takes into account all goals, plans, expectations, preferences, and so on; and somehow generates the M1 output. This pathway is not used to make any predictions, and so we do not need to model it.

## *Population Analysis*

Our goal is to explain average population (or subpopulation) responses rather than individual response types (Kalaska et al., 1989). Because of the redundancy in the M1-to-muscle mapping, the same pattern of muscle activity can be generated with an infinite family of M1 activation patterns. How the brain chooses one of them is an interesting question, which I address separately in the sections "Cosine Tuning" and "The Model in Perspective." For the most part, however, I will not distinguish between M1 activity patterns that result in the same EMG pattern.

Schematic Illustration                          Detailed Muscle Model

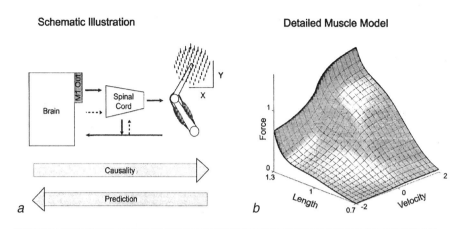

**Figure 6.1**   Model overview. *(a)* Solid arrows denote pathways explicitly taken into account; dashed arrows correspond to pathways that I argue can be neglected in a first-order model. The force field illustrates the static, position-dependent endpoint forces produced by an elbow flexor when the endpoint of a two-link arm with 30-cm links is moved over a 20 × 20 cm work space (not drawn to scale). Note that the forces are roughly parallel and become smaller when the endpoint is displaced in the force direction. *(b)* Force output of the nonlinear muscle model at maximal activation, shown as a function of physiological length and velocity.

Figure 6.1a reprinted from Todorov (2000a). Figure 6.1b reprinted from Todorov (2000b).

## Simplifications

A number of simplifications allow us to avoid curve fitting and ad hoc assumptions about poorly understood mechanisms (see the later section "From M1 Output to Motor Behavior"). In particular, the model uses linear approximations to the spinal circuitry, muscle force production mechanisms, and kinematics of the multijoint arm. The effects of other descending systems are ignored, although there is evidence that rubrospinal projections can be modeled similarly (Miller and Sinkjaer, 1998). Sensory feedback through spinal pathways is assumed to modulate the muscle activity generated by descending signals (see the later section "The Model in Perspective"). While such feedback modulation is very important for achieving stability, its effect is washed out in the trial-averaged analyses used in the M1 literature, and so I do not model it explicitly here.

## Muscle State Dependence

It is well established that for a fixed activation level, the force generated by a muscle varies with its length and velocity (Joyce et al., 1969; Zajac, 1989; Brown et al., 1999). The force-length-velocity surface at maximum (tetanic) activation is illustrated in figure 6.1b, using the state-of-the-art muscle model of Brown et al. (1999); details are given in table 6.1 and the section "From M1 Output to Motor

**Table 6.1   Detailed Muscle Model**

| Functions | Parameters |
|---|---|
| $f(a,l,v) = AF_{\mathrm{L}}F_{\mathrm{V}} + F_{\mathrm{P1}} + AF_{\mathrm{P2}}$ | |
| $A(a,l) = 1 - \exp\left(-\left(\dfrac{a}{a_{\mathrm{f}}N_{\mathrm{f}}}\right)^{N_{\mathrm{f}}}\right)$ | $a_{\mathrm{f}} = 0.56$ |
| $N_{\mathrm{f}}(l) = n_{\mathrm{f0}} + n_{\mathrm{f1}}\left(\dfrac{1}{l}-1\right)$ | $N_{\mathrm{f0}} = 2.11;\ n_{\mathrm{f1}} = 4.16$ |
| $F_{\mathrm{L}}(l) = \exp\left(-\left\lvert\dfrac{l^{\beta}-1}{\omega}\right\rvert^{\rho}\right)$ | $\beta = 1.93;\ \rho = 1.87;\ \omega = 1.03$ |
| $F_{\mathrm{V}}(l,v) = \begin{cases} \dfrac{v_{\max} - v}{v_{\max} + (c_{\mathrm{v0}} + C_{\mathrm{v1}}l)v}, & v \le 0 \\[2mm] \dfrac{b_{\mathrm{v}} - \left(a_{\mathrm{v0}} + a_{\mathrm{v1}}l + a_{\mathrm{v2}}l^{2}\right)v}{b_{\mathrm{v}} + v}, & v > 0 \end{cases}$ | $v_{\max} = -5.72;\ b_{\mathrm{v}} = 0.62$ <br> $c_{\mathrm{v0}} = 1.38;\ c_{\mathrm{v1}} = 2.09$ <br> $a_{\mathrm{v0}} = -3.12;\ a_{\mathrm{v1}} = 4.21;\ a_{\mathrm{v2}} = -2.67$ |
| $F_{\mathrm{P1}}(l) = c_{1}k_{1}\ln\left(\exp\left(\dfrac{l-l_{\mathrm{r1}}}{k_{1}}\right)+1\right)$ | $c_{1} = 104.25;\ k_{1} = 0.052;\ l_{\mathrm{r1}} = 1.42$ |
| $F_{\mathrm{P2}}(l) = c_{2}\exp\left(k_{2}\left(l-l_{\mathrm{r2}}\right)-1\right)$ | $c_{2} = -0.02;\ k_{2} = -18.7;\ l_{\mathrm{r2}} = 0.$ |

The first equation shows the muscle force as a function of activation, length, and velocity. The remaining equations define the different terms in the first equation and the corresponding parameter values.

Behavior." Note that for the same activation level and within the physiological range of muscle lengths and velocities, the force output varies from almost 0 to above maximum isometric force (defined as 1). Clearly the neural circuits controlling muscle activation have to take this state dependence into account if the resulting behavior is to resemble the desired one even remotely. The M1 signal compensating for the state dependence illustrated in figure 6.1b plays a central role in our model since it correlates with position and velocity and thus explains the observations that appear most problematic.

# From M1 Output to Motor Behavior

The relationship between M1 output and motor behavior is no doubt complex. If we incorporate every detail whose existence is currently suspected, the resulting model will probably have enough free parameters to fit every available observation. The usefulness of a model, however, comes not from incorporating all proposed mechanisms and fitting all existing data but from illuminating the underlying principles whose interplay gives rise to, or at least can give rise to, the data. My strategy is to avoid free parameters and the curve fitting associated with them. I do so with the help of simplifying assumptions: linearizing functions that are mildly nonlinear, assuming quantities that vary slightly to be constant, ignoring terms that tend to average out, linking together parameters that have similar values. Every simplification is justified when first introduced, with the exception of cosine tuning, which is addressed separately in the section "Cosine Tuning."

It is important to realize that the simplifications themselves do not give rise to the phenomena the model is trying to explain. Therefore the model's ability to reproduce these phenomena indicates that they arise from the underlying principle behind the model: direct cortical control of muscle activation that takes into account the basic properties of the musculoskeletal system.

## *From M1 Output to Muscle Activation*

Let $t$ denote time, $c_j(t)$ the mean firing rate of the $j$th pyramidal tract neuron relative to its baseline, $a_i(t)$ the EMG activity of the $i$th muscle relative to its baseline, $w_{ij}$ the net effect that neuron $j$ has on muscle $i$, and $d$ the average delay between movement-related activity in M1 and movement onset.[1] Baseline is defined as the mean activity during posture in the center of the work space. To relate M1 output to muscle activation, use the first-order model

$$a_i(t) = \sum_j w_{ij} c_j(t-d) + \varepsilon_i(t) \qquad (6.1)$$

where $\varepsilon_i(t)$ denotes the effects of other descending systems and spinal feedback. The model does not impose any restrictions on the pattern of weights $w_{ij}$; that is, each neuron can excite or inhibit any combination of muscles. The weights $w_{ij}$ represent not only monosynaptic projections from pyramidal tract neurons to motoneurons but a linear approximation to the input-output behavior of the spinal cord. Similarly the delay $d$ corresponds to transmission delays and also approximates the net effect of any low-pass filtering or recurrent processing in the spinal cord.

Note that equation 6.1 is used to describe the relationship between M1 and muscle activity during natural voluntary behaviors such as reaching or pushing. During instructed delay periods, during sleep, or after a subject was trained to control a cursor with signals recorded in M1 (Helms Tillery et al., 2001), the descending activity may somehow be gated at the spinal level. Anatomically, the M1 output is not the only descending source of activation: There are other descending systems, and the pyramidal tract itself originates from multiple cortical areas (Dum and Strick, 1991). It is not yet known, however, whether the pyramidal tract neurons in premotor and supplementary motor areas behave more similarly to the mixed population in their respective area or to the pyramidal tract neurons in M1 (in which case the present model applies to them as well). Recordings from the red nucleus indicate that equation 6.1 may be a reasonable approximation of the effects of other descending systems (Miller and Sinkjaer, 1998). It should also be noted that lesions in M1 produce more profound deficits than lesions in any other supraspinal motor area (Johnson, 1992), further justifying the emphasis on M1. As discussed earlier and in the later section "The Model in Perspective," the spinal feedback contributions are assumed to average out over repeated trials.

## *From Muscle Force to Endpoint Force*

Let $f_i(t)$ be the force (tension) that muscle $i$ generates, and $e_i(t)$ the corresponding endpoint force in the 2D work space of the hand. While the direction of $e_i(t)$ depends on joint configuration, that dependence (see figure 6.1a) is negligible for the small work spaces and stereotyped postures adopted in M1 experiments, so we can ignore it. Then

$$\mathbf{e}_i(t) = \mathbf{p}_i f_i(t) \qquad (6.2)$$

where $\mathbf{p}_i$ is a constant 2D vector whose length determines the scaling from muscle force to endpoint force. Note that the present formulation ignores the effects of muscle forces causing redundant joint rotations. If we take this redundant subspace into account as outlined in Todorov (2000a), we could derive additional constraints on the M1 population activity (without affecting the constraints derived later). However, M1 data has traditionally been analyzed in endpoint space, so these additional constraints could not be compared with existing experimental results.

## *Arm Dynamics in Endpoint Space*

Let $M$ be the $2 \times 2$ matrix expressing arm inertia in endpoint space, $\mathbf{f}_{ext}(t)$ the endpoint force that the hand applies against external objects, and $\mathbf{x}(t)$ the hand position in endpoint space (the origin of the 2D coordinate system is defined as the center of the work space). We assume that changes in inertia are negligible for the small movement extents and velocities used in the M1 literature and approximate the arm dynamics with an anisotropic point mass. Making explicit the dependence of muscle force on activation, length, and velocity (the latter two being functions of $\mathbf{x}$ and $\dot{\mathbf{x}}$), the endpoint dynamic is

$$\sum_i \mathbf{p}_i f_i(a_i(t), \mathbf{x}(t), \dot{\mathbf{x}}(t)) = \mathbf{f}_{\text{ext}}(t) + M\ddot{\mathbf{x}}(t) \tag{6.3}$$

We now encounter a redundancy problem: There are many more muscle activations $a_i$ (and even more cell activations $c_j$) than constraints given by equation 6.3. We can proceed in two ways: (1) linearize the left-hand side of equation 6.3 to obtain a first-order approximation of the M1-to-behavior mapping or (2) introduce further assumptions that resolve redundancy and allow us to use the detailed muscle model illustrated in figure 6.1b. I pursue the first approach (described in the next section, "Using a Linearized Muscle Model") throughout this chapter. The second approach (described in the section "Using a Detailed Muscle Model") is used only when conclusions reached on the basis of the linearization might seem sensitive to details of the muscle model.

### Using a Linearized Muscle Model

Assembling all $a_i$'s in the vector $\mathbf{a}$, all $c_j$'s in the vector $\mathbf{c}$, all $f_i$'s in the vector $\mathbf{f}$, all $w_{ij}$'s in the matrix $W$, and all $\mathbf{p}_i$'s in the columns of the matrix $P$, equation 6.3 can be written in matrix form:

$$Pf(a, x, \dot{x}) = f_{ext} \lessgtr M\ddot{x} \tag{6.3a}$$

Linearizing $\mathbf{f}$ around the baseline $\mathbf{f(0,0,0)} = \mathbf{0}$ yields an approximation of the left-hand side of equation 6.3a: $Pf(\mathbf{a}, \mathbf{x}, \dot{\mathbf{x}}) = PS\mathbf{a} - K\mathbf{x} - B\dot{\mathbf{x}}$. Here $K$ and $B$ are the endpoint

stiffness and damping by definition, and the scaling matrix $S = \partial \mathbf{f}/\partial \mathbf{a}$ is diagonal because each muscle is affected only by its own activation. From equation 6.1 we have $PS\mathbf{a} = PSW\mathbf{c}$, and so $PSW\mathbf{c} = \mathbf{f}_{\text{ext}} + M\ddot{\mathbf{x}} + B\dot{\mathbf{x}} + K\mathbf{x}$.

We can now approximate $PSW$ with $FU$, where the column vector $\mathbf{u}_j$ of the matrix $U$ is a 2D unit vector pointing in the same direction as the $j$th column vector of $PSW$. Thus, the $j$th neuron activates a linear combination of muscles that generate endpoint force in the direction $\mathbf{u}_j$. The $2 \times 2$ matrix $F = PSWU^T(UU^T)^{-1}$, chosen to minimize the norm of the approximation error $PSW - FU$, can be thought of as fitting an ellipse to the direction-dependent variation of the lengths of the column vectors in $PSW$. Since the scaling from firing rates to forces is arbitrary, we can assume without loss of generality that $|F| = 1$. Summarizing the derivation so far,

$$FU\mathbf{c}(t - d) = \mathbf{f}_{\text{ext}}(t) + M\ddot{\mathbf{x}}(t) + B\dot{\mathbf{x}}(t) + K\mathbf{x}(t) \tag{6.4}$$

The $2 \times 2$ matrices $M$, $B$, $K$, and $F$ all reflect the geometry of the arm in roughly the same way. Consider a four-degree-of-freedom arm, with the elbow pointing down and the hand constrained to a horizontal plane at about shoulder level. Endpoint inertia is clearly larger along the forward-backward $y$ axis than the lateral $x$ axis. Stiffness and damping are known to be larger along the hand-shoulder axis (Tsuji et al., 1995), which in this configuration coincides with the $y$ axis. Assuming that the weights $W$ and the activation-to-force scaling terms $S$ do not vary systematically with direction, the only anisotropy in $F$ comes from the matrix $P$ and is due to the fact that generating endpoint force along the $y$ axis requires joint torques of smaller magnitude.[2] Then the ellipse corresponding to $F$ is also elongated along the $y$ axis, and since the aspect ratios of the four ellipses are similar, we assume that the four matrices are proportional to each other: $M = mF$, $B = bF$, $K = kF$. Since $|F| = 1$, the scalars $m$, $b$, and $k$ are the direction-averaged inertia, damping, and stiffness. Multiplying equation 6.4 by $F^{-1}$ yields

$$U\mathbf{c}(t-d) = F^{-1}\mathbf{f}_{\text{ext}}(t) + m\ddot{\mathbf{x}}(t) + b\dot{\mathbf{x}}(t) + k\mathbf{x}(t) \tag{6.5}$$

Equation 6.5 is the relationship between M1 population activity $\mathbf{c}$ and motor behavior $\mathbf{f}_{\text{ext}}, \ddot{\mathbf{x}}, \dot{\mathbf{x}}, \mathbf{x}$ that we wanted to derive. The left-hand side is the sum of neuronal activities $c_j$ multiplied by the corresponding vectors $\mathbf{u}_j$, or in other words, a population vector (Georgopoulos et al., 1983). Note that, unlike the PV methods used in the M1 literature, the vector $\mathbf{u}_j$ assigned to neuron $j$ is a force direction rather than a physiological preferred direction. These two directions, however, are similar (Fetz and Cheney, 1980). Even if the difference between them is substantial for some neurons, the PV defined in the M1 literature is an unbiased estimate of the quantity $U\mathbf{c}$ as long as that difference is zero on average. Once we fix the parameters $m$, $b$, $k$, and the aspect ratio of $F$, we can generate predictions regarding population vectors *without* resolving the redundancy in equation 6.5. The parameter values I use everywhere—$m = 1$ kg, $b = 10$ Ns/m, $k = 50$ N/m, $F$ aspect ratio = 2:1—are derived from the human psychophysics literature (see Todorov, 2000a). Since the model predictions depend on the relative rather than absolute magnitudes of $m$, $b$, and $k$, the present conclusions should not be affected if these constants were scaled down to values appropriate for the monkey arm.

The constraint given by equation 6.5 is sufficient to model the PV, but the redundancy mentioned earlier has not yet been resolved (i.e., equation 6.5 does not tell us how individual neurons behave). Since several of the phenomena we want to address require such a model, let us augment equation 6.5 with the assumption of cosine tuning to obtain individual neuron responses:

$$c_j(t-d) = \frac{\mathbf{u}_j^T}{2}\left(F^{-1}\mathbf{f}_{\text{ext}}(t) + m\ddot{\mathbf{x}}(t) + k\mathbf{x}(t)\right) + b\left\lfloor \mathbf{u}_j^T\dot{\mathbf{x}}(t)\right\rfloor \tag{6.6}$$

This equation is essentially the dot product of $\mathbf{u}_j$ with the right-hand side of equation 6.5 (resulting in cosine tuning). The reason we treat the damping term differently is that muscle damping is known to be asymmetric—predominantly present during shortening (see figure 6.1b). The truncated cosine term $\lfloor \mathbf{u}_j^T\dot{\mathbf{x}}(t)\rfloor$ implies that neuron $j$ compensates for damping only when the hand is moving within 90° of its force direction $\mathbf{u}_j$ (corresponding to shortening of the muscles it activates).

Note that equation 6.6 prescribes an "ideal" response that does not capture the diversity of real neuronal responses (Kalaska et al., 1989) and should be thought of as the average response of all cells whose force directions are close to $\mathbf{u}_j$. To obtain an explicit model of response variability, we replace the endpoint impedance parameters $m$, $k$, and $b$ in equation 6.6 with cell-specific $m_j$, $b_j$, and $k_j$. These constants are sampled independently from uniform distributions between zero and twice the average value: $m_j \in [0;2]$, $b_j \in [0;20]$, $k_j \in [0;100]$. Multiplying by 2 and adding a cell-specific baseline $\bar{c}_j$ sampled uniformly from $\bar{c}_j \in [0;34]$ yields an average response of 45 Hz in the preferred direction and 5 Hz in the opposite direction, which is close to the range observed experimentally (Crammond and Kalaska, 1996).

Equation 6.6 can also be used to analyze one-degree-of-freedom movements or to compute the average firing of all neurons in their preferred direction ($\mathbf{u}_A$) and the direction opposite to it ($\mathbf{u}_N$). In either case, there are only two directions of interest, $\mathbf{u}_A$ and $\mathbf{u}_N$, which simplifies equation 6.6 to

$$c_A(t-d) = \frac{1}{2}\left(f_{\text{ext}}(t) + m\ddot{x}(t) + kx(t)\right) + b\dot{x}(t)$$

$$c_N(t-d) = -\frac{1}{2}\left(f_{\text{ext}}(t) + m\ddot{x}(t) + kx(t)\right)$$

$$(6.7)$$

## Using a Detailed Muscle Model

We now return to equation 6.3 and rederive the M1-to-behavior mapping using the detailed muscle model illustrated in figure 6.1b. That model is identical to Brown et al. (1999), except for the effects of sag, yielding, low-pass filtering, and tendon elasticity, which we ignore. The muscle force $f(a, l, v)$ given in table 6.1 is a function of activation $a$, length $l$, and velocity $v$. All parameters are set to the average values for fast-twitch and slow-twitch muscles, which account for data from a wide range of experiments (Brown et al., 1999). The activation $a$ is normalized so that $a = 0$ corresponds to the recruitment threshold and $a = 1$ to the frequency at which the force output saturates. Length $l$ and velocity $v$ are expressed in units of $l_0$ and $l_0$/sec, where $l_0$ is the length at which maximum isometric force is generated. Force output $f$ is in units of maximum isometric force.

The results from this section are applied only to movement tasks where the directional asymmetries cancel each other (see equation 6.5), so equation 6.3 becomes

$$e_{\max}\sum_i \mathbf{p}_i f_i\left(a_i(t) + \bar{a}_i,\ l_i(\mathbf{x}(t)),\ v_i(\mathbf{x}(t))\right) = m\ddot{\mathbf{x}}(t) \qquad (6.8)$$

The vectors $\mathbf{p}_i$ now have unit length, $l_i$ and $v_i$ denote the length and velocity of muscle $i$, $\bar{a}_i$ is the baseline activity corresponding to posture at the center of the work space, and $e_{\max}$ is the maximum isometric force each muscle can contribute in endpoint space. The baseline $\bar{a}_i$ is needed here because the muscle model is nonlinear and requires the total muscle activation.

The direction of hand movement for which muscle $i$ shortens most rapidly is very close to the direction $\mathbf{p}_i$ in which it produces endpoint force, and its orientation varies little over a small work space (see figure 6.1a). We approximate[3] this direction as constant and equal to the (constant) line of action $\mathbf{p}_i$. Then the length $l_i$ is proportional to the projection $\mathbf{p}_i^T \mathbf{x}$ of the endpoint position $\mathbf{x}$ on $\mathbf{p}_i$. The relationship between endpoint and muscle kinematics becomes

$$l_i = r_i - h\mathbf{p}_i^T \mathbf{x}$$

$$v_i = -h\mathbf{p}_i^T \dot{\mathbf{x}}$$

$$(6.9)$$

The negative sign is due to the fact that muscles shorten when the hand moves in the direction in which they produce force. The constants $r_i$ specify the muscle lengths when the hand is at the center $\mathbf{x} = (0, 0)$ of the work space, and $h$ is a scaling constant that relates endpoint distance to muscle length.

To resolve the redundancy in equation 6.8, we again use the assumption of cosine tuning. The total force $m\ddot{\mathbf{x}}$ that needs to be generated will be distributed among individual muscles as

$$\text{dis}_i(\ddot{\mathbf{x}}) = \frac{1}{ne_{\text{max}}} \left\lfloor co + 2m\mathbf{p}_i^T \ddot{\mathbf{x}} \right. \tag{6.10}$$

where $n$ is the number of muscles, the co-contraction level co is the scalar sum of the magnitudes of endpoint forces contributed by individual muscles, and the dot product $\mathbf{p}_i^T \ddot{\mathbf{x}}$ corresponds to cosine tuning. For a uniform distribution of $\mathbf{p}_i$'s and co large enough to ensure that the functions $\text{dis}_i(\ddot{\mathbf{x}})$ are full cosines, it can be verified that setting $f_i = \text{dis}_i(\ddot{\mathbf{x}})$ satisfies equation 6.8.

Given motor behavior $(\ddot{\mathbf{x}}, \dot{\mathbf{x}}, \mathbf{x}$, we can use equations 6.9 and 6.10 to compute muscle forces $f_i = \text{dis}_i(\ddot{\mathbf{x}})$, lengths $l_i(\mathbf{x})$, and velocities $v_i(\dot{\mathbf{x}})$. Let $\text{act}(f_i, l_i, v_i)$ be the activation level at which a muscle at length $l_i$ and velocity $v_i$ generates force $f_i$. This function is uniquely defined because muscle force increases monotonically with activation for fixed length and velocity. The function act is found by inverting the muscle model $f$ given in table 6.1, that is, by numerically solving the equation $f(\text{act}, l_i, v_i) = f_i$ with respect to act. The baselines and time-varying activations relative to the baselines can now be computed:

$$\bar{a}_i = \text{act}\left(\frac{co}{ne_{\text{max}}}, 0, 0\right)$$

$$a_i(t) = \text{act}\left(\text{dis}_i(\ddot{\mathbf{x}}(t)), l_i(\mathbf{x}(t)), v_i(\dot{\mathbf{x}}(t))\right) - \bar{a}_i \tag{6.11}$$

Equation 6.11 is the relationship between muscle activation and motor behavior that we wanted to derive. The population vector computed from muscle activations is $\sum_j \mathbf{p}_i a_i(t)$. Under the assumption that weight magnitudes $|w_{ij}|$ do not vary systematically with direction (see the section "Using a Linearized Muscle Model"), it can be verified that the population vector computed from cell firing rates is identical (apart from the delay $d$).

The parameters of the model were set as follows: mass $m = 1$ kg, number of muscles $n = 10$, maximum endpoint isometric force per muscle $e_{\text{max}} = 30$ N, and scaling constant $h = 0.6$, mapping a 1-m range of motion in $\mathbf{x}$ to a [0.7; 1.3] physiological range of normalized muscle lengths. The co-contraction level was adjusted to $co = 30$ N, which resulted in empirical stiffness $k = 76$ N/m and damping $b = 9$ Ns/m. The empirical stiffness and damping were identified via perturbation experiments applied to the model. Note that unlike the linearized muscle model discussed earlier, stiffness and damping cannot be set independently here. Instead, they are implicitly determined by the time-varying muscle activations computed in equation 6.11. The muscle lengths $r_i$ at the center of the work space were chosen randomly in the interval [0.9;

1.1]. Ten sets of random $r_i$'s were generated and the results averaged over the 10 simulation runs.

## Basic Results

Many experiments have been designed to identify what parameter of motor behavior is being represented in M1. Instead of a clear-cut answer, however, this effort has produced a long list of correlations. Our model predicts that such a list should indeed accumulate, because muscle activation is correlated with all the candidate representations that have been considered.

### *Position*

The postural activity of individual neurons predicted by the model (equation 6.6) is illustrated in figure 6.2a for eight hand positions arranged in a circle around the center of the work space. The gradient of the response surface is oriented along the neuron's preferred direction, and the slope is determined by the amount of stiffness that needs to be compensated. Such monotonically increasing and roughly linear postural responses have been well documented (Georgopoulos et al., 1984; Kettner et al., 1988).

### *Load*

The predicted M1 activity in isometric force conditions (figure 6.2b) is a linear function of the force being generated. In the one-degree-of-freedom case (equation 6.7), the response increases linearly with force magnitude for neurons whose force vector $\mathbf{u}$ is within 90° of the isometric force $\mathbf{f}_{ext}$ and decreases otherwise. In the two-degree-of-freedom case (equation 6.6), the response varies linearly with the cosine of the angle between $\mathbf{u}$ and $\mathbf{f}_{ext}$. Such monotonically increasing and roughly linear load responses have been well documented (Fetz and Cheney, 1980; Kalaska et al., 1989).

### *Movement*

The average activity of all M1 neurons in their preferred and opposite directions (equation 6.7) is illustrated in figure 6.2c for a typical 10-cm movement of 500-ms duration and bell-shaped speed profile. The M1 signal predicted from the linearized muscle model (figure 6.2c, left panel) is the sum of position, velocity, and acceleration terms weighted by the direction-averaged stiffness, damping, and inertia, respectively. When the detailed muscle model is used instead (equation 6.11), the individual contributions of these terms can no longer be separated. The composite M1 signal, however, remains similar (figure 6.2c, right panel).

The predicted movement response closely resembles the speed profile and varies with direction, which explains why the activity of M1 neurons has often been interpreted as an encoding of movement direction (Georgopoulos et al., 1982) or velocity (Schwartz, 1994). In our model this phenomenon occurs simply because the damping that needs to be compensated dominates the other terms making up the M1 response. Note that the time-varying fluctuations relative to baseline are

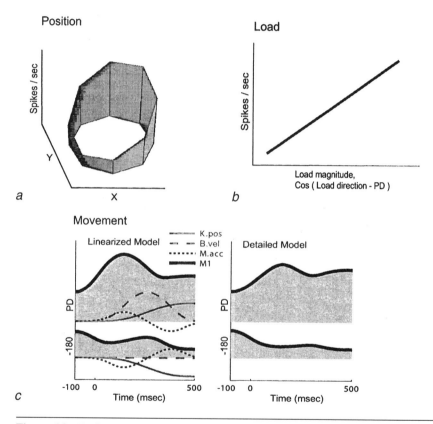

**Figure 6.2** Basic results. *(a)* The predicted postural response for targets arranged in a circle is a planar surface. *(b)* The predicted response for increasing load magnitude in a constant direction is linear. A linear response is also predicted when the direction of a constant-magnitude load is varied; in this case, the response is linear in the cosine of the angle between preferred and actual direction. *(c)* Predicted movement-time response. Note that the compound response *(left)* is a sum of positional, velocity, and acceleration terms weighted by system-level stiffness, damping, and inertia, respectively. In the nonlinear model *(right)* these components can no longer be separated, but the overall response is similar. *(d)* Predicted response when both the movement direction and imposed load direction are varied independently. *(e)* Population vector predictions for displacements or movements in different directions, loads in different directions, and movements in different directions in the presence of a constant load.

Figures 6.2c *(left)* and 6.2e reprinted from Todorov (2000a).

Movement + Load

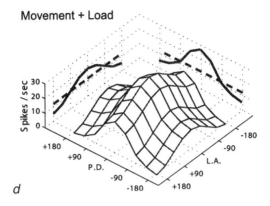

d

Population Vectors

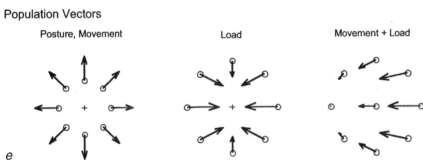

e

**Figure 6.2**   *(continued)*

different in the preferred and opposite directions, which is a direct consequence of the fact that muscle damping is asymmetric. The asymmetry seen in figure 6.2c has been observed experimentally (Kalaska et al., 1989; Crammond and Kalaska, 1996; Moran and Schwartz, 1999b). In comparison to the predicted response during an isometric force ramp, the signal in figure 6.2c has a more elaborate temporal structure, in agreement with experiments comparing movement and isometric force conditions (Sergio and Kalaska, 1998).

One might wonder why the predictions in figure 6.2c do not resemble the classic triphasic burst pattern of muscle activity. The reason is that this pattern is typical for large ballistic movements (Brooks, 1986), which are much faster than the movements studied in the M1 literature. If we apply our model (equation 6.7) to a movement that is $x$ times faster, the magnitude of the position component remains the same, the velocity component scales by $x$, and the acceleration component scales by $x^2$. Thus, for faster movements the model predicts that the acceleration component of the M1 signal will become more pronounced, causing PV reversals consistent with the triphasic burst pattern.

One might ask whether maintaining a position away from the center always requires a substantial increase in agonist activity (as shown in figure 6.2c). This is indeed a side effect of the linearized model, in which muscle stiffness is constant, but is no longer true in the detailed muscle model. As table 6.1 shows, the stiffness of realistic muscles scales with activation. Therefore, the peripheral position can be maintained by substantially lower muscle activations. In the model, reducing muscle co-contraction is accomplished by reducing the co-contraction parameter co in equation 6.10 and 6.11, and the prediction is that the overall activity in M1 will also decrease. The relationship between overall M1 activity and muscle co-contraction is further discussed in the section "Muscle Co-contraction."

## Movement With External Load

If a constant load is added during movement, the model prediction (equation 6.6) is the sum of the corresponding movement and load responses, as observed experimentally (Kalaska et al., 1989). The predicted response as a function of movement and load direction is shown in figure 6.2d.

If an isotropic inertial load $m_{ext}$ is added during movement, the model prediction (equation 6.6) is the sum of the movement response and the term $F^{-1}m_{ext}\ddot{x}(t)$. This added term accentuates the acceleration-dependent component of the signal shown in figure 6.2c, especially in lateral directions where $F^{-1}$ is larger. Thus, our model predicts that in the presence of inertial loads of increasing magnitude, reversals of PV direction during the movement will begin to be observed, first in lateral movement directions. This is indeed the case (Kalaska et al., 1992).

## Population Vectors

Figure 6.2e shows the population vectors (equation 6.5) for different postures, movements, loads, and movements in the presence of a constant load. In movement conditions the PV prediction was averaged over the movement time. For posture and movement, the PV successfully recovers the target direction, as it does in experimental data (Georgopoulos et al., 1983).

This is no longer the case during load compensation and movement with load. The load compensation PV is systematically distorted, so that vectors pointing in lateral directions are elongated and vectors pointing at 45° are rotated toward the lateral axis. These distortions result from the anisotropy of the matrix $F^{-1}$ in equation 6.5 (which captures the anisotropy of the Jacobian transformation that relates endpoint forces and joint torques). Very similar distortions in load PVs have been observed experimentally (Kalaska et al., 1989). It has also been observed that PVs computed in a mixed movement and load condition completely fail to reconstruct the movement direction and show the same pattern of distortions as figure 6.2e (Kalaska and Crammond, 1992). This failure of the PV in the model is, of course, due to the added load-related signal.

## Muscle Co-contraction

A number of studies have found systematic differences in M1 activity recorded during movements made in identical directions under varying experimental conditions (Caminiti et al., 1991; Scott and Kalaska, 1995; Kakei et al., 1999; Li et al., 2001). While these studies contradict the hypothesis of abstract directional encoding and are generally consistent with our model (see the opening paragraphs of this chapter and the later section "The Model in Perspective"), they do not point directly to a muscle-based representation in M1. To provide direct evidence for a muscle-based representation, one would have to compare experimental conditions in which both kinematic and kinetic parameters are identical but muscle activity is different. It is possible to design such an experiment by instructing, training, or otherwise provoking a subject to modulate the level of muscle co-contraction. Apart from some interesting early results (Humphrey and Reed, 1983), the control of muscle co-contraction has received surprisingly little attention in the M1 literature.

We analyzed the changes in M1 activity associated with different levels of muscle co-contraction in both monkeys and humans (Todorov et al., 2000). Monkeys trained in force field adaptation experiments show increased muscle co-contraction during the movement time, even in the baseline condition before any forces are applied (Li et al., 2001). In that condition their movements are kinematically and kinetically indistinguishable from the typical movements that monkeys make in center-outward reaching tasks, yet the M1 activity is markedly different. Both the directionally tuned and nontuned populations of neurons increase their firing rates after movement onset, for all movement directions. In contrast, previous studies have found that, after movement onset, responses increase in the preferred direction and *decrease* in the antipreferred direction (Crammond and Kalaska, 1996; Moran and Schwartz, 1999b), as our model predicts in the absence of co-contraction. Thus, increased muscle co-contraction is accompanied by a nonspecific increase of M1 activity.

We also conducted a functional MRI experiment in which human subjects were asked to co-contract their forearm and wrist muscles while maintaining posture (Todorov et al., 2000). In agreement with the monkey data, activation over M1 was significantly elevated in the co-contraction condition compared with rest in the same posture. Since subjects were not producing movements or isometric forces in any direction, the observed change in M1 activity cannot correspond to any directional command. This converging evidence from monkeys and humans provides strong evidence against the directional coding hypothesis and fits naturally in our framework.

## Trajectory Reconstruction

Given the correlations between M1 activity and various behavioral parameters illustrated in figure 6.2, it should be possible to reconstruct the movement trajectory more or less accurately from a population of M1 responses. The potential for neuroprosthetic applications has recently generated substantial interest in this topic (Wessberg et al., 2000; Helms Tillery et al., 2001). Here I propose a simple reconstruction method that takes advantage of the multiple correlations. I also explain within the framework of our model why trajectory reconstructions based on the population vector hypothesis (Schwartz, 1994; Moran and Schwartz, 1999a) are systematically distorted.

## *Reconstruction Methods*

Since the M1 signal most closely resembles movement velocity (figure 6.2c), the simplest viable method is to integrate the PV over time, yielding a reasonably accurate trajectory reconstruction (Schwartz, 1994; Moran and Schwartz, 1999a). We applied this method to the PV predicted by our model (equation 6.5) for the spiral movements used experimentally (1.5- to 7.5-cm spiral radius, traced in 2.5 s according to the two-thirds power law). The reconstruction we obtained is very similar to the results reported by Schwartz (1994) and Moran and Schwartz (1999a) and displays the same distortion near the center of the spiral (figure 6.3a; the reason for the distortion is discussed later). An alternative method that has been studied is fitting a multilinear regression model (or

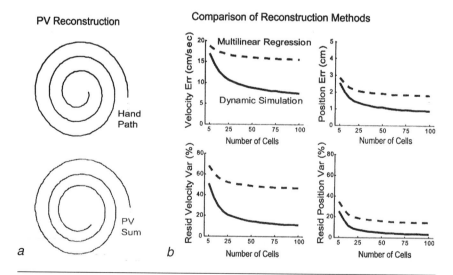

**Figure 6.3**    Trajectory reconstruction. *(a)* Comparison of simulated hand kinematics *(top)* and the sum of population vectors predicted by the model *(bottom)*. *(b)* Comparison of the reconstruction errors (*y* axis) of different methods. *(c)* Analysis of the variable time-lag effect in the linearized model. *(d)* Demonstration that the conclusions of the simple analysis hold for the detailed nonlinear muscle model.

Figures 6.3a and 6.3c reprinted from Todorov (2000a)

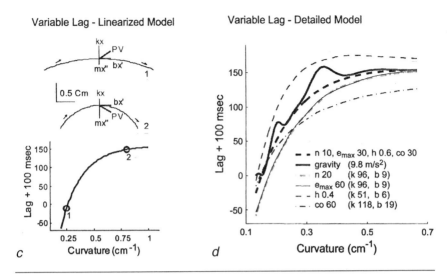

Figure 6.3    *(continued)*

a neural network) that maps cell firing rates to hand trajectories (Wessberg et al., 2000).

These methods implicitly assume that cell firing contains information about a *single* movement parameter: velocity in Schwartz (1994) and Moran and Schwartz (1999a) and position in Wessberg et al. (2000). Empirically, this is not the case, and it is therefore possible to develop better methods that take advantage of the multiple correlations that have been documented (as well as the regularities of hand kinematics). Optimal reconstruction can be achieved by a Bayesian method that involves (1) a generative model of how neural activity depends on arm state, (2) a dynamic model predicting the current arm state from the previous one, and (3) a recursive estimator that computes the posterior distribution of the arm state given the distribution inferred previously and the current neural activity. Although steps toward building such a method are already being taken (Gao et al., 2001), this is a difficult estimation problem, and the optimal solution is not likely to be found in the immediate future.

Here we propose a simple reconstruction method that is related to PV integration (Schwartz, 1994) but also takes advantage of the correlations with hand position and acceleration (or load). According to our model (equation 6.5), the population vector $U\mathbf{c}(t - d)$ can be interpreted as the force acting on a point mass that moves in a viscoelastic environment. Therefore, we can reconstruct the hand trajectory by simulating such a point mass and driving it with the (instantaneously computed) population vector. The state of the simulation is our prediction regarding the state of the hand. As in the PV integration method, the initial state has to be known. Endpoint impedance and external loads also have to be known (or fitted to optimize performance).

To assess the performance of our method, we generated a synthetic database containing 200 minimum-jerk trajectories (100 straight, 100 curved) of 300- to 600-ms duration and 5- to 10-cm extent. Each trajectory was executed in four dynamic conditions: normal, external load, external friction, and external spring. For each execution we simulated the responses of 100 Poisson-spiking cells with mean firing rates given by equation 6.6 (using the model of response variability), binned the spike data into 20-ms bins, and smoothed it with a fourth-order Butterworth filter whose parameters were optimized separately for each reconstruction method. Figure 6.3b shows that the reconstruction error of our method (dynamic simulation) is lower than that of multilinear regression. As expected, prediction error decreases with the number of cells in the data set. Note that our method generates simultaneous predictions about position and velocity, while the regression model is different in each case. An explicit comparison to the PV integration method is not shown because it is a special case of multilinear regression applied to velocity prediction.

The reconstruction method described here may appear to be tailored to our model of M1 responses, but this is not quite true. It is a very generic method, applicable to any population that (for whatever reason) happens to correlate with position, velocity, and force. Such simultaneous correlations in M1 are an empirical fact, and therefore they can be taken advantage of by using similar reconstruction methods.

## Variable Time Lag

The distortion seen in figure 6.3a and reported by Schwartz (1994) and Moran and Schwartz (1999a) is due to an interesting phenomenon described by Schwartz (1994). The time lag between the M1 population vector and hand velocity is not constant but increases with the curvature of the hand path. The increase observed experimentally is quantitatively similar to the model predictions (figure 6.3, c and d) in the spiral movements of figure 6.3a. In the linearized muscle model (equation 6.5), this increase can be computed analytically (Todorov, 2000a). The answer is $\mathrm{atan}((m\omega - k/\omega)/b)/\omega$, where the angular velocity $\omega$ is related to the curvature $\kappa$ by the two-thirds power law $\omega = 12\kappa^{2/3}$, and the scaling constant $12 \text{ rad} \cdot \text{cm} \cdot \text{s}^{-1}$ is extracted from the data in Schwartz (1994).

An intuitive explanation of why the model produces this effect is given in figure 6.3c (top). In the outer part of the spiral the curvature is small (thus the acceleration component $m\ddot{x}$ is small), while the distance from the center of the work space is large (thus the position component $kx$ is large). As a result, the PV direction is biased in a way that matches the direction of hand movement at some earlier point in time (i.e., the PV appears time-advanced). In the inner part of the spiral, the interplay between the position and acceleration components causes the opposite bias, making the PV appear time-delayed. Note that the instantaneous speeds in the inner and outer parts of the spiral are also different; this is not visible in the intuitive plot but is taken into account in the analytical calculation.

My explanation of the variable time-lag phenomenon (Todorov, 2000a) has been challenged on the basis that the model is too simple (Moran and Schwartz, 2000). It is not clear how the striking similarity between the model predictions and the experimental data could be an artifact of the simplifications used in the model, but to rule out that possibility, I repeated the analysis with the detailed muscle model (Todorov, 2000b). Figure 6.3d shows the time lag between the PV and hand movement direction computed from equation 6.11. The four parameters of the detailed model were each varied by a factor of 2, demonstrating the robustness of the phenomenon. In one simulation I added gravity compensation, which caused fluctuations of the curvature–time lag function that were similar to those observed experimentally (Moran and Schwartz, 1999a) but that did not alter its underlying shape. It is not surprising that the detailed and linearized muscle models produce almost identical results: The variable time-lag phenomenon in the detailed model is due to the compensation for viscoelasticity, and the linearized model captures that viscoelasticity to the first order.

# Evidence for Direction Encoding?

According to the hypothesis of directional control, M1 encodes predominantly the direction, rather than the magnitude, of movement velocity (Georgopoulos et al., 1982) and isometric force (Taira et al., 1996; Ashe and Georgopoulos, 1994). Apart from the damping asymmetry in equations 6.5, 6.6, and 6.7 (which makes the encoding of speed more difficult to detect), our model treats velocity and force as vectors whose direction and magnitude are nowhere separated. Thus, it is important to examine in detail the results that have been interpreted as encoding direction irrespective of magnitude. After examining six such results (discussed later), I conclude that none of them is convincing evidence for direction encoding and, in fact, they are all consistent with our model.

Note that the magnitude of both velocity (Schwartz, 1994) and force (Fetz and Cheney, 1980) is clearly being encoded in M1. Thus, the question here is whether the encoding of direction dominates the encoding of magnitude in a way inconsistent with treating either force or velocity as a vector.

## *Force Magnitude Versus Direction*

Let $k$ denote the trial number; $r(k)$, the magnitude of the 3D isometric force vector $\mathbf{f}_{ext}(k)$; $x(k)$, $y(k)$, and $z(k)$, the coordinates of the unit vector that points in the same direction as $\mathbf{f}_{ext}(k)$; and $mfr(k)$, the rate at which a given neuron fires in trial $k$. To assess the relative contributions of force magnitude and direction to the firing rate of that neuron, it might seem reasonable to compare the two regression models

$$M:\ mfr(k) = b_0 + b_r r(k)$$
$$D:\ mfr(k) = b_0 + b_x x(k) + b_y y(k) + b_z z(k)$$

For 79% of the M1 neurons studied by Taira et al. (1996), only regression model D provided a significant fit. Can we then conclude that 79% of the neurons in M1 do not encode force magnitude, and if we reach such a conclusion, how can we reconcile it with earlier studies showing the opposite (Fetz and Cheney, 1980)?

All we can conclude from the results of Taira et al. (1996) is that the majority of M1 neurons do not encode force magnitude in the way prescribed by regression model M. Note, however, that model M prescribes a rather unnatural encoding of magnitude: The response of the neuron is supposed to increase when the force magnitude increases, even when the force direction is opposite to the neuron's preferred direction. Consider instead a more natural encoding (equation 6.6), in which the response of the neuron is simply the dot product of its preferred direction and the force vector. Geometrically, such a response is a plane (figure 6.4a, left panel). The regression models used by Taira et al. (1996) attempt to fit the surfaces shown in figure 6.4a (right panel) to M1 data. If M1 neurons encode force as we predict, regression model D would clearly provide a significant (although not perfect) fit,

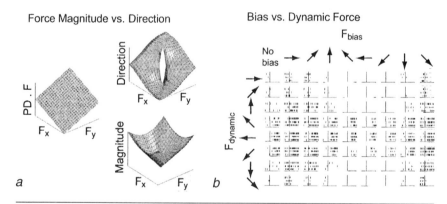

**Figure 6.4**  Apparent evidence for direction encoding. *(a)* The predicted response for 2D isometric force is planar *(left)*. Attempts to fit such responses by separating the contributions of force magnitude and direction are expected to fail, because the corresponding surfaces *(right)* are inappropriate for fitting planar responses. *(b)* Model predictions of firing-rate modulation due to independently varying the directions of dynamic and bias force. *(c)* The problems associated with classifying cells as position, velocity, acceleration, or direction related. Thin solid lines mark correct classification boundaries; thick solid lines mark the classification boundaries generated by linear regression classifiers; thin dashed lines mark the correct classification boundaries when the movement is made two times faster. *(d)* Both cortical activation and muscle activation are known to be more phasic than the resulting torque pattern, which can be due to low-pass filtering. *(e)* How simple summation of cortical signals at the muscle level can lead to very different modulation ratios of cortical and muscle tuning (2:1 vs. 8:1). *(f)* When targets at different distances are used, speed profiles scale both in magnitude and duration *(left)*. As a result, the initial portion of the trajectory is roughly invariant with regard to target distance, so the predicted cortical signal is best correlated with direction early in movement *(right)*.

Figure 6.4c reprinted from Todorov (2000b). Figure 6.4f reprinted from Todorov (2000a).

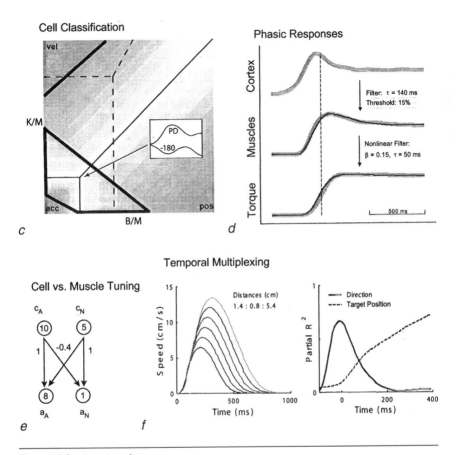

**Figure 6.4** *(continued)*

while regression model M would not fit at all. We have confirmed this using synthetic responses generated from equation 6.6 (Todorov, 2000a).

## Bias Versus Dynamic Force

To assess the relative contributions of static and dynamic isometric force, monkeys were trained to maintain a static (bias) force in a specified direction and then produce an additional (dynamic) force pulse in the direction of a randomly chosen target (Georgopoulos et al., 1992). The finding that the preferred direction for dynamic force does not depend on the direction of bias force (and vice versa) was taken as evidence that bias and dynamic forces are somehow encoded separately in M1. This finding was illustrated with a plot almost identical to figure 6.4b.

Our model predicts the same effect (figure 6.4b) without explicitly separating bias and dynamic force. Consider a neuron whose firing *mfr* is given by the dot product of its preferred direction **u** and the total isometric force $\mathbf{f}_{total}$. Since $\mathbf{f}_{total}$ is the sum of $\mathbf{f}_{dynamic}$ and $\mathbf{f}_{bias}$, we have

$$mfr = \mathbf{u}^T\mathbf{f}_{total} = \mathbf{u}^T(\mathbf{f}_{dynamic} + \mathbf{f}_{bias}) = \mathbf{u}^T\mathbf{f}_{dynamic} + \mathbf{u}^T\mathbf{f}_{bias}$$

If we now fix $\mathbf{f}_{bias}$ and determine the preferred direction by varying $\mathbf{f}_{dynamic}$, the term $\mathbf{u}^T\mathbf{f}_{bias}$ simply acts as a baseline, and the preferred direction is **u**. If we change the direction or magnitude of $\mathbf{f}_{bias}$ (or remove it completely) and repeat the same procedure, the only difference is in the baseline, so the preferred direction remains unchanged. The same holds for fixing $\mathbf{f}_{dynamic}$ and computing the preferred direction with respect to $\mathbf{f}_{bias}$.

## Cell Classification

Although it is clear that the responses of individual neurons are correlated with multiple movement parameters, neurons could be classified according to the movement parameter showing the strongest correlation. This was done in a 2D movement task in which the time-varying mean firing rate of each neuron was correlated with target direction (which does not vary within a trial), hand position, velocity, and acceleration (Ashe and Georgopoulos, 1994). The responses classified as direction related were most common (47%), while the acceleration-related responses were least common (6%). Does this finding contradict our model, which contains no explicit representation of movement direction? The answer turns out to be negative: The same classification scheme applied to equation 6.6 (with response variability) yields up to 30% direction-related responses and only 2% acceleration-related responses.

How can a seemingly reasonable classification scheme find a large percentage of direction-related responses in a model without any explicit encoding of target direction? This is possible because a weighted sum of position, velocity, and acceleration (equation 6.6) does not necessarily resemble any one of these signals, as illustrated in figure 6.4c. The family of synthetic response types given by equation 6.6 is parameterized by the cell-specific constants $m_j$, $b_j$, $k_j$, and $\bar{c}_j$. The baseline and overall scale do not affect the outcome of the classification, so it is sufficient to study the family of responses parameterized by $k_j/m_j$ and $b_j/m_j$. Each point in that two-parameter family corresponds to a response type, one of which is shown as an inset in figure 6.4c. The classification boundaries induced by the procedure of Ashe and Georgopoulos (1994) are marked with thick lines, while the correct classification boundaries (computed in the model by identifying the component signal with largest contribution) are marked with thin lines. The correlation-based classification boundaries are substantially different from the correct ones. In particular, a direction region (the trapezoid surrounded by thick lines) that should not exist has been created. This region is centered around the point where the correct boundaries meet, which corresponds to the synthetic response type most difficult to classify as either position, velocity, or acceleration related. The correlation-based procedure misclassifies the responses in this region as directional simply because they do not fit well in any of the alternative categories. For example, the response in the middle of the misclassified region resembles the velocity profile in the preferred direction and the acceleration profile in the opposite direction.

The results in figure 6.4c are obtained using the mean firing rates given by equation 6.6 and do not reflect any classification biases due to data transformations. Smoothing single-trial spike trains can cause further biases, as demonstrated on synthetic data (Todorov, 2000a). Georgopoulos and Ashe (2000) showed that smoothing does not affect the results of Ashe and Georgopoulos (1994), but that may happen in other data sets.

A deeper problem with classifying cells into discrete categories is that even if we had access to the correct classification, it is likely to change between task conditions. That problem is illustrated in figure 6.4c, where the dashed lines show the correct classification boundaries for a movement two times faster than the original. As explained previously in subsection "Movement" of "Basic Results," executing the movement faster increases the relative contribution of the acceleration component, shifting the classification boundaries substantially. What does it mean then to label a cell as "velocity related" if it can become "acceleration related" in a faster movement, "position related" in a slower movement, and "direction related" in a condition where the response is too complex to fit in any of the alternative categories?

## Phasic Responses

The simple relationship between M1 and EMG activity given by equation 6.1 does not strictly hold, as Fetz et al. (1989) showed by averaging the activity of all corticomotoneuronal cells and muscles they recorded (figure 6.4d). In particular, the M1 response at the onset of an isometric force ramp is more phasic than muscle activation. Is this evidence for abstract directional encoding? The answer is obviously negative. As figure 6.4d illustrates, EMG activity is more phasic than joint torque, just as M1 activity is more phasic than EMG activity. If we agree to interpret such differences as evidence for directional encoding, we must conclude that muscle activation carries an abstract directional component, which is quite absurd. The EMG-force difference is to be expected, given that muscles act as low-pass filters (Zajac, 1989; Brown et al., 1999). This suggests a similar explanation for the M1-EMG difference: If the processing in the spinal cord (which we approximated with a fixed delay in equation 6.1) has the effect of a low-pass filter, the descending M1 signal has to be more phasic in order to generate the necessary EMG activity. The black lines in figure 6.4d show that the M1 signal given in Fetz et al. (1989) can be filtered and thresholded to yield a close match to the EMG signal and filtered again (using the nonlinear muscle filter from Zajac, 1989) to match the force trace.

An alternative explanation is that the phasic M1 signal serves a "priming" role, such as bringing near to threshold the spinal networks that activate the group of agonist muscles. The difference between a signal designed to compensate for the effects of low-pass filtering and a signal designed to overcome thresholds is that the former should always be present, while the latter should be present only around the onset of EMG activity. The fact that phasic responses have not been reported in drawing tasks of longer duration (Moran and Schwartz, 1999a; Schwartz, 1994) makes the priming explanation more likely.

Note that phasic responses found in movement tasks (Kalaska et al., 1989) are most common in superficial-layer neurons, which we are not concerned with here (since they do not project to the spinal cord). This may explain why recordings from a mixed M1 population show an unusually strong phasic component, leading to a large population vector for dynamic force and an almost nonexistent population vector for bias force (Georgopoulos et al., 1992). The latter result is difficult to interpret, however; it is not clear how the population vector method could fail to reconstruct the bias force, given that the majority of M1 neurons were significantly tuned for bias force (Georgopoulos et al., 1992). One possible explanation for this puzzling result is that the preferred directions for dynamic force (which were used in computing the bias-force population vector) were not sufficiently close to the preferred directions for bias force (which should ideally be used). Even if the difference between the dynamic and bias preferred directions averaged over the population is zero, the bias population vector computed in this way scales down by an amount related to the circular variance of the distribution of differences.

### Cell Versus Muscle Tuning Modulation

To assess how directly M1 neurons control muscles, we can compute the ratio of maximal to minimal activation (which is a measure of directional modulation) and compare these ratios for M1 neurons and muscles. It has been shown that M1 tuning curves are less modulated by the direction of bias force than muscle tuning curves are (Georgopoulos et al., 1992). Is that finding inconsistent with equation 6.1? Not at all—in fact, such a difference is to be expected if M1 output controls the activation of muscle groups directly. One possible mechanism is illustrated in figure 6.4e: If we have just two neurons driving two muscles with both excitatory and inhibitory weights, an M1 tuning modulation of 2:1 can be transformed into a muscle tuning modulation of 8:1. Suppression of muscles pulling opposite to the neurons' preferred direction—which is essential for this mechanism—has been documented (Fetz and Cheney, 1980). Another mechanism that can change the tuning modulation is simply the subtraction of some "baseline," which physiologically could correspond to descending activity that results in subthreshold spinal activation. If we modify the setup in figure 6.4e to have only excitatory projections and subtract a baseline of 4, an M1 tuning modulation of 2:1 can be transformed into a muscle tuning modulation of 6:1. Therefore, differences in tuning modulation are consistent with our model.

## Temporal Multiplexing

An interesting possibility suggested by Fu et al. (1995) is that the nature of the M1 encoding changes in different phases of the movement (although it is not clear what "phase" means in continuous movements of longer duration). In the case of reaching, it was shown that M1 activity is best correlated with target direction around movement onset, and correlations with other parameters (such as target location and distance) peak later in the movement (Fu et al., 1995). Does that imply an encoding of target direction in extrapersonal space around movement onset? It does not, for two reasons.

The first explanation (already mentioned in the section "Phasic Responses") is that M1 may have to send a signal that brings spinal neurons to their thresholds. This signal depends on which muscle groups need to be activated (and that depends on the movement direction) but is not affected by how far away the target is. Note that varying the arm posture should affect such a compensation signal (Scott and Kalaska, 1997), so it can be distinguished experimentally from an abstract direction encoding.

The second explanation is even simpler, in the sense that it does not require additional assumptions. In the study of Fu et al. (1995), monkeys made movements of different extents in each direction. As expected from Fitts' law, both the duration and speed of the movement scaled with distance. Such scaling (figure 6.4f) tends to make the initial portions of the trajectories indistinguishable; that is, it is difficult to tell how far away the indented target is, given the arm kinematics around movement onset. Therefore our model (equation 6.6) predicts a weak correlation with target distance or location at the beginning of the movement and a stronger correlation with target direction (see figure 6.4f). The details of the partial $R^2$ calculation can be found in Todorov (2000a).

# Cosine Tuning

Cosine tuning of both M1 neurons (Georgopoulos et al., 1982; Kettner et al., 1988; Kalaska et al., 1989; Caminiti et al., 1991) and muscles (Turner et al., 1995; Herrmann and Flanders, 1998; Hoffman and Strick, 1999) has been observed repeatedly. The robustness of this phenomenon suggests that cosine tuning curves must be appropriate in a rather fundamental way, yet a satisfactory explanation is lacking. In a historical context dominated by single-joint studies, the broad directional tuning of M1 neurons could have been interpreted as a principle of cortical computation. But the fact that muscles (as well as muscle spindles) have the same tuning curves as cortical neurons suggests that the explanation is more likely to involve known peripheral properties rather than unknown computational principles (see also the later section "The Origin of Directional Tuning").

Muscle length and velocity vary with the cosine of hand displacement and velocity (equation 6.9), as first pointed out by Mussa-Ivaldi (1988). That would, of course, explain cosine tuning of spindle afferents, but is it an adequate explanation of cosine tuning in the motor output? We do not believe so, for the following reasons: (1) Cosine tuning is present in isometric force tasks and before movement onset. (2) Muscle preferred directions can be systematically different from their lines of action (Cisek and Scott, 1998; Hoffman and Strick, 1999). (3) Many tuning curves are sharper than cosine (Hoffman and Strick, 1999; Amirikian and Georgopoulos, 2000). (4) The arm musculature is redundant, so any set of net joint torques can be achieved with an infinite variety of EMG patterns (i.e., each muscle does not have to compensate for its own viscoelasticity or mimic the activity of its own spindle afferents).

Why is it then that the motor system tends to choose one out of the infinitely many activation patterns that would generate the same behavior? I argue that the apparent redundancy is due only to the traditional emphasis on average behavior (see also Loeb, 2000). If factors such as robustness to noise and fatigue are taken into account, it can be shown that cosine tuning is the unique muscle activation pattern that optimizes expected performance. Observed deviations from cosine tuning also fall outside of this minimization (Todorov, 2002). This argument is summarized next.

## Consequences of Multiplicative Noise

It is well established that neuromotor noise is multiplicative, in the sense that the standard deviation of the net force increases linearly with its mean. Such scaling has been demonstrated for tonic isometric force (Sutton and Sykes, 1967; McAuley et al., 1997) as well as for brief isometric force pulses (Schmidt et al., 1979). These empirical results lead to a neuromotor noise model in which each muscle contributes endpoint force with standard deviation $\sigma$ linear in the mean $\mu$: $\sigma = \lambda\mu$. Incorporating this scaling law into a minimum variance model of trajectory planning provides an explanation of Fitts' law and the smoothness of arm trajectories (Harris and Wolpert, 1998).

The preceding scaling law has another interesting consequence, which is the basis for our explanation of cosine tuning. Suppose we have two identical muscles pulling in the same direction, and we want them to produce average net force $\mu$. If we activate only one muscle so that it generates average force $\mu$, the variance of the net force will be $\lambda^2\mu^2$. If instead we activate both muscles so that each one of them generates average force $\mu/2$, the force output of each muscle will have variance $\lambda^2\mu^2/4$. Assuming uncorrelated noise, the variance of the net force will be $\lambda^2\mu^2/2$, which is two times smaller! I have confirmed experimentally both the scaling law and the predicted noise reduction due to redundancy (Todorov, 2002). Figure 6.5a shows that the standard deviation of isometric grip force is linear in the mean. As predicted, the noise magnitude decreases when subjects use both hands (instead of the dominant hand alone) to generate the same instructed force.

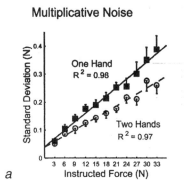

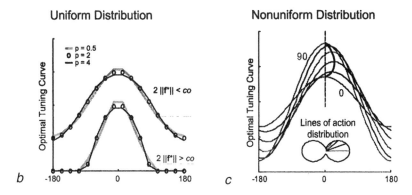

**Figure 6.5** Cosine tuning. *(a)* Measured isometric force fluctuations (*y* axis) are a linear function of instructed grip force. Each subject gripped the force sensor in two conditions: with one hand and with both hands. *(b)* Optimal tuning curves can be full cosines or truncated cosines, depending on the ratio between specified co-contraction and force magnitude. *p* is the exponent of the cost function. The similarity of the curves for the three values of *p* indicates that our analytical results are not sensitive to the square cost (*p* = 2) used to derive them. *(c)* Optimal tuning curves when the distribution of pulling directions (illustrated at the bottom) is nonuniform. The preferred directions are misaligned relative to the lines of action, so that the gap in the distribution is filled.

Figures 6.5a, 6.5b, and 6.5c reprinted from Todorov (2002).

Thus, it is advantageous to activate all muscles that pull in the direction of desired net force. What about muscles pulling in slightly different directions? If all of them are recruited simultaneously, the noise in the net force direction still decreases, but at the same time extra noise is generated in orthogonal directions. In other words, the advantage of activating redundant muscles decreases with the angle away from the net force direction. Because of this systematic decrease, there exists a unique tuning curve for which the average net force is generated with minimum expected error. To identify that optimal tuning curve, we need a formal model.

## A Model of Noisy Force Production

As in the section "Using a Detailed Muscle Model," muscle $i$ generates endpoint force along a fixed line of action given by the unit vector $\mathbf{p}_i$. The muscle force (or tension) $f_i$ is now divided into two components: $f_i = \mu_i + z_i$. The mean force $\mu_i$ is assumed to be under the control of the nervous system, while the zero-mean term $z_i$ combines all sources of noise affecting the force output of muscle $i$. The net endpoint force is then $\sum_i (\mu_i + z_i)\mathbf{p}_i$. The cost of using the vector of mean muscle forces $\mu = [\mu_1,\ldots,\mu_n]$ to generate the desired net endpoint force $\mathbf{f}^*$ is defined as

$$\text{Cost}(\mu, \mathbf{f}^*) = \mathrm{E}_{z|\mu}\left\|\mathbf{f}^* - \sum_i (\mu_i + z_i)\mathbf{p}_i\right\|^2 \leq \eta \sum_i \mu_i^2 \qquad (6.12)$$

The first term in equation 6.12 penalizes the expected difference between the desired and realized endpoint force, the second term is an effort cost, and the weighting parameter $\eta$ sets the tradeoff between accuracy and effort. We use a supralinear (i.e., quadratic) function to approximate effort because larger muscle forces are produced by larger and more rapidly fatiguing motor units (according to Henneman's size principle). The expectation is taken over the probability distribution of the noise terms $z_i$ conditional on the mean forces $\mu_i$. Since the quantity whose expectation we have to compute is quadratic in the random variables $z_i$, all we need to specify is the mean and covariance of the conditional distribution $p(\mathbf{z} \mid \mu)$. The mean is zero by definition, and the conditional covariance is modeled as

$$\text{Cov}(z_k, z_s \mid \mu_k, \mu_s) = \left(\lambda_1 \mu_k \mu_s + \lambda_2 (\mu_k + \mu_s)\right)\left(\delta(k,s) + \lambda_3 + \lambda_4 \mathbf{p}_k^T \mathbf{p}_s\right) \quad (6.13)$$

The quadratic function parameterized by $\lambda_1$ and $\lambda_2$ generalizes the scaling law discussed earlier. The linear term $\lambda_2(\mu_k + \mu_s)$ is needed because of the nonzero intercept in figure 6.5a (a constant term is also needed to model the nonzero intercept, but it does not affect the minimization with respect to $\mu$, so we ignore it). The second multiplicative term in equation 6.13 does not depend on $\mu$ but instead models the effects of the angle between the lines of action: The delta function $\delta(k, s)$ corresponds to independent noise in the output of each muscle; $\lambda_3$ is a noise term common to all muscles; $\lambda_4 \mathbf{p}_k^T \mathbf{p}_s$ is a noise correlation whose strength varies with the angle between the two lines of action. The latter term is needed to capture the observation that muscles with similar lines of action show correlated EMG fluctuations (Stephens et al., 1999).

The constraints we impose on the mean forces $\mu_i$ are

$$\mu_i \geq 0 \text{ for all } i$$
$$\sum_i \mu_i = co \text{ (optional)} \qquad (6.14)$$

The nonnegativity constraint is needed because muscles can only pull. The co-contraction constraint is optional and allows us to specify the desired arm impedance (see the section "Using a Detailed Muscle Model"). Note that generating muscle forces that cancel each other is always suboptimal according to the cost function in equation 6.12 because it increases both the noise and energy consumption without affecting the net force. Ideally, the cost function would take into account the advantages of higher impedance (allowing us to derive the optimal impedance and tuning function simultaneously), but that leads to technical complications, which we leave for future work. For the purpose of deriving the optimal tuning curve, it is sufficient to minimize equation 6.12, subject to equations 6.13 and 6.14, for every possible setting of the parameters $\mathbf{f}^*$, $\eta$, $co$, $\lambda_1, \ldots, \lambda_4$.

## Cosine Tuning Is Optimal

The general minimization problem defined earlier was solved for many cases of interest in Todorov (2002). The main results are summarized here.

When the distribution of lines of action $\mathbf{p}_i$ is uniform, it can be shown analytically that the optimal tuning curve is either a cosine or a truncated cosine. If the optional co-contraction constraint is specified, the tuning curve is a cosine for $2\|\mathbf{f}^*\| \leq co$ and a truncated cosine otherwise (figure 6.5b, $p = 2$). If co-contraction is not specified, this condition becomes $2\|\mathbf{f}^*\| \leq -\lambda_2 / 2\lambda_1$. While analytical results could be derived only for a square cost (equation 6.12), I also solved the minimization problem numerically for a variety of cost functions in which the force error term was raised to the power $p \in [0.5; 4]$. As figure 6.5b shows, the optimal tuning curves were very similar to those derived analytically for $p = 2$. Both cosine and truncated cosine tuning curves have been observed experimentally (Hoffman and Strick, 1999). Our model predicts that the tuning curves will become broader when the co-contraction level is increased. Indeed, we have obtained indirect evidence supporting this prediction (Todorov et al., 2000).

For a nonuniform distribution of lines of action $\mathbf{p}_i$, the optimal tuning curves are not exactly cosine but very close (figure 6.5c). The direction of net force for which a muscle is maximally active (i.e., its preferred direction) is no longer aligned with its line of action. Instead, the optimal preferred direction is rotated to fill in gaps in the distribution of lines of action. This effect is illustrated for a bimodal distribution in figure 6.5c. Such systematic misalignment has been observed experimentally for both arm (Cisek and Scott, 1998) and wrist muscles (Hoffman and Strick, 1999).

Another prediction of the model is a negative force bias (or undershoot) that increases with force level. This is because both the error and effort terms in equation 6.12 are minimized when the net force is smaller than desired. The predicted magnitude of the effect depends on the error–effort tradeoff specified by $\eta$. In an isometric force experiment, I observed such a negative bias (Todorov, 2002). As predicted, it increased with the force level and was larger in the one-hand condition.

## The Model in Perspective

There is an interesting parallel between the M1 model presented here and the classic model of orientation selectivity in the primary visual cortex (V1): Both models

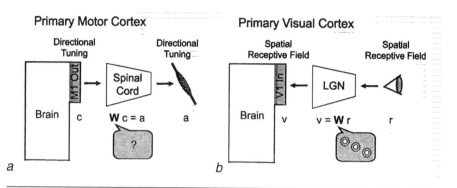

**Figure 6.6**  Mechanistic models of M1 and V1. Schematic comparison of the model proposed here for the primary motor cortex M1 *(a)* and the classic model of orientation selectivity in the primary visual cortex V1 *(b)*. The structure of the weight matrix *W* in the case of V1 is known and explains how orientation selectivity can emerge on the cortical level. In contrast, the M1-to-muscle weight matrix has unknown structure; as a result, our model can presently address only those phenomena that reflect basic properties of the musculoskeletal system. Directional tuning is such a phenomenon and closely corresponds to the spatial localization of receptive fields in the visual system.

involve a primary cortical area (M1 or V1), a corresponding peripheral organ (muscle or retina), and an intermediate processing stage (spinal cord or lateral geniculate nucleus [LGN]) approximated with a linear mapping (figure 6.6). Making this parallel explicit can help us place the issues discussed earlier within the broader context of computational neuroscience and identify directions for future research.

## *The Origin of Directional Tuning*

The defining feature of a muscle is its line of action (determined by the fixed attachment to the skeleton), while the defining feature of a photoreceptor is its location on the retina. In any given posture, a fixed line of action implies a preferred direction, just as a fixed retinal location implies a spatially localized receptive field. Therefore, directional tuning in the motor system is no more surprising than spatial tuning in the visual system, in that both types of tuning reflect fundamental peripheral properties. Of course, directional tuning of muscles does not necessitate such tuning in M1. Similarly, V1 neurons do not have to display spatial tuning: We can imagine, for example, a spatial Fourier transform[4] in the retina or LGN that completely abolishes the localized receptive fields of photoreceptors. But perhaps the nervous system avoids such drastic changes in representation, so the tuning properties that arise at one level propagate to neighboring levels, regardless of the direction of connectivity. The same argument may apply with regard to topographic organization: 2D topography arises in the retina and is found in V1, whereas muscle lines of action are not topographically organized (at least not in a sufficiently low-dimensional space) and correspondingly no detailed topography has been found in M1 (Schieber, 2001).

Proponents of the directional coding hypothesis have criticized the idea of muscle control on the basis that M1 neurons cannot possibly be "just higher-level motoneurons." The parallel with V1 illustrates how unreasonable such arguments are. Consider criticizing the related V1 model on the basis that V1 neurons cannot possibly be "just higher-level retinal ganglion neurons." Indeed they are not: V1 neurons display robust orientation tuning that emerges at the cortical level and does not reflect any peripheral properties (Hubel and Wiesel, 1962). But that phenomenon is perfectly consistent with the simple linear model in figure 6.6b, where V1 layer 4 neurons are driven by sets of retinal ganglion neurons with coaligned center-surround receptive fields. This parallel emphasizes the potential of structured high-dimensional mappings to generate interesting physiological responses and the importance of elaborating the structure of the M1-to-muscle weight matrix $W$ in future research. The latter would be much easier if a purely cortical phenomenon, comparable in robustness to V1 orientation selectivity, was discovered in M1. In contrast, all the phenomena addressed in this chapter reflect the basic properties of the musculoskeletal system, which is why we could account for them without specific assumptions regarding the structure of $W$.

## The Organization of Muscle Synergies

Each column of the M1-to-muscle weight matrix $W$ corresponds to the "muscle field" of a pyramidal tract neuron. Are these muscle fields composed of arbitrary subsets of muscles, or is there some organizing principle, as is the case with V1?

The short-latency contributions of corticomotoneuronal (CM) neurons to muscle activity, as measured by spike-triggered averaging, clearly have some structure: It is known that individual neurons tend to facilitate groups of muscles pulling in similar directions (i.e., agonists) and to suppress their antagonists (Fetz and Cheney, 1980). This evidence, however, comes from single-joint studies; in a multijoint setting, the notion of agonists and antagonists is much more elusive, and a quantitative description of the biomechanical features that cofacilitated muscles share is yet to come. An interesting step toward a multijoint description of cofacilitated muscle groups is the recent finding that some CM neurons facilitate proximal muscles, others facilitate both proximal and distal muscles, but very few CM neurons facilitate distal muscles alone (McKiernan et al., 1998). This observation makes sense biomechanically because the hand can exert forces against external objects only if those forces are transmitted via the proximal joints. Thus, muscle fields appear to be organized along some principles, but such principles are not nearly as clear as those underlying V1 organization. Furthermore, the CM neurons facilitating hand muscles appear to have rather uninterpretable muscle fields (Schieber, 2002); this is somewhat disturbing, given that the CM pathway is most prominent in hand control.

The preceding discussion focuses on muscle fields as defined by spike-triggered averaging. But M1 neurons exert most of their effects through spinal interneurons, and therefore a more proper definition of a muscle field would include both direct and indirect contributions. Unfortunately, the indirect contributions are hard to quantify. One approach is to rely on long-term correlations between neuronal and EMG activity, keeping in mind that the results are likely to be affected by correlations with other neurons. Using that approach, it was recently shown that the muscle fields so defined appear to be grouped in a small number of clusters (Holdefer and Miller, 2002). But a somewhat different analysis of hand-related neurons showed no evidence of clustering or any other easily interpretable form of organization (Poliakov and Schieber, 1999). Note also that the correspondence between a neuron's direct and indirect contributions—as measured by spike-triggered averages and long-term correlations, respectively—is somewhat loose (McKiernan et al., 2000).

In summary, the experimental literature on muscle synergies is far from conclusive, and the issues could probably be clarified if the empirical work was complemented by formal models. Is there a modeling approach that could yield specific predictions regarding the structure of muscle synergies? The parallel with V1 again turns out to be illuminating. The discovery of orientation tuning and its simple mechanistic explanation have generated great theoretical interest about why the mapping illustrated in figure 6.6b should have that particular structure and why V1 neurons should be orientation tuned. Several models have led to the same general answer, which is that the V1 encoding is optimized to capture the statistical regularities of natural images (Olshausen and Field, 1996). In other words, orientation tuning cannot be predicted from properties of the visual periphery alone but makes sense only when the properties of the visual world are also taken into account. By analogy, theoretical predictions regarding the structure of muscle synergies might come from analysis of the dynamic interactions between the musculoskeletal system and the natural environments in which it operates. We have began to develop a model of sensorimotor synergies (Todorov and Ghahramani, 2003) based on the same general idea: using unsupervised learning algorithms to capture the statistical regularities in the sensorimotor flow. Such an approach may also be useful in modeling the experience-dependent reorganizations in M1 (Nudo et al., 1996). This work will be presented in another publication.

## *Using the Redundancy of Population Codes*

The field of motor control has long suffered from the misconception that redundancy is a problem. It certainly is a problem from the point of view of the researcher trying to understand why a specific motor pattern is being chosen. But from the point of view of the motor system, redundancy is a solution rather than a problem because the existence of multiple acceptable patterns can only make the discovery of one of them easier. Our recent theory of motor coordination clarifies why musculoskeletal redundancy is useful and summarizes a number of psychophysical results demonstrating that such redundancy is being utilized by the motor system (Todorov and Jordan, 2002).

Redundancy is also present, to a much greater extent, at the level of neurophysiology. Any muscle activation pattern can be generated by a large set of cortical activation patterns,[5] and therefore we might expect this flexibility to be somehow taken advantage of. Indeed, a number of studies have shown that individual neuronal responses, and the way they change between experimental conditions, can be hard to interpret, and yet the population of such responses generally behaves in accordance with our model. The change of preferred directions, when averaged over the M1 population, matches (1) the amount of shoulder rotation in 3D reaching (Caminiti et al., 1991) and (2) the average rotation of muscle preferred directions in 2D force field adaptation (Li et al., 2001). In both cases, however, the changes displayed by individual neurons span a wide spectrum and are generally uninterpretable. Similarly, adding the muscle fields of a number of hand-related cortical neurons provides reasonable reconstructions of the pattern of observed muscle activity (Schieber, 2002), despite the fact that the relationship between the activity of individual M1 neurons and the muscles they directly facilitate or suppress is rather complex (McKiernan et al., 2000) and probably task specific (Kilner et al., 2000). Finally, linear regression models that reconstruct movement trajectories from cortical population activity can work quite well in the face of substantial trial-to-trial fluctuations of single-neuron activity (Wessberg et al., 2000).

The preceding examples indicate that the motor cortex may take advantage of the redundancy of population codes, but they do not clarify the nature of that advantage. A rare case where the latter is possible is the center-outward wrist movement task of Kakei et al. (1999), who measured the changes of M1 responses caused by changing the forearm posture. While the preferred directions of one M1 subpopulation rotated as much as muscle preferred directions (and lines of action), another subpopulation showed smaller rotations accompanied by changes in overall firing rate (or gain). Such changes are clearly inconsistent with an abstract encoding of direction, which predicts no effect of posture on any aspect of neural activity. The observed changes can be consistent with our model, as follows. Consider a muscle whose activation $a$ is generated by two cosine-tuned neurons, with gains $b_{1,2}$ and preferred directions $\mathbf{u}_{1,2}$. Under isometric force $\mathbf{f}$, we have $a = b_1 \mathbf{f}^T \mathbf{u}_1 + b_2 \mathbf{f}^T \mathbf{u}_2 = \mathbf{f}^T(b_1 \mathbf{u}_1 + b_2 \mathbf{u}_2)$; that is, the muscle activity is cosine-tuned with preferred direction $b_1 \mathbf{u}_1 + b_2 \mathbf{u}_2$. The latter vector can be rotated by rotating $\mathbf{u}_{1,2}$ but also by keeping $\mathbf{u}_{1,2}$ fixed and varying only $b_{1,2}$. Therefore, the same rotation in muscle space (required to perform the task in a different forearm posture) can be accomplished by two different changes of cortical output: a rotation of preferred directions or a change in gains.

Why would M1 employ a mix of the two mechanisms? We offer the following intuitive answer. It is reasonable to assume that, in the wrist movement task of interest, there are at least two relevant inputs to M1: one specifying the target location in extrapersonal space and possibly originating in ventral premotor area (Kakei et al., 2001) and the other one specifying the current arm posture irrespective of the task. If these two input signals are combined additively, they will produce gain changes without preferred direction changes, resembling the "extrinsic-like" neurons of Kakei et al. (1999). How should M1 transform such an input pattern into an output pattern appropriate for the task, given that many output patterns are task appropriate? We might expect the transformation to be accomplished with the least amount of work, which means that the output should resemble the input as much as possible, subject to the constraint that the necessary rotation in muscle space is implemented. We have performed a number of neural network simulations in which recurrent networks were trained to transform the input just described into any task-appropriate output. The learning algorithm always converged to networks whose output patterns were a mix of "intrinsic" and "extrinsic" responses, as observed by Kakei et al. (1999). These network models will be described in detail in a later publication.

## *The Role of the Spinal Cord*

Our model does not clarify how the spinal cord works but rather how it does not work. The fact that so many M1 phenomena can be explained using the simple feedforward transformation in equation 6.1 indicates that the spinal cord does not isolate or hide the basic properties of the musculoskeletal system from the rest of the brain. Indeed that would be a poor strategy, because primate arms (and especially hands) are used in a wide range of tasks with different dynamic requirements, so a peripheral detail that is a nuisance in one task may become a crucial feature in another. The spinal cord could, however, augment musculoskeletal properties in a way consistent with the model. For example, short-latency stretch reflexes can compensate for muscle yielding and thus maintain springlike behavior on longer time scales (Nicols and Houk, 1976). To incorporate such a mechanism, we simply have to modify the stiffness and damping terms in our model. (In fact, the psychophysical estimates we relied on probably reflect both muscle and reflex impedance.)

More generally, we can think of the spinal cord as integrating two sources of activity: descending and afferent. The effects of the (pyramidal tract) descending signal on muscle activity are modeled to first order by our linearization. Our results imply that the spinal cord generates the bulk of the muscle activity as a feedforward transformation of the descending signal, and that transformation is sufficiently smooth to appear linear over the small range of displacements, velocities, and loads typically used in the M1 literature. In this scheme, spinal feedback is used not to drive the movement or to translate abstract directional commands but to counteract undesirable deviations by modulating muscle activity on short time scales.

This contrasts with the view that afferent signals play the leading role in generating muscle activity, while descending signals play the modulatory role of setting thresholds or gains for the spinal circuits. I disagree with this view for two general reasons. (1) Following deafferentation, both monkeys (Bizzi et al., 1984) and humans (Ghez and Sainburg, 1995) can produce substantial and quasi-normal muscle activity, although a leading role of afferent signals would seem to predict a lack of muscle activity in that condition. (2) The large network of supraspinal areas has all the information needed to compute the average muscle activations that propel the arm, especially in simple and overtrained tasks, where all the internal models underlying this computation have presumably been formed. The only thing that the supraspinal system is known to be incapable of is generating very rapid corrections for undesirable deviations. Such corrections are crucial for ensuring stability, and since the spinal cord is ideally suited to generating them, we do not see why it should be burdened with other computations that are best performed elsewhere.

To make this discussion more concrete, we introduce some ideas from stochastic optimal feedback control that are relevant here (Davis and Vinter, 1985). Consider a system with (unobservable) state $\mathbf{x}_t$, control $\mathbf{u}_t$, noisy feedback $\mathbf{y}_t = H\mathbf{x}_t + \xi_t$, and stochastic dynamics $\mathbf{x}_{t+1} = A\mathbf{x}_t + B\mathbf{u}_t + \omega_t$. Such systems are controlled optimally by computing an internal state estimate $\hat{\mathbf{x}}_t$ using the Kalman filter $\hat{\mathbf{x}}_{t+1} = A\hat{\mathbf{x}}_t + B\mathbf{u}_t + K_t(\mathbf{y}_t - H\hat{\mathbf{x}}_t)$ and mapping this estimate (rather than the raw feedback) into a control signal $\mathbf{u}_t = -L_t\hat{\mathbf{x}}_t$. It is not presently clear how this should be implemented in a sensorimotor hierarchy containing multiple feedback loops that operate simultaneously. Nevertheless, the preceding equations emphasize two important points. (1) Estimation and control are computationally separate processes and involve separate sets of time-varying parameters ($K$ and $L$, respectively). The sensory gains $K$ reflect the reliability of the afferent signal. When that signal becomes infinitely unreliable (or absent), the optimal $K$ becomes zero, which automatically transforms the system into an open-loop controller with similar average behavior, in agreement with deafferentation studies. (2) The short-term contribution of the afferent signal $\mathbf{y}$ to the control $\mathbf{u}$ is given by the term $L_{t+1}K_t(H\hat{\mathbf{x}}_t - \mathbf{y}_t)$, which is proportional to the difference between the expected and observed feedback. Since the difference is zero on average, that contribution is washed out in analyses that average data over trials—even in tasks where rapid, single-trial feedback corrections are large and crucial for achieving stability and overall performance.

## Equilibrium-Point Control?

The equilibrium-point (EP) hypothesis (Feldman and Levin, 1995) has not been extensively applied to the M1 literature, but I include here a brief discussion of it because EP control is a rare example of a coherent theoretical framework of the kind that I argue for. Unfortunately, I do not see how it can be reconciled with the M1 literature. Although the presence of positional gradients and co-contraction-related signals in M1 correspond naturally to the R and C commands postulated by the EP hypothesis, a number of other well-established facts appear inconsistent with it:

1. The most salient finding from center-outward reaching tasks is that movement-time activity is dominated by a velocity-related signal. In particular, most neurons (during movement in their preferred direction) show an increase in firing followed by a decrease. In contrast, neural activity that encodes positional shifts should display monotonic changes in the course of reaching movements. The only way around that problem seems to be a proportional-derivative modification along the lines of McIntyre and Bizzi (1993), who proposed that both positional and velocity reference signals may be needed. This still does not explain why the M1 encoding of velocity is strongly asymmetric in the same way that muscle damping is asymmetric.

Note also that including a transient velocity command results in a mode of control that is neither "equilibrium" nor a "point."

2.  Straight reaching movements produced under curl-viscous forces (Li et al., 2001) are encoded differently from kinematically identical movements produced in the absence of such forces. As mentioned earlier, the average rotation of muscle preferred directions coincides with the average rotation of M1 preferred directions. The only way to reconcile EP control with such observations is to admit that, after all, the control signal takes dynamics into account (Gribble and Ostry, 2000). Then one would also have to admit that the reference trajectory for reaching movements can exhibit reversals, because such reversals have been observed in M1 (Kalaska et al., 1992). Note that, in general, dynamic additions to EP control eliminate one of the main advantages of such control: the avoidance of (either explicit or implicit) dynamic calculations. At the same time, such additions bring EP control closer to being an irrefutable hypothesis.

3.  Finally, the ability of deafferented subjects to generate quasi-normal muscle activity (Bizzi et al., 1984; Ghez and Sainburg, 1995) seems fundamentally inconsistent with any view in which afferent signals play the leading role in activating muscles. We could postulate that, following deafferentation, both the spinal cord and M1 are reorganized so profoundly that they begin to function according to our model, but that would be merely a way to dismiss these important observations rather than deal with them.

It should be noted that the apparent difficulties and lack of parsimony are not necessarily real: Since the EP command signals do not directly correspond to any one behavioral parameter, they may in principle be correlated with all parameters in the ways observed. I look forward to a specific neural implementation of EP control that addresses the M1 literature in detail. In the meantime, however, I remain skeptical, for the reasons just outlined.

## Conclusions

This chapter summarized a series of recent studies that developed a simple, mechanistic model of M1 control. The model accounts for a large number of experimental results, indicating that, in the absence of major unpredictable events, the trial-averaged M1 signal contains sufficient information to specify the trial-averaged pattern of muscle activations. This descending signal, which is the major output of the large supraspinal network of motor areas, takes into account peripheral properties such as muscle state dependence and perhaps spinal reflex gains. Therefore, the essential dynamic properties of the motor periphery are not "hidden" by the spinal cord, as the directional coding hypothesis has suggested. In retrospect, this is hardly surprising: It would be a waste of resources if the entire supraspinal system were devoted to computationally trivial tasks such as calculating 3D vectors and if the much more difficult problem of controlling complex musculoskeletal dynamics in real time were left to the ancient spinal circuits.

# Notes

[1]Notation: x is a scalar, $\mathbf{x}$ is a column vector, $\mathbf{x}^T$ is a transposed (row) vector, $\mathbf{x}^T \mathbf{y}$ is the dot-product of $\mathbf{x}$ and $\mathbf{y}$, $X$ is a matrix, $\dot{\mathbf{x}}$ and $\ddot{\mathbf{x}}$ are the temporal derivatives of x, $\|\mathbf{x}\|$ is the vector length, $|X|$ is the matrix determinant, $X^{-1}$ is the matrix inverse, $\lfloor x \rfloor = x$ for $x > 0$ and 0 otherwise, $\delta(k,s) = 1$ for $k = s$ and 0 otherwise.

[2] In other words, the Jacobian that relates endpoint force to joint torque is anisotropic.

[3] This approximation is very similar to the linearization used in Mussa-Ivaldi (1988).

[4] A Fourier transform is a linear mapping and therefore can be implemented by the connectivity illustrated in figure 6.6.

[5] In our linear model, that redundant set is a linear subspace. The population vector is a projection that maps the entire redundant subspace into a point; this is why in the linear case we could predict population vectors without having to resolve redundancy.

# Acknowledgments

I would like to thank Anatol Feldman and Gerald Loeb for their extensive comments on the manuscript. This work was supported by the Gatsby Charitable Foundation and the Alfred Mann Institute for Biomedical Engineering.

# References

Amirikian B, Georgopoulos A (2000) Directional Tuning Profiles of Motor Cortical Cells. *Neurosci Res* 36: 73-79.

Ashe J, Georgopoulos AP (1994) Movement Parameters and Neural Activity in Motor Cortex and Area 5. *Cereb Cortex* 6: 590-600.

Bizzi E, Accornero N, Chapple W, Hogan N (1984) Posture Control and Trajectory Formation During Arm Movement. *J Neurosci* 4: 2738-2744.

Brooks V (1986) *The Neural Basis of Motor Control*. New York: Oxford University Press.

Brown IE, Cheng EJ, Loeb GE (1999) Measured and Modeled Properties of Mammalian Skeletal Muscle: II. The Effects of Stimulus Frequency on Force-Length and Force-Velocity Relationships. *J Muscle Res Cell Motil* 20: 627-643.

Caminiti R, Johnson PB, Galli C, Ferraina S, Burnod Y (1991) Making Arm Movements Within Different Parts of Space: The Premotor and Motor Cortical Representation of a Coordinate System for Reaching to Visual Targets. *J Neurosci* 11: 1182-1197.

Cisek P, Scott SH (1998) Cooperative Action of Mono- and Bi-articular Arm Muscles During Multijoint Posture and Movement Tasks in Monkeys. *Soc Neurosci Abstr* 164.4.

Conway BA, Halliday DM, Farmer SF, Shahani U, Maas P, Weir AI, Rosenberg JR (1995) Synchronization Between Motor Cortex and Spinal Motoneuronal Pool During the Performance of a Maintained Motor Task in Man. *J Physiol (Lond)* 489: 917-924.

Crammond DJ, Kalaska JF (1996) Differential Relation of Discharge in Primary Motor Cortex and Premotor Cortex to Movements Versus Actively Maintained Postures During a Reaching Task. *Exp Brain Res* 108: 45-61.

Davis MHA, Vinter RB (1985) *Stochastic Modelling and Control.* London: Chapman and Hall.

Dum RP, Strick PL (1991) The Origin of Corticospinal Projections From the Premotor Areas in the Frontal Lobe. *J Neurosci* 11: 667-669.

Evarts EV (1968) Relations of Pyramidal Tract Activity to Force Exerted During Voluntary Movements. *J Neurophysiol* 31: 14-27.

Evarts EV (1981) Role of Motor Cortex in Voluntary Movements in Primates. In: *Handbook of Physiology* (Brooks VB, ed), pp 1083-1120. Baltimore: Williams and Wilkins.

Feldman AG, Levin MF (1995) The Origin and Use of Positional Frames of Reference in Motor Control. *Behav Brain Sci* 18: 723-744.

Fetz EE (1992) Are Movement Parameters Recognizably Coded in the Activity of Single Neurons? *Behav Brain Sci* 15: 679-690.

Fetz EE, Cheney PD (1980) Postspike Facilitation of Forelimb Muscle Activity by Primate Corticomotoneuronal Cells. *J Neurophysiol* 44: 751-772.

Fetz EE, Cheney PD, Mewes K, Palmer S (1989) Control of Forelimb Muscle Activity by Populations of Corticomotoneuronal and Rubromotoneuronal Cells, Chap. 36. *Prog Brain Res* 80: 437-449.

Fu QG, Flament D, Coltz JD, Ebner TJ (1995) Temporal Encoding of Movement Kinematics in the Discharge of Primate Primary Motor and Premotor Neurons. *J Neurophysiol* 73: 836-854.

Gao Y, Bienenstock E, Black M, Shoham S, Serruya M, Donoghue J (2001) Encoding/Decoding of Arm Kinematics From Simultaneously Recorded MI Neurons. *Soc Neurosci Abstr* 63.3.

Georgopoulos AP, Ashe J (2000) One Motor Cortex, Two Different Views. *Nat Neurosci* 3: 963-965.

Georgopoulos AP, Ashe J, Smyrnis N, Taira M (1992) The Motor Cortex and the Coding of Force. *Science* 256: 1692-1695.

Georgopoulos AP, Caminiti R, Kalaska JF (1984) Static Spatial Effects in Motor Cortex and Area 5: Quantitative Relations in a Two-Dimensional Space. *Exp Brain Res* 54: 446-454.

Georgopoulos AP, Caminiti R, Kalaska JF, Massey JT (1983) Spatial Coding of Movement: A Hypothesis Concerning the Coding of Movement Direction by Motor Cortical Populations. *Exp Brain Res Suppl* 7: 327-336.

Georgopoulos AP, Kalaska JF, Caminiti R, Massey JT (1982) On the Relations Between the Direction of Two-Dimensional Arm Movements and Cell Discharge in Primate Motor Cortex. *J Neurosci* 2: 1527-1537.

Ghez C, Sainburg R (1995) Proprioceptive Control of Interjoint Coordination. *Can J Physiol Pharmacol* 73: 273-284.

Gribble PL, Ostry DJ (2000) Compensation for Loads During Arm Movements Using Equilibrium-Point Control. *Exp Brain Res* 135: 474-482.

Harris CM, Wolpert DM (1998) Signal-Dependent Noise Determines Motor Planning. *Nature* 394: 780-784.

Helms Tillery SI, Lin WS, Schwartz AB (2001) Training Non-human Primates to Use a Neuroprosthetic Device. *Soc Neurosci Abstr* 63.4.

Herrmann U, Flanders M (1998) Directional Tuning of Single Motor Units. *J Neurosci* 18: 8402-8416.

Hoffman DS, Strick PL (1999) Step-Tracking Movements of the Wrist: IV. Muscle Activity Associated With Movements in Different Directions. *J Neurophysiol* 81: 319-333.

Holdefer R, Miller LE (2002) Primary Motor Cortical Neurons Encode Functional Muscle Synergies. *Exp Brain Res.* 146(2): 233-243.

Hubel DH, Wiesel TN (1962) Receptive Fields, Binocular Interaction and Functional Architecture in the Cat's Visual Cortex. *J Physiol (Lond)* 160: 106-154.

Humphrey DR, Reed DJ (1983) Separate Cortical Systems for Control of Joint Movement and Joint Stiffness: Reciprocal Activation and Coactivation of Antagonist Muscles. In: *Advances in Neurology: Motor Control Mechanisms in Health and Disease* (Desmedt JE, ed), pp 347-372. New York: Raven Press.

Johnson PB (1992) Toward an Understanding of the Cerebral Cortex and Reaching Movements: A Review of Recent Approaches. In: *Control of Arm Movement in Space: Neurophysiological and Computational Approaches* (Caminiti R, Johnson PB, Burnod Y, eds). Berlin: Springer-Verlag.

Joyce GC, Rack PMH, Westbury DR (1969) The Mechanical Properties of Cat Soleus Muscle During Controlled Lengthening and Shortening Movements. *J Physiol (Lond)* 204: 461-474.

Kakei S, Hoffman D, Strick P (1999) Muscle and Movement Representations in the Primary Motor Cortex. *Science* 285: 2136-2139.

Kakei S, Hoffman DS, Strick PL (2001) Direction of Action Is Represented in the Ventral Premotor Cortex. *Nat Neurosci* 4: 1020-1025.

Kalaska JF, Cohen DAD, Hyde ML, Prud'homme M (1989) A Comparison of Movement Direction–Related Versus Load Direction–Related Activity in Primate Motor Cortex, Using a Two-Dimensional Reaching Task. *J Neurosci* 9: 2080-2102.

Kalaska JF, Crammond DJ (1992) Cerebral Cortical Mechanisms of Reaching Movements. *Science* 255: 1517-1523.

Kalaska JF, Crammond DJ, Cohen DAD, Prud'homme M, Hyde ML (1992) Comparison of Cell Discharge in Motor, Premotor, and Parietal Cortex During Reaching. In: *Control of Arm Movement in Space: Neurophysiological and Computational Approaches* (Caminiti R, Johnson PB, Burnod Y, eds). Berlin: Springer-Verlag.

Kettner RE, Schwartz AB, Georgopoulos AP (1988) Primate Motor Cortex and Free Arm Movements to Visual Targets in Three-Dimensional Space: III. Positional Gradients and Population Coding of Movement Direction From Various Movement Origins. *J Neurosci* 8: 2938-2947.

Kilner JM, Baker SN, Salenius S, Hari R, Lemon RN (2000) Human Cortical Muscle Coherence Is Directly Related to Specific Motor Parameters. *J Neurosci* 20: 8838-8845.

Lemon RN, Mantel GW, Muir RB (1986) Corticospinal Facilitation of Hand Muscles During Voluntary Movement in the Conscious Monkey. *J Physiol* 381: 497-527.

Li CS, Padoa-Schioppa C, Bizzi E (2001) Neuronal Correlates of Motor Performance and Motor Learning in the Primary Motor Cortex of Monkeys Adapting to an External Force Field. *Neuron* 30: 593-607.

Loeb G (1999) What Might the Brain Know About Muscles, Limbs and Spinal Circuits? In: *Progress in Brain Research 123: Peripheral and Spinal Mechanisms in the Neural Control of Movement* (Binder MD, ed), pp 405-409. Amsterdam: Elsevier.

Loeb GE (2000) Overcomplete Musculature or Underspecified Tasks? *Motor Control* 4: 81-83.

McAuley JH, Rothwell JC, Marsden CD (1997) Frequency Peaks of Tremor, Muscle Vibration and Electromyographic Activity at 10 Hz, 20 Hz and 40 Hz During Human Finger Muscle Contraction May Reflect Rhythmicities of Central Neural Firing. *Exp Brain Res* 114: 525-541.

McIntyre J, Bizzi E (1993) Servo Hypotheses for the Biological Control of Movement. *J Mot Behav* 25: 193-202.

McKiernan BJ, Marcario JK, Karrer JH, Cheney PD (1998) Corticomotoneuronal Postspike Effects in Shoulder, Elbow, Wrist, Digit, and Intrinsic Hand Muscles During a Reach and Prehension Task. *J Neurophysiol* 80: 1961-1980.

McKiernan BJ, Marcario JK, Karrer JH, Cheney PD (2000) Correlations Between Corticomotoneuronal (CM) Cell Postspike Effects and Cell-Target Muscle Covariation. *J Neurophysiol* 83: 99-115.

Miller LE, Sinkjaer T (1998) Primate Red Nucleus Discharge Encodes the Dynamics of Limb Muscle Activity. *J Neurophysiol* 80: 59-70.

Moran DW, Schwartz AB (1999a) Motor Cortical Activity During Drawing Movements: Population Representation During Spiral Tracing. *J Neurophysiol* 82: 2693-2704.

Moran DW, Schwartz AB (1999b) Motor Cortical Representation of Speed and Direction During Reaching. *J Neurophysiol* 82: 2676.

Moran DW, Schwartz AB (2000) One Motor Cortex, Two Different Views. *Nat Neurosci* 3: 963-965.

Mussa-Ivaldi FA (1988) Do Neurons in the Motor Cortex Encode Movement Direction? An Alternative Hypothesis. *Neurosci Lett* 91: 106-111.

Nicols TR, Houk JC (1976) Improvement in Linearity and Regulations of Stiffness That Result From Actions of Stretch Reflex. *J Neurophysiol* 39: 119-142.

Nudo RJ, Milliken GW, Jenkins WM, Merzenich MM (1996) Use-Dependent Alterations of Movement Representations in Primary Motor Cortex of Adult Squirrel Monkeys. *J Neurosci* 16: 785-807.

Olshausen BA, Field DJ (1996) Emergence of Simple-Cell Receptive Field Properties by Learning a Sparse Code for Natural Images. *Nature* 381: 607-609.

Poliakov AV, Schieber MH (1999) Limited Functional Grouping of Neurons in the Motor Cortex Hand Area During Individuated Finger Movements: A Cluster Analysis. *J Neurophysiol* 82: 3488-3505.

Schieber MH (2001) Constraints on Somatotopic Organization in the Primary Motor Cortex. *J Neurophysiol* 86: 2125-2143.

Schieber, MH (2002) Controlling the Hand: A Complex Journey From Motor Cortex to Finger Movements. In: *Peripheral and Spinal Mechanisms in the Neural Control of Movement* (Binder MD, ed). Oxford: Elsevier.

Schmidt RA, Zelaznik H, Hawkins B, Frank JS, Quinn JT Jr (1979) Motor-Output Variability: A Theory for the Accuracy of Rapid Motor Acts. *Psychol Rev* 86: 415-451.

Schwartz AB (1994) Direct Cortical Representation of Drawing. *Science* 265: 540-542.

Scott SH (1997) Comparison of Onset Time and Magnitude of Activity for Proximal Arm Muscles and Motor Cortical Cells Before Reaching Movements. *J Neurophysiol* 77: 1016-1022.

Scott SH, Gribble PL, Graham KM, Cabel DW (2001) Dissociation Between Hand Motion and Population Vectors From Neural Activity in Motor Cortex. *Nature* 413: 161-165.

Scott S, Kalaska J (1995) Changes in Motor Cortex Activity During Reaching Movements With Similar Hand Paths but Different Arm Postures. *J Neurophysiol* 73: 2563-2567.

Scott S, Kalaska J (1997) Reaching Movements With Similar Hand Paths but Different Arm Orientation: I. Activity of Individual Cells in Motor Cortex. *J Neurophysiol* 77: 826-852.

Sergio LE, Kalaska JF (1998) Changes in the Temporal Pattern of Primary Motor Cortex Activity in a Directional Isometric Force Versus Limb Movement Task. *J Neurophysiol* 80: 1577-1583.

Stephens JA, Harrison LM, Mayston MJ, Carr LJ, Gibbs J (1999) The Sharing Principle. In: *Peripheral and Spinal Mechanisms in the Neural Control of Movement* (Binder MD, ed). Oxford: Elsevier.

Sutton GG, Sykes K (1967) The Variation of Hand Tremor With Force in Healthy Subjects. *J Physiol* 191(3): 699-711.

Taira M, Boline J, Smyrnis N, Georgopoulos A, Ashe J (1996) On the Relations Between Single Cell Activity in the Motor Cortex and the Direction and Magnitude of Three-Dimensional Static Isometric Force. *Exp Brain Res* 109: 367-376.

Todorov E (2000a) Direct Cortical Control of Muscle Activation in Voluntary Arm Movements: A Model. *Nat Neurosci* 3: 391-398.

Todorov E (2000b) Reply to "One Motor Cortex, Two Different Views." *Nat Neurosci* 3: 963-964.

Todorov E (2002) Cosine Tuning Minimizes Motor Errors. *Neural Comput* 14: 1233-1260.

Todorov E, Ghahramani Z (2003) Unsupervised learning of sensory-motor primitives. In Proceedings of the 25th IEEE International Conference on Engineering in Medicine and Biology.

Todorov E, Jordan M (2002) Optimal Feedback Control as a Theory of Motor Coordination. *Nat Neurosci* 5(11): 1226-1235.

Todorov E, Li R, Gandolfo F, Benda B, DiLorenzo D, Padoa-Schioppa C, Bizzi E (2000) Cosine Tuning Minimizes Motor Errors: Theoretical Results and Experimental Confirmation. *Soc Neurosci Abstr* 785.6.

Tsuji T, Morasso PG, Goto K, Ito K (1995) Human Hand Impedance Characteristics During Maintained Posture. *Biol Cybern* 72: 475-485.

Turner RS, Owens J, Anderson ME (1995) Directional Variation of Spatial and Temporal Characteristics of Limb Movements Made by Monkeys in a Two-Dimensional Work Space. *J Neurophysiol* 74: 684-697.

Wessberg J, Stambaugh CR, Kralik JD, Beck PD, Laubach M, Chapin JK, Kim J, Biggs SJ, Srinivasan MA, Nicolelis MA (2000) Real-Time Prediction of Hand Trajectory by Ensembles of Cortical Neurons in Primates. *Nature* 408: 361-365.

Zajac FE (1989) Muscle and Tendon: Properties, Models, Scaling, and Application to Biomechanics and Motor Control. *Crit Rev Biomed Eng* 17: 359-411.

# Changes
# in Motor Control
# With Age
# or Neurological
# Disorder

# 7

# Postural Responses Triggered by Surface Perturbations Are Task Specific and Goal Directed

*Joyce Fung, Rumpa Boonsinsukh, and Margherita Rapagna*

McGill University and Jewish Rehabilitation Hospital
Montreal and Laval, Quebec

Automatic postural responses are triggered by unexpected surface perturbations to maintain equilibrium during both static and dynamic tasks. However, it remains unclear how the responses are organized with respect to task goals and postural constraints in the maintenance of static or dynamic equilibrium. The purpose of this study is to compare and contrast kinematic responses triggered by unexpected, multidirectional surface tilts during quiet stance and walking. Subjects were exposed to different axial combinations of pitch and roll surface perturbations during the double-limb support phase of walking and comparable posture in quiet stance.

Results showed that the kinematic responses were, in general, much larger in standing than in walking. During standing, kinematic adjustments were made in a distal-to-proximal progression through the ankle, knee, and hip joints, with trunk motions interspersed. The trunk and pelvis moved in the same direction in response to pitch surface perturbations, whereas they moved in opposite directions during roll surface perturbations. Minimal kinematic responses were triggered by the same surface perturbations during walking, except for the ankle joint in the front limb, which increased dorsiflexion or plantarflexion to adapt to the surface inclination. These responses were associated with the displacement of the body center of mass (CM) during surface perturbations. Kinematic responses are thus organized differently, depending on the task and the maintenance of the body CM with respect to the base of support. The equilibrium demands seem to be much higher during quiet stance than during walking.

Two important behavioral goals that need to be accomplished in the control of posture are the maintenance of postural orientation and equilibrium (Horak and Macpherson, 1996). Postural orientation is the alignment or relative positioning of the body segments with respect to each other and with respect to the environment, whereas postural equilibrium is the state in which all the forces acting on all the joints are balanced in such a way that the body remains in the desired position and orientation (static equilibrium) or moves in a controlled fashion (dynamic equilibrium). The body CM is the point at which the entire mass of the body is balanced and on which the resultant of the external forces acts. Unexpected displacements of a support surface trigger automatic postural responses that aim to maintain equilibrium during both static and dynamic tasks.

Although the circuitry for generating the rhythmic pattern of locomotion is organized in the spinal cord (see the review by Rossignol, 2000), recent studies suggest that the control of balance is much more complex and that the postural responses that are triggered require multiple levels of control in the neuraxis of the central nervous system (CNS), especially supraspinal circuitries (Fung and Macpherson, 1999; Macpherson and Fung, 1999). Apart from rhythmic pattern generation, postural equilibrium has to be maintained during propulsion, and the CNS must be able to adapt the locomotor pattern to the environment and to the needs and goals of the animal. Different variables of postural orientation and equilibrium are controlled simultaneously during locomotion, including trunk orientation and position of the CM. Although the CM is rarely within the base of support during locomotion, its trajectory is controlled to maintain dynamic equilibrium (Jian et al., 1993). The trunk oscillates no more than 2° in the sagittal plane through the active control of hip musculature (Thorstensson et al., 1984), whereas stabilization of the trunk in the frontal plane is achieved primarily through foot placement and action of the axial musculature (Winter et al., 1993). More recent research showed that, in quiet stance with feet together, balance in the sagittal plane is achieved mainly by the control of ankle torque, whereas balance in the frontal plane is controlled predominantly by changing hip torque (Winter et al., 1996). New findings on multidirectional surface translations in humans show similar control mechanisms with complex central and peripheral organization of the postural responses (Henry et al., 1998a, 1998b). However, it remains unclear how these responses are organized with respect to task goals and postural constraints in the maintenance of dynamic equilibrium. The present study was undertaken to characterize the kinematic responses triggered by unexpected, multidirectional surface tilts during quiet stance and walking in healthy subjects.

## Methods

A total of seven healthy subjects between 20 and 70 years of age (three male, four female) participated in the study. None of the subjects had any history of neurological or musculoskeletal disorders affecting balance. Subjects were instructed to stand on or walk over a movable platform powered by electrohydraulic actuators (Fung and Johnstone, 1998). Eight different axial combinations of pitch and roll plane surface tilts (ramp amplitude 10°, peak velocity 53°/s) and catch trials with no surface perturbations were randomly presented to each subject during the double-limb support phase of walking and during quiet stance in a step stance posture to mimic double-limb support (see table 7.1 and figure 7.1).

Three-dimensional body kinematics were captured at 120 Hz by a six-camera Vicon 512 system. Reflective markers were affixed to 23 anatomical landmarks, and anthropometric measures were taken from each subject. Ground reaction forces were acquired at 1080 Hz by two AMTI force plates mounted within the movable platform in the middle of a 10-m walkway.

Four standing and four walking trials in each direction of surface perturbation were analyzed. Four parameters of interest were calculated after perturbation onset (figure 7.1): (1) center of pressure (CP); (2) CM; (3) bilateral angular displacements of the hip, knee, and ankle; and (4) displacement of the trunk and pelvis segments.

## Results and Discussion

Figure 7.2 shows segmental and joint angular traces in the sagittal plane from one representative subject in response to combinations of toes-up and toes-down perturbations during standing. In general, the kinematic strategies used during pitch perturbations (toes-up and toes-down tilts) involve increased sagittal movement of the trunk (6°) and pelvis (6°) opposite to the direction of the surface tilt, that

**Table 7.1 Testing Conditions and Total Number of Testing Trials**

| Task | Directions | Tests | Total trials |
|------|-----------|-------|--------------|
| Standing | Surface rotations through 8 directions in the pitch and roll planes | 8 tilts, 8 no tilts | 16 × 4 blocks = 64 |
| Walking | | 8 tilts, 8 no tilts | 16 × 4 blocks = 64 |

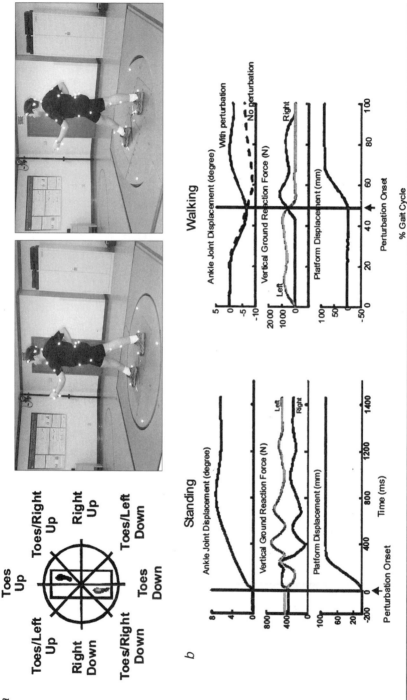

**Figure 7.1** (*a*) Eight directions of surface perturbation were introduced during semitandem stance posture and double support phase of walking with the right foot in front of the left foot. (*b*) Examples of platform and ankle joint trajectories and ground reaction forces in standing and walking during toes-up tilt.

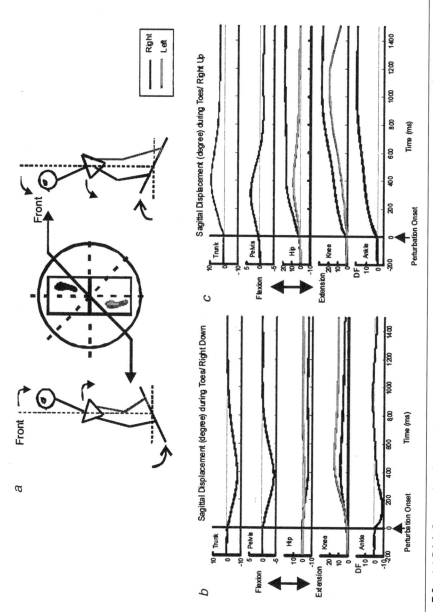

**Figure 7.2** (*a*) Stick figures showing the kinematic strategies used during combinations of pitch and roll plane tilts. (*b*) Trajectories of trunk and pelvic segmental angles and hip, knee, and ankle joint angles in the sagittal plane from one representative subject during toes-down/right-down tilt and (*c*) toes-up/right-up tilt.

173

is, forward bending when the surface tilts up and vice versa. The lower-limb joint angular adjustments during toes-up rotation of the support surface in standing consisted of dorsiflexion of both ankles (8°), increased knee flexion in the front stance limb (16°) as compared with the rear (3°), and flexion of the front (13°) and rear (8°) hip. Similar kinematic adjustments were found in other directions during perturbations with an upward pitch component (i.e., toes-up/right-up and toes-up/left-up perturbations). During toes-down rotation of the support surface, the postural responses included plantarflexion of both ankles (6°), increased knee flexion in the rear stance limb (16°) as compared with the front (3°), and bilateral hip extension (7°). Similar adjustments were observed for surface perturbations in other pitch directions (toes-down/right-up and toes-down/left-up). In contrast, during roll surface perturbations, the trunk and pelvic segments displaced more in the frontal plane and in opposite directions, while more flexion occurred on the stance limb that was tilted up (figure 7.3). The main distinguishing feature between pitch and roll rotations was that the pelvis moved in the same direction as the surface and opposite to the trunk during roll perturbations, whereas both trunk and pelvis moved opposite to the surface during pitch perturbations.

Despite differences in postural responses to perturbations in the pitch and roll planes, the kinematic strategy is organized by the same principle with respect to the direction of trunk movement to restore balance when quiet stance is perturbed. This strategy involves moving the trunk opposite to the surface and flexing the knee of the stance limb that is tilted upward by the perturbation. It has been suggested that the movement of the knee is aimed to displace the body CM, mainly in the vertical direction (Ko et al., 2001). Thus, this strategy may be used to counteract the undesirable movement of the body CM due to surface tilts. For example, to prevent the CM from being displaced upward and backward during a toes-up surface tilt, knee flexion quickly lowers the CM, and transferring weight onto the front stance limb displaces it forward. Trunk movements opposite to the surface perturbations also assist in rapidly correcting the CM and preventing it from being displaced outside the base of support. It can be seen that trunk verticality is not the primary control variable in response to surface tilts. The movement of the trunk is also a part of the hip strategy during surface translation (Horak and Nashner, 1986). Such trunk motion in the hip strategy is suggested to be more effective for counteracting large disturbances (Kuo and Zajac, 1993).

Figure 7.4 shows the onset latency of joint and segment movements from one representative subject during the same four axes of surface rotations presented in figures 7.2 and 7.3. There was a distal to proximal sequencing of joint excursion changes (from ankle to hip), with the onset of trunk displacement occurring between knee and hip movements. This pattern of coordination is similar to the response obtained from surface translations (Henry et al., 1998a).

Figure 7.5 shows the average excursions of the trunk, pelvis, and front stance limb joint angles of all seven subjects during standing and contrasts the same kinematic outcomes during walking after perturbed profiles were subtracted from the average unperturbed profile normalized to the gait cycle. The kinematic responses were much

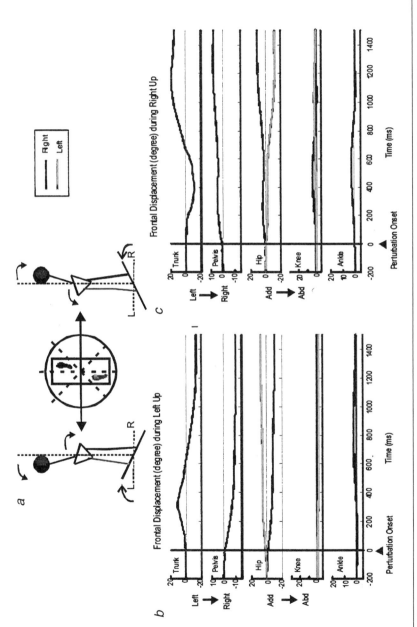

**Figure 7.3a-c** (a) Stick figures showing the kinematic strategies used during left-up (or right-down) and right-up tilts. (b) Trajectories of trunk and pelvic segmental angles and hip, knee, and ankle joint angles in the frontal plane tilt from one representative subject during left-up tilt and (c) right-up tilt.

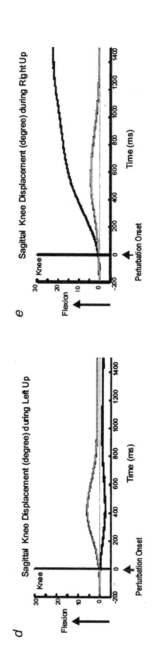

**Figure 7.3d-e** *(d)* Trajectories of the knee joint angles in the sagittal plane during left-up tilt and *(e)* right-up tilt from the same subject show more knee flexion on the side of the surface that was tilted up.

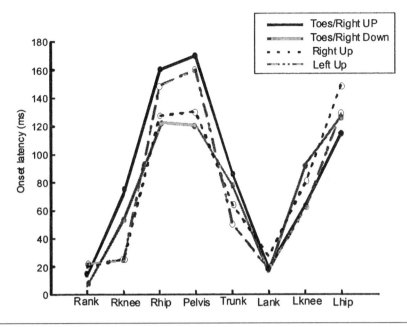

**Figure 7.4**  Onset latency of bilateral lower-limb joints and trunk and pelvic movements from one representative subject during four different combinations of surface tilts.

smaller when surface perturbations occurred during walking than during standing. Minimal kinematic responses (< 1°) were triggered by surface perturbations during walking, except for the ankle joint in the front stance limb, which increased dorsiflexion or plantar flexion (~6°) to adapt to the final surface inclination. This finding is in accordance with the study of automatic postural adjustments during surface translation by Tang et al. (1998). They found that the distal muscles (i.e., leg and thigh muscles) of the stance limb participated in balance corrections during distally perturbed gait at heel strike, whereas the proximal muscles (i.e., hip and trunk muscles) did not contribute significantly to balance corrections. Tang et al. (1998) indicated that activities from the leg and thigh muscles were the principal elements for regaining balance after surface perturbations during walking. Thus, it can be seen that balance correction to surface perturbation during walking can be adequately accomplished by adjustments of distal limb segments without adjustments from the proximal limb and trunk segments. In contrast, during standing, both proximal and distal segments are involved in the postural corrections to surface perturbations. Thus, the equilibrium demand seems to be much higher during quiet standing than during forward locomotion, since the task goals are different. Locomotion itself creates a perturbation of the CM, as each stepping motion leads to moving and projecting the CM outside the base of support. In contrast, the CM must be controlled to stay within the base of support during perturbation in quiet standing.

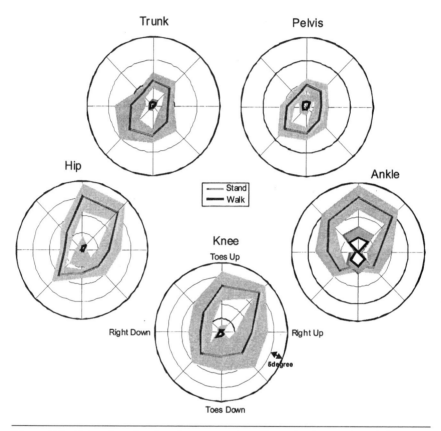

**Figure 7.5**   Polar plots showing the average ($n = 7$) maximal excursion of the trunk, pelvis, hip, knee, and ankle in standing and walking during all eight directions of surface tilt. The gray zone represents ±1 SD, and the distance between each concentric ring is 5° of movement.

Figure 7.6a shows an individual example of the CP and CM trajectories in the anteroposterior (AP) and mediolateral (ML) directions during perturbations in standing. Figure 7.6b shows polar plots of the average CP and CM changes from all seven subjects in both the AP and ML directions across all eight perturbation axes. In general, the CP excursions encompassed the CM excursions, and the magnitude of change was largest for the AP response to pitch perturbation. Figure 7.7a shows the CP and CM trajectories of one representative subject during walking with and without surface perturbations. Figure 7.7b shows polar plots of the average CP and CM changes in all seven subjects after subtracting the normal walking displacements. In general, CP and CM displacements were much smaller in walking and they were modulated with the maximal excursions which were limited to the plane of forward progression (the pitch directions, toes-up or toes-down tilts). These changes paralleled the observed kinematic adjustments in which the

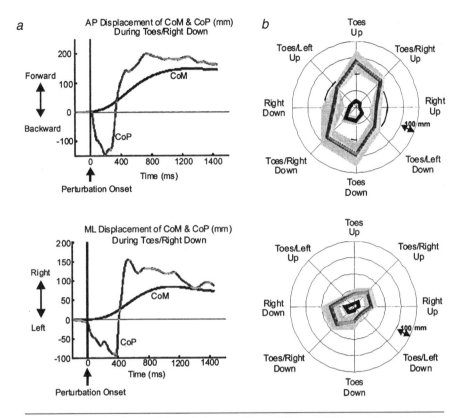

**Figure 7.6** *(a)* Sagittal and frontal plane profiles of CM and CP in standing during the maximal-excursion tilt direction (toes-down/right-down tilt) from one representative subject. *(b)* Polar plots showing the average (*n* = 7) peak excursions of the CM and CP in standing during all eight directions of surface tilt. The distance between each concentric ring equals 100 mm, and the gray zone is ±1 SD.

maximal adjustments were seen at the ankle joint during toes-up and toes-down tilts. During standing, maximal excursions of the CP or the CM were found in the diagonal plane during toes-down/right-down and toes-up/right-up tilts. This constraint may be related to the step stance posture (with right foot leading) to maintain the same safety margin of the CP or CM throughout. In contrast, during walking, the safety margin is limited by the location of the leading foot (front limb) during forward progression, thus constraining the excursion of the CP or CM in the sagittal plane (toes-up and toes-down tilts). Forward progression, as revealed by CM velocity, was not affected by most perturbations except those that involved toes-up tilts. Forward progression velocity during combinations of toes-up tilts was slower (by about 30%) than walking with no perturbations. This result is in accordance with our previous findings that characteristics of ground reaction force manifested a delayed and increased load acceptance to counteract sudden toes-up

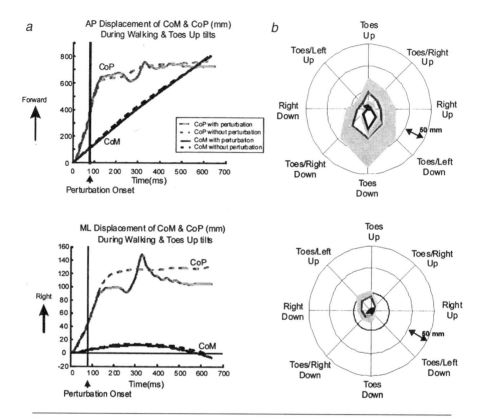

**Figure 7.7** *(a)* Sagittal and frontal plane profiles of CM and CP in walking during the maximal-excursion tilt direction (toes-up tilt) and during no surface perturbation from one representative subject. *(b)* Polar plots showing the average (*n* = 7) maximal excursion of the CM and CP in walking during all eight directions of surface tilt. The distance between each concentric ring equals 50 mm, and the gray zone is ±1 SD.

tilts during walking (Fung et al., 2000). Taken together, the findings indicate that the prime goal is to maintain walking velocity during surface perturbations unless the dynamics of the perturbation itself, such as a pure toes-up surface tilt, opposes forward progression of the body CM.

## Conclusions

Unexpected rotation of a support surface during quiet standing triggers similar kinematic strategies, regardless of the direction of rotation. The strategy involves trunk movement opposite to the direction of surface rotation and some flexion of the knee. Knee flexion movements are always larger on the side that is tilted up. In terms of latency, the movement onsets progress from distal to proximal, from the ankle and knee to the hip, with trunk movement interposed between knee and hip motions.

Maximal excursions of the CP or CM are found during surface tilts in the toes-down/right-down and toes-up/right-up directions. This constraint may be related to the step stance posture (with right foot forward) to maintain the same safety margin of the CP or CM throughout.

Minimal kinematic adjustments are triggered by surface perturbations during walking, except for the ankle joint in the front limb, which adapts to the surface inclination. This suggests that postural responses are task-dependent and the equilibrium demand is much higher when surface perturbation occurs during forward locomotion, since the task goals are different.

# References

Fung, J., and Johnstone, E. (1998) Lost in space: Multi-axial and multi-dimensional surface perturbations delivered by a novel motion base device. *Soc Neurosci Abstr* 24: 455.410.

Fung, J., and Macpherson, J.M. (1999) Attributes of quiet stance in the chronic spinal cat. *J Neurophysiol* 82: 3056-3065.

Fung, J., Rapagna, M., Boonsinsukh, R., and Galiana, L. (2000) Effects of multi-axial surface perturbations on posture and gait. *Soc Neurosci Abstr* 26: 785.10.

Henry, S.M., Fung, J., and Horak, F.B. (1998a) Control of stance during lateral and anterior/posterior surface translations. *IEEE Trans Rehabil Eng* 6: 32-42.

Henry, S.M., Fung, J., and Horak, F.B. (1998b) EMG responses to maintain stance during multidirectional surface translations. *J Neurophysiol* 80: 1939-1950.

Horak, F.B., and Macpherson, J.M. (1996) Postural orientation and equilibrium. In Shepard, J., and Rowell, L. (Eds.), *Integration of motor, circulatory, respiratory and metabolic control during exercise*, pp. 255-292. New York: Oxford University Press.

Horak, F.B., and Nashner, L.M. (1986) Central programming of postural movements: Adaptation to altered support-surface configurations. *J Neurophysiol* 55: 1369-1381.

Jian, Y., Winter, D.A., Ishac, M.G., and Gilchrist, L. (1993) Trajectory of the body COG and COP during initiation and termination of gait. *Gait Posture* 1: 9-22.

Ko, Y., Challis, J.H., and Newell, K.M. (2001) Postural coordination patterns as a function of dynamics of support surface. *Hum Mov Sci* 20: 737-764.

Kuo, A.D., and Zajac, F.E. (1993) Human standing posture: Multi-joint movement strategies based on biomechanical constraints. *Prog Brain Res* 97: 349-358.

Macpherson, J.M., and Fung, J. (1999) Weight support and balance during perturbed stance in the chronic spinal cat. *J Neurophysiol* 82: 3066-3081.

Rossignol, S. (2000) Locomotion and its recovery after spinal injury. *Curr Opin Neurobiol* 10: 708-716.

Tang, P., Woollacott, M., and Chong, R.K.Y. (1998) Control of reactive balance adjustments in perturbed human walking: Roles of proximal and distal postural muscle activity. *Exp Brain Res* 119: 141-152.

Thorstensson, J., Nilsson, J., Carlson, H., and Zomlefer, M.R. (1984) Trunk movement in human locomotion. *Acta Physiol Scand* 121: 9-22.

Winter, D.A., MacKinnon, C.D., Ruder, G.K., and Wieman, C. (1993) An integrated EMG/biomechanical model of upper body balance and posture during human gait. *Prog Brain Res* 97: 359-367.

Winter, D.A., Prince, F., Frank, J.S., Powell, C., and Zabjek, K.F. (1996) Unified theory regarding A/P and M/L balance in quiet stance. *J Neurophysiol* 75: 2334-2343.

# 8

# Balance Control and Protective Arm and Trunk Movements in the Elderly: Implications for Fall Prevention

*John H.J. Allum*
University Hospital, Basel

*Mark G. Carpenter*
University Hospital, Basel,
and University of Waterloo

*Bastiaan R. Bloem*
University of Nijmegen

The pathophysiology underlying age-related falls and injuries remains incompletely understood. We used unpredictable, multidirectional balance perturbations to provide information on how the central nervous system (CNS) corrects falls in different directions. For this purpose, we perturbed the stance of healthy subjects divided equally into three age groups: young (20-34 years), middle-aged (35-55 years), and elderly (60-75 years). Outcome measures included electromyographic (EMG) and biomechanical responses.

We observed three types of age-related changes in balance corrections. First, amplitudes of balance-correcting responses (over 120-220 ms) in the ankle muscles were smaller in the elderly than in the young for all perturbation directions. This reduced early activity was compensated by increased lower-leg activity after 240 ms in the elderly. These EMG changes were paralleled by comparable differences in ankle torque responses. Second, stimulus-induced trunk roll, but not trunk pitch, changed dramatically with age. Young subjects responded with early and large roll movements of the trunk in the opposite direction to platform roll. The elderly had very little initial trunk roll modulation and balance-correcting responses in hip and trunk muscles were reduced in amplitude. Following the onset of balance corrections, trunk roll was in the same direction as support-surface motion for all groups but resulted in overall trunk roll toward the fall side in the elderly but not in the young. Finally, protective arm movements changed with age. Arm roll movements were largest in the young, smaller in the middle-aged, and smallest in the elderly. Initial arm roll movements were in the same direction as initial trunk motion in the young and middle-aged but in the opposite direction in the elderly.

We conclude that decreased trunk roll flexibility is a key biomechanical change with age. This interferes with early compensatory trunk movements, leads to trunk displacements in the direction of the impending fall, and may contribute to the genesis of hip fractures. The uniform delay and amplitude reduction of balance-correcting responses that we observed across many segments (legs, hips, and arms) suggests a neurally based alteration in processing times and response modulation with age. These results help explain the mechanisms underlying fall-related injuries in the elderly and offer possible approaches for their prevention.

Aging can influence balance corrections in many ways and lead to falls. Indeed, recurrent falls and fall-related injuries are common among elderly persons, and this is an important determinant of a reduced quality of life. Better insight into the complex and multifactorial pathophysiology underlying falls in the elderly is required to reduce the incidence of falls and, even if falls cannot be prevented entirely, to minimize the associated injuries.

Many investigators have used posturography (quantified assessment of balance control, with either a fixed or moving force plate) to elucidate the mechanisms associated with falls in the elderly. Although assessment of quiet stance can show clear changes in elderly persons (e.g., an increase in trunk sway; see Brocklehurst et al., 1982; Gill et al., 2001; Lord et al., 1991), many researchers feel that postural control is best probed using perturbations of upright stance (Furman et al., 1993). The majority of these dynamic posturography studies used controlled postural perturbations in a single direction, usually the anterior-posterior plane. The results of these studies revealed a host of postural changes in elderly subjects, including an increase in induced sway (Stelmach, Phillips, et al., 1989; Stelmach, Teasdale, et al., 1989), delayed onsets and amplitude changes in automatic postural responses in ankle muscles (Maki, 1993), delayed and slightly weaker torques about the ankle joint (Keshner et al., 1993; Rivner et al., 2001; Shepard et al., 1993), abnormal compensatory stepping reactions (Maki and McIlroy, 1998), a narrowing of the limits of stability (Murray et al., 1975), and impaired habituation across serial trials (Stelmach, Teasdale, et al., 1989).

Despite these advances, various questions remain unanswered, particularly about lateral sway control. First, posturography studies in the anterior-posterior plane may have revealed statistical differences between populations of young and elderly persons, or between elderly fallers and nonfallers, but the evidence that such changes can be used to identify individuals at risk of falls is much less convincing. Indeed, age-related changes in automatic postural responses of ankle muscles were generally modest (Stelmach, Teasdale, et al., 1989; Woollacott, 1986), and it has been disputed whether these small changes in the pitch plane are sufficient to produce instability and possibly cause a fall (Alexander et al., 1992). The associations between posturography findings and faller status were often weak or even absent in most studies (Baloh et al., 1995, 1998; Bartlett et al., 1986; Brocklehurst et al., 1982; Campbell et al., 1989; Fernie et al., 1982; Fife and Baloh, 1993; Imms and Endhold, 1981; Lichtenstein et al., 1988, 1990; Maki et al., 1990, 1991; Overstall et al., 1977). Analysis of spontaneous or induced sway in the mediolateral plane appears to correlate better with faller status than anteroposterior sway (Lord et al., 1999; Maki et al., 1994; Williams et al., 1997), yet reliable predictors of falls remain to be identified. Some investigators failed to find a relationship between mediolateral sway and falls in daily life (Baloh et al., 1995, 1998). Second, the pathophysiology underlying postural changes in the elderly for the lateral (roll) plane is still largely unclear. One significant complicating factor is the ability of the nervous system to effectively adjust its motor programs to accommodate some age-related changes and thus mask possible abnormalities. This compensation is facilitated when the postural perturbations become predictable through repetition of identical stimuli, as was the case in many previous studies. Finally, some puzzling clinical observations still require explanation. For example, it remains unclear why the incidence of hip fractures increases exponentially with age, whereas the incidence of wrist fractures appears to level off or even decrease with age (Melton et al., 1988). Such phenomena are possibly explained by changes in postural strategies, but just how this occurs remains to be clarified.

Some answers to these questions may be provided by modified posturography protocols. First, because falls in daily life are typically unpredictable and can occur in any possible direction, better insights might be expected from the use of randomly mixed perturbations in multiple directions. An advantage of such an experimental setting is that stimulus predictability is reduced, compared with the serial use of identical perturbations in a single plane. The imposed stimulus directions should include a roll component, because laterally directed falls are common in daily life (Maki et al., 1994, 1996; O'Neill et al., 1994). Moreover, lateral falls are associated with the genesis of hip fractures (Greenspan et al., 1994). Unpredictable perturbations in lateral directions also require more complex coordination of muscle responses in the left and right sides of the body (Carpenter et al., 1999). For example, when the support surface tilts, the "downhill" leg must extend and the "uphill" leg must flex to regain upright stance. The CNS must additionally coordinate pitch and roll motion of the trunk (Carpenter et al., 2001). Inclusion of pitch stimuli is also relevant because forward falls occur in daily life as well, for example, during ambulation (Nevitt and Cummings, 1993). Backward falls are apparently more common than forward falls, possibly because the limits of stability are relatively narrow in this direction or because vision is less helpful to prevent a backward fall. Combinations of all these different fall directions offer an opportunity to examine a more complete spectrum of fall types and can also provide insight into the possibility of a directional preponderance for falls in daily life. Indeed, earlier experiments suggested that use of multidirectional perturbations may reveal postural abnormalities that would have been missed using perturbations restricted to a single plane (Carpenter et al., 1999; Maki et al., 1996).

A second improvement would be to expand the analysis of postural responses beyond the traditionally emphasized ankle muscle responses. Restriction of the analysis to ankle muscles ignores the contribution of both trunk muscle activity and compensatory arm movements to balance corrections. Rapid trunk movements are required to compensate for roll-directed falls (Carpenter et al., 1999). If the elderly are inflexible in lateral bending, then a study of lateral perturbations would provide better insights on changes in body mechanics with age than studies of pitch-plane perturbations, especially as the trunk appears to be more flexible in roll than pitch in young subjects (Carpenter et al., 1999). Rapid arm movements are also important components of the natural defense against falls. Preliminary work indicates that arm muscle responses can in fact precede those of leg muscles and effectively help to prevent a fall or to cushion the impact (McIlroy and Maki, 1994). Analysis of such arm movements is also clinically relevant because wrist fractures are typically due to a fall on the outstretched hand (Chiu and Robinovitch, 1998; Melton et al., 1988). A study of aging effects on the ability to execute appropriate trunk motion and protective arm responses to multidirectional perturbations could provide insights into the effects of CNS slowing on the generation of balance commands.

## Methods

We investigated the balance-correcting responses of 36 healthy subjects (18 male, 18 female) divided equally into young (20-34 years of age), middle-aged (35-55), and elderly (60-75) groups. All subjects gave witnessed informed consent to participate in the experiment according to the Declaration of Helsinki. The Institutional Review Board of the University Hospital in Basel approved the study.

### Outcome Measures

We obtained EMG and biomechanical outcome measures using previously described techniques (Carpenter et al., 1999). Many of the techniques we used are described elsewhere (Bloem et al., 2002) and therefore are stated only briefly here. EMG signals were recorded from the left tibialis anterior, left soleus, and bilaterally on gluteus medius, paraspinal, and medial deltoid muscles. Support-surface reaction forces of the left foot were measured from strain gauges embedded within the rotating support. From these forces, the anteroposterior and mediolateral ankle torques were calculated for the left foot. Trunk angular velocity in the pitch and roll planes was collected using transducers at the level of the sternum. Two similar angular velocity transducers (Systron Donner, Inglewood, California) measured velocity of the left upper arm in the pitch and roll directions.

## Procedure

The subject's feet were lightly strapped into heel guides fixed to the top surface of the dual-axis rotating platform. The experiment consisted of two series of 44 perturbations, each a randomized combination of six different perturbation directions and two different perturbation velocities (either 30°/s or 60°/s), all at a constant amplitude of 7.5°. The six perturbation directions included two that were purely in the pitch plane (forward, or 0° in our notation, and backward, or 180°; see figure 8.1). For the four additional perturbation directions, pitch stimuli were combined with leftward and rightward roll components to make forward right (45°), backward right (135°), backward left (225°), and forward left (315°) perturbations. In response to each rotational perturbation, subjects were instructed to recover their balance as quickly as possible. Three handrails (80 cm high) were located at a distance of 40 cm to the sides and to the front of the platform center. Subjects were informed that they were allowed to grasp the handrails if needed. Two assistants (one behind and one to the side of the subject) were present to lend support in case of a fall.

## Data Analysis

Following analog-to-digital conversion of the data, all biomechanical and EMG signals were averaged off-line across each perturbation direction and velocity. Subject averages were pooled to produce population averages for a single direction and velocity combination (as shown in figures 8.2 and 8.3). All angular velocities (two each for the trunk and arm) were integrated off-line using trapezoid numerical integration to yield angular displacement. The difference between the angle value at 0 ms (the start of the perturbation) and at 700 ms was employed as a measure of a body-link angular change caused by the support-surface rotation. Angular displacements of the arm were calculated relative to the trunk by subtracting the arm position from the trunk position.

Small differences in muscle background EMG activity (BGA) prior to the onset of the stimuli were noted between the age groups (see figure 8.4). Effects of prestimulus BGA may confound between-group comparisons of response amplitudes (Bloem et al., 1993). Therefore, EMG areas were corrected by subtracting the average amount of BGA (measured over a 100-ms period prior to perturbation onset) from the overall response amplitude. This approach largely eliminates influences of prestimulus BGA (Bloem et al., 1993). Corrected EMG areas were calculated

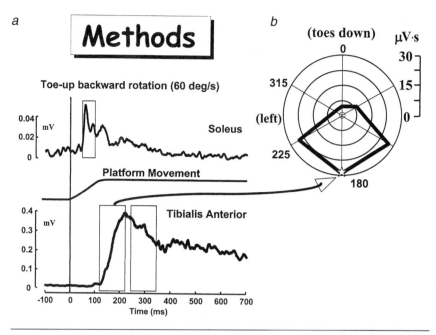

**Figure 8.1**   Schematic to illustrate methods. *(a)* The directions of support-surface tilt are indicated by the plots taken looking down on the platform. *(b)* The intervals used to measure EMG activity are shown for leg muscle responses of the elderly population to tilt in the 180° direction (toe-up).

using trapezoid integration within predetermined time intervals associated with stretch reflex (40-100 or 80-120 ms from stimulus onset) and balance-correcting responses (120-220 ms; see figure 8.1 and Carpenter et al., 1999). We also analyzed secondary balance-correcting responses (240-340 ms) and stabilizing responses (350-700 ms).

## Results

Although we found changes with age in the outcome measure at the ankle joints, these were not as profound as those at the trunk. Ankle muscle responses to support-surface toe-up displacements (i.e., to backward pitch rotations), however, form the overwhelming majority of descriptions in the literature concerning the effect of age on balance corrections. For this reason our description of changes with age commences with a brief description of aging effects at the ankle joint. We have extended prior knowledge on age-related effects on muscles and torques at this joint to off-pitch directions. Trunk rotations in response to support-surface roll proved to be markedly age dependent. These changes, as well as accompanying alterations in the responses of the trunk and hip muscles, constitute the main part

# Backward Left Rotation (60°/s)

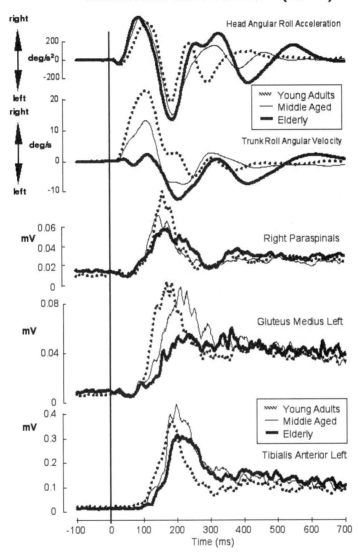

**Figure 8.2**  Trunk and leg muscle and velocity population responses to a backward left rotation of 60°/s. Each of the traces shown is the average of 12 subjects' responses to seven randomized repetitions of the stimulus, yielding a total of 84 responses to the average curve. The vertical line at 0 ms represents the onset of the support-surface rotation, which lasted 120 ms (until 7.5°). The movement directions for head and trunk roll are indicated to the left of the respective trace. Note the decreased muscle response amplitudes and delays in the tibialis anterior and gluteus medius muscles in the elderly. Note also the negligible initial trunk roll velocity in the direction opposite to the support-surface tilt and the final trunk roll displacement in the same direction as the tilt in the elderly.

189

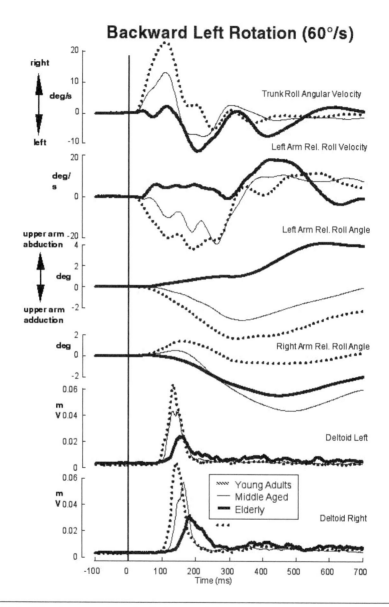

**Figure 8.3** Arm muscle and velocity population responses to a backward left rotation of 60°/s. The trunk velocity trace is the same as shown in figure 8.2. The relative angular velocity of the arm shown in the roll direction was computed from the difference of the measured angular velocity of the left upper arm and that of the trunk. Left and right roll angular position of the arm are the numerical integral of these traces. Note the different directions of the arm roll movements and the delayed and smaller deltoid responses for the elderly compared to the young.

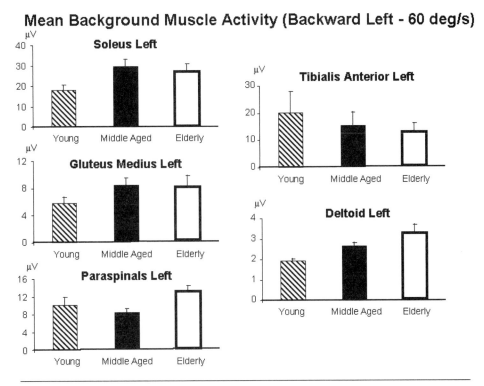

**Figure 8.4** Comparisons of background EMG activity. The height of columns represents the mean value. Error bars are the standard error of the mean.

of our description of human balance corrections. Finally, because arm responses are highly dependent on initial trunk roll movement in each group we tested, these results form the concluding part of the description of our results.

## Changes in Pitch-Plane Sensitivity of Ankle Joint Responses With Age

Balance-correcting responses to support-surface rotations have larger amplitudes in unloaded than in stretched lower-leg muscles (Carpenter et al., 1999). These responses, captured in the 120- to 220-ms measurement interval, had three characteristic changes with age, which can also be observed in tibialis anterior traces in figure 8.2. First, the response onset was delayed some 20 to 35 ms in the elderly; second, the primary balance-correcting response amplitude (between 120 and 220 ms) was smaller in the elderly; and third, the secondary response (between 240 and 340 ms) is larger in the elderly. These three characteristics were observed for all directions of support-surface tilt, with the strongest effects in tibialis anterior for backward tilt and soleus for forward tilt. This result is not unexpected because we found that the maximal activity direction is aligned along the pitch plane for tibialis anterior and 30° off-pitch for soleus (Carpenter et al., 1999). Differences with age also occurred for secondary balance corrections (240-340 ms). These later responses were larger in the elderly than in the young, not smaller. Backward right and forward tilts caused larger amplitudes in the elderly and middle-aged than the young in the left tibialis anterior and soleus, respectively, over the 240- to 340-ms period.

These differences in early and late balance-correcting responses with age (smaller early responses in the elderly apparently compensated by larger later responses) cannot be ascribed to differences in muscle background activity (BGA) with age. Figure 8.4 shows the levels of BGA in all three age groups just prior to the displacements shown in figures 8.2 and 8.3. The soleus BGA is larger in the elderly, compared to the young, whereas the tibialis anterior BGA is smaller. A dependence of balance-correcting responses on these levels should have led to smaller early soleus responses in the young, not larger, as we observed.

The interaction of age and direction on balance-correcting torques was consistent with the differences in ankle muscle responses with age. Torque changes were initially smaller in amplitude for the elderly, as measured between 160 and 260 ms (i.e., delayed 40 ms with respect to muscle response measurements to take into account muscle electromechanical activation coupling). Lower initial torque changes were partially compensated by a larger later (between 280 and 380 ms) amplitude of torque in the elderly, so that the sum of the torque changes between 160 and 380 ms was approximately constant with age. The directional orientation of ankle torques (the vector direction of anteroposterior and laterally directed torques) was not different between the young and the elderly over the two measurement periods we used.

The pitch-plane orientation of ankle torque responses implies that these torques will generate changes in angular displacements of leg and trunk segments in the pitch plane. Although significant differences in ankle muscles responses and ankle torques were observed in early and late balance-correcting responses between young and elderly subjects, the opposite direction of the age differences in the early and late periods yielded no major differences in the final pitch rotation of the ankle joint or trunk. Thus, the pitch-plane orientation of ankle muscle responses across all age groups and the compensation for smaller early ankle torques by larger later torques in the elderly caused no major age differences in the amount of trunk pitch at 700 ms (figure 8.5).

## Changes in Roll-Plane Sensitivity of Trunk Responses With Age

Major age-related differences in trunk roll angular velocity as well as trunk and hip muscle responses were observed over the first 300 ms. As figures 8.2, 8.5, and 8.6 show, age-related differences in balance corrections became very apparent when a roll component was added to the postural disturbance. Figure 8.2 provides an example of the striking age differences in the early amplitudes of trunk roll angular velocity for a backward left rotation at 60°/s. In the young and middle-aged, the trunk

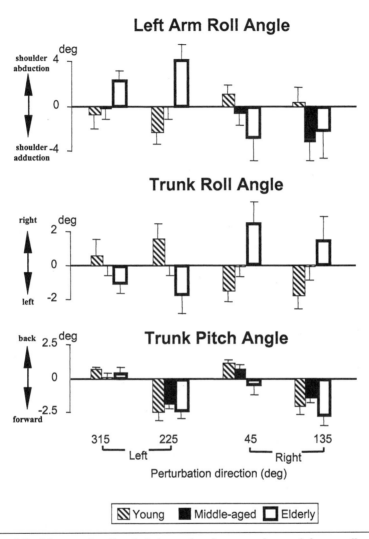

**Figure 8.5** Mean trunk roll and pitch angular changes and mean left arm roll angular changes (relative to the trunk) from stimulus onset to 700 ms later, when trunk velocities have stabilized. Mean and standard errors of the means are shown for each age group. The direction of support-surface rotation causing the changes is indicated by the plot abscissa: leftward directions on the left, rightward on the right. Note that the trunk and arm roll changes are in the opposite direction in young and elderly subjects, but trunk pitch rotations are in similar directions.

rolls in the opposite direction within 30 ms of platform tilt. In the elderly, there is a very small early excursion of trunk velocity in the same direction as the young, followed by a small motion in the opposite direction. The main change in trunk roll velocity in the elderly occurred around 180 ms, coinciding with a slowing of trunk

# Proximal Muscle Balance Correcting Responses
## Paraspinals over 120-220 ms

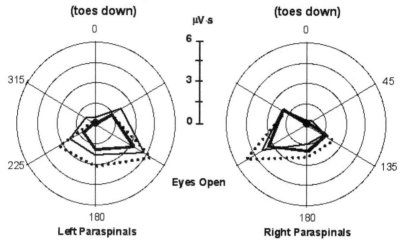

## Gluteus Medius over 120-220 ms

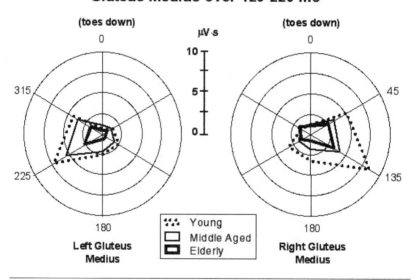

**Figure 8.6** Polar plots for areas of left and right paraspinal and gluteus medius EMG responses averaged over a time interval (120-220 ms) consisting of balance-correcting reactions. Each radial line represents one of the six directions of support-surface rotation (0°, 45°, 135°, 180°, 225°, and 315°). Mean population values are plotted for each direction, with amplitude represented as distance from the center. The response amplitude is scaled between the set of plots according to the different vertical scales for the two recording sites. Note the roll-plane orientation of the responses and the smaller response amplitudes in the elderly. The maximum activity directions do not change with age.

roll velocity in the young and middle-aged. The traces in figure 8.2 show that the main trunk roll in the elderly was in the same direction as the support-surface tilt (left for left tilt). The middle-aged have trunk roll velocity profiles between those of the young and the elderly. They roll in the direction somewhat opposite support-surface tilt with velocity amplitudes approximately one-half those of the young. Using the average velocity over 40 ms—20 ms before and after the time when peak velocities occurred on average (110 ms for roll, shown in figure 8.2, and 200 ms for pitch, not shown)—we captured how trunk velocities change with age for each direction. In every direction of roll, the young exhibit the greatest early trunk roll velocities, the middle-aged less, and the elderly low velocities, consistent with a more rigid trunk response. This effect was very significant ($p < 0.0001$, $F = 27.8$). On average, roll velocity between 90 and 130 ms for 60°/s stimuli was 21°/s for the young, 12°/s for the middle-aged, and 1°/s for the elderly.

Despite their stiffer roll-directed trunk response, the elderly were more unstable in terms of velocity than the young only prior to 600 ms. As shown in figure 8.2, trunk roll velocities in the young and the elderly are both near zero after 600 ms, so 700 ms was a suitable time point to measure trunk angular displacement from stimulus onset. The age differences in the early roll velocity and the lack of a compensatory movement by the elderly yielded a final trunk orientation tilted toward the direction of support-surface movement in the elderly. The trunk orientation was in the opposite direction—away from the support-surface movement—in the young and hardly tilted at all in the middle-aged (see trunk roll means in figure 8.5b). The average mean difference in trunk roll in response to roll stimuli between the elderly and the young was 3° to 4°, or about two thirds of the tilt stimulus roll angle (see figure 8.5b). Thus, as depicted by the schematic of figure 8.7 and the measurement means of figure 8.5b, trunk roll amplitudes changed with age. The elderly respond to roll displacements with trunk movements more like those of a stiff inverted pendulum, with motion in the same direction as the tilt. The young responded instead with considerably more flexible roll rotation of the trunk about the pelvis and lumbar spine.

Head roll accelerations in the elderly, like trunk movements in the young, were always in the direction opposite platform rotation over the first 100 ms (see traces in figure 8.2). That is, despite the age differences in early roll velocities of the trunk, head roll accelerations, regardless of age, followed a pattern expected as a result of the body being pushed in the direction opposite of that of support-surface roll. Consistent with stiffer trunk motion, however, the head accelerations of the elderly were more rapid in onset and peaked earlier than those of the young (see traces in figure 8.2).

Roll perturbations cause stretch and unloading reflexes in both paraspinals and gluteus medius muscles. This action occurs because the pelvis tilts in the direction of platform tilt and the upper trunk tilts in the opposite direction or, in the case of the elderly, in the same direction as but less than the pelvis (see figure 8.7). Thus, backward left perturbations cause a stretch of the right gluteus medius and left paraspinal muscles, as shown schematically in figure 8.7. Likewise, backward left

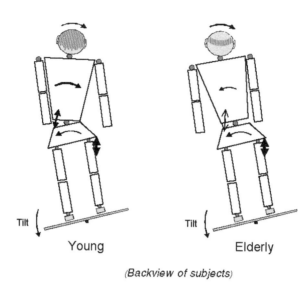

Young                  Elderly

*(Backview of subjects)*

**Figure 8.7** Schematic of the roll movements of the young and the elderly to a left tilt of the support surface. The curved arrows on the body segments indicate the initial velocities 100 ms after tilt onset. The thickness of the arrows represents their velocities. The vertical arrows indicate muscle stretch directions at the lower gluteus medius and upper parts (paraspinal muscles) of the pelvis. Smaller stretch is indicated by the thinner arrow for the paraspinals of the elderly.

perturbations unload the left gluteus medius and the right paraspinal muscles, as shown by the decreases in activity at 30 ms on the traces of figure 8.2. Analyses of the amplitudes of paraspinal reflex responses for stretch and unloading measured over the interval from 40 to 100 ms revealed both age and age-by-direction interactions; amplitudes were larger in the young than in the elderly for backward roll stimuli. We presume that these early paraspinal responses are highly dependent on the amplitude of early trunk roll velocity. Thus, the reduced responses in the elderly are consistent with their reduced early trunk roll motion. There were no significant differences in the amplitudes of gluteus medius muscle activity, suggesting that there are fewer age-related changes in pelvis movement than in trunk movement (however, this was not directly measured).

As described earlier, the tilt of the support surface causes the upper body of the young to tilt in the opposite direction (Carpenter et al., 1999). The pelvis tilts in the same direction as the support surface tilts. Elderly persons tilt the trunk in the same direction as the support surface rotation. To achieve a measure of stability despite this disadvantageous trunk lean, they should activate their hip and trunk muscles more than the young. Figures 8.2 and 8.6 show that this is not the case.

The most prominent age-related response of the trunk muscles was the reduced amplitude of the gluteus medius response between 80 and 220 ms in the elderly as compared with both the young and the middle-aged (see figures 8.2 and 8.6b).

Response amplitude reductions with age were very significant in both left and right gluteus medius muscles for all backward directions (see figure 8.6). The left gluteus response amplitudes shown in figure 8.6 were smaller in the elderly than in the young for all roll directions except forward right. The significant differences over the 80- to 120-ms period in gluteus medius can be ascribed to latency differences among the age groups. The left gluteus medius balance-correcting responses commenced at 109 ms on average and were 20 ms earlier in the young than in the elderly or middle-aged. Paraspinal balance-correcting responses showed no latency differences with age. As figure 8.6 documents, paraspinal responses had less age effect than gluteus medius responses over the 120- to 220-ms measurement period. The polar plots in figure 8.6 illustrate the interaction of age and direction on gluteus medius and paraspinal EMG response amplitudes. The direction of maximal activity in these muscles did not change with age. An alternative means of achieving stability would be to adjust the ratio of activation levels of left and right hip and trunk muscles. The asymmetry ratios that were calculated on the basis of values plotted in figure 8.6 indicate that there is a trend for the elderly to increase the paraspinals' right-to-left asymmetry and decrease the gluteus medius muscles' left-to-right asymmetry, thereby achieving a body-tilting effect counter to the support-surface tilt.

Yet another way for the elderly to compensate for weaker initial responses in trunk muscles would be to increase later activity as in the leg muscles. In contrast to leg muscles, the hip and trunk muscles whose activity we recorded did not demonstrate continued phasic activity after 250 ms. Rather, as can be seen in figure 8.2, the dynamic pulse of the balance-correcting response was followed after 250 ms by tonic activity, which presumably held the body in the tilted position. These tonic activity levels did not differ between young and elderly. Thus, following the initial lean of trunk that was directed differently in the young and the elderly (see figure 8.7), only a change in trunk and hip muscle response asymmetry for early 120- to 220-ms activity appeared to have some of the metrics necessary to shift the downhill lean of the elderly more uphill. Neither the absolute amplitude of this asymmetry nor the ongoing, stabilizing tonic activity in hip and trunk muscles of the elderly that we measured between 350 and 700 ms provided an uphill shift of the trunk.

## *Compensatory Arm Movements*

When subjects were perturbed by support-surface tilt, rapid arm movements occurred. These arm movements have different roll characteristics, depending on the age of the subject (see figure 8.3). We showed earlier that the trunk rolls in different directions with age. We discovered that differences in arm movements with age were highly dependent on the greater initial trunk roll flexibility in the young, as shown by the traces of figure 8.3. The arm roll velocity traces shown in figure 8.3 show profiles and age effects over the first 200 ms that are markedly similar to the trunk velocity traces. The amplitude of initial roll velocity of the arms is much greater in the young, less in the middle-aged, and least in the elderly. Furthermore, the direction of arm velocity over the first 300 ms in the elderly was opposite to that of the other age groups. The net result of these age differences in early roll veloci- ties is illustrated in figure 8.3 by the left-arm roll angle traces, which are plotted relative to the trunk for a left roll. The roll angle traces of the arm for the different age groups clearly diverge from one another. The left arm for the rightward tilt is moving uphill in the young and downhill in the elderly. For a backward right tilt, the left arm moves as the right arm presumably would move for a left tilt. We show this as the "right arm" in figure 8.3. For this "right arm," however, the difference with age is not as large nor as significant as the left-arm movement for the backward left direction (also compare the 225° and 135° columns for the left arm in figure 8.5a). Thus, the initial roll velocities for the young and middle-aged place the arms in a statically more stable position. There were no observable age differences in the early (before 200 ms) pitch velocities of the arms relative to the trunk.

The arm muscle responses shown in figure 8.3 are stronger and earlier in the young than in the elderly, and the middle-aged show amplitudes between the other two age groups. These deltoid responses were delayed in the elderly for backward left and right roll directions but not for the pure backward pitch direction. The average onset for backward left and right roll directions was 105 ms in the young, 110 ms in the middle-aged, and 129 ms in the elderly. These differences occurred despite a significant increase in deltoid background muscle activity in the elderly compared with the young (see figure 8.4).

The effect of the activation of the arm muscles is to create a reactive torque on the trunk that tends to move the trunk in the direction opposite to the arm accel- eration. As figure 8.3 shows, after the onset of deltoid activity, the left arm of the young subjects rapidly decelerated (i.e., accelerated in the abduction direction), and there was some minor movement of the arm back toward the trunk. The left arm of the middle-aged subjects moved in a similar manner. Motion of the left arm of the elderly subjects consisted of an increase in velocity to place the arm more in abduction, that is, more downhill than it was already. Thus, across all age groups, a righting torque was imposed on the trunk due to the arm's acceleration into abduction, but in the case of the elderly, the arm movement placed the arm even more downhill and forward than initially.

As a result of both the early stimulus-induced movement of the arms and trunk and the balance-correcting activity in shoulder muscles, such as the deltoid, the arms of both young and elderly subjects in general ended up at 700 ms in a position ahead of that of the trunk (see figures 8.3 and 8.5). Important differences, which presumably affect the overall stability of the elderly, underlie this observation, however. First, because the trunk and the arms relative to the trunk moved toward the downhill side in the elderly and toward the uphill side in the young (see the arm relative roll angles in figure 8.3), these arm movements placed the body's center of mass more downhill in the elderly. The plots of relative arm roll induced by 700 ms (figure 8.5) indicate that both the young and elderly had moved their arms by this time point in the direction of trunk motion but that these directions, like those for the trunk motion, were different with age. For example, for the left arm roll shown in figure 8.3 (direction 225° in figure 8.5), the average arm abduction in the elderly was 3.9°, significantly different from the adduction of 2.3° in the young. Figure 8.5a shows that this difference between the young and elderly in the direction of arm roll at 700 ms was observed for all perturbation directions with a roll component (315°, 225°, 45°, and 135°). The more extended final position of the arms in the elderly for backward roll directions was correlated with the tendency for increased tonic activity in deltoid muscles of the elderly after 350 ms (see figure 8.3). In summary, differences in arm movements with age, like those in trunk movements, and the inherent instabilities that these movements produced in the elderly were revealed readily by combinations of roll and pitch support-surface rotations.

# Discussion

In our studies we examined changes with age in trunk balance corrections, directions of protective arm movements, and central processing delays. We concluded our studies with an outlook for preventive treatment.

## Changes in Trunk Balance Corrections With Age

By employing roll perturbations of the support surface, we were able to focus on two aspects of movement synergies that differed fundamentally between the elderly and the young. Both these differences underlying balance corrections appeared to be linked to inherent changes in roll flexibility of the trunk with aging. The first age-related characteristic concerns the initial movement of the trunk. In the young the trunk is tilted uphill when the support surface is tilted, and the legs and pelvis are turned downhill (see figure 8.7). We showed that hardly any initial trunk rotation occurs in the elderly, and if it does, the rotation is in the same direction as the support-surface tilt. Because the trunk movement in the young provides a counterweight to the downhill displacement of the body's center of mass, a logical response for the elderly might seem to be a balance-correcting response to achieve the same end stability as the young. It appears from our results, however, that from the initial position of hardly any trunk movement, the elderly subsequently move the trunk further downhill, as do the young. Thus, our observations indicate that the elderly use the same balance-correcting movement synergy as the young, albeit with smaller amplitudes of hip and trunk muscle responses, and in a sense they do not adapt their movement strategy to deal with the changed biomechanical response of the body to the disturbance.

The significance of our findings about these aspects of trunk movement is reinforced by the results for the middle-aged, which were observed exactly between results for the young and the elderly. The findings for the middle-aged imply that the changes with age that we observed occur gradually. We expected that the elderly, being in a downhill position initially, would have responded more effectively by increasing trunk and hip muscle responses more, not less, than the young. In this way the trunk would have been forced uphill, compensating for the lack of initial stimulus-induced uphill trunk roll. The only evidence we found for some adaptation was a change in the activation ratios of left- and right-side trunk and hip muscles so as to rotate the trunk more in the desired uphill direction. If the trunk muscles cannot be activated more strongly in the elderly, changing such activation ratios would be one means of achieving more stability. Another means would be to increase the amplitude of later bursts of activity. Leg muscles, but not the trunk and hip muscles from which we recorded, showed such a pattern change. In the leg muscles the second part of the balance-correcting response (240-340 ms) and ankle torques were larger in the elderly, indicating a compensation for the early (120-220 ms), weaker part of the balance-correcting response. In trunk muscles we found no evidence for a similar adaptation. It is thus an open question why the elderly achieve considerable adaptation in the leg muscles but not in the trunk muscles.

The major question that arises from our work is why the elderly do not employ a balance-correcting strategy for trunk and hip muscles that is more well adjusted to trunk inflexibility. One reason could be that, in contrast to the changed early stretch reflexes in leg muscles, upper-body motion sensors provide insufficient or conflicting indications that the elderly trunk will roll significantly less than it used to. The proprioceptive reflexes we were able to record as stretch and unloading reflexes in gluteus medius and paraspinal muscles provided some evidence for differences with age, but only in the paraspinal muscles. The earliest (around 30 ms) stretch and unloading reflexes we observed in the gluteus medius were quite similar for the different age groups; that is, the activation and deactivation of background activity by these reflexes seemed consistent with the initial counterrotations of the pelvis segment with respect to the rotation of the trunk, which was similar for all age groups (see figure 8.7). The differences among age groups appeared first, around 50 ms, in paraspinal stretch and unloading reflexes; decreased trunk velocities with age were presumably due to increased trunk stiffness in the elderly. Because we observed stretch reflex amplitudes that were reduced in paraspinal muscles but normal in gluteus medius muscles, we must assume that proprioceptive systems in the trunk and hips provided information on the differences in velocities of the pelvis and trunk segments to the CNS. Furthermore, amplitudes of early stretch and unloading reflexes would presumably be reduced in more trunk muscles than just the paraspinal muscles. Nonetheless, it is unusual that the balance correction generated by the CNS failed to take into account the lack of initial trunk roll in the elderly. Our recordings of head roll accelerations support acceleration of the trunk that is initially in the same direction for all age groups but then is slowed down in the elderly by trunk stiffness. As a result, the head is whipped into roll angular acceleration faster in the elderly (see head acceleration traces in figure 8.2), thus, in conjunction with reduced proprioceptive input at the trunk, providing the CNS a clear indication of an initially slower-moving trunk compared with a faster-moving head. The CNS of the elderly appears unable to take this differing proprioceptive and vestibular information into account when planning and executing balance corrections.

## Directions of Protective Arm Movements Differ With Age

The second fundamentally different movement response of the elderly compared with the young that our results showed was changed compensatory arm movements. Arm movements can perform a number of static and dynamic functions, including acting as a counterweight, providing a dynamic righting force, or cushioning a possible fall. For someone on the verge of a possible fall, choosing between placing the arms as a counterweight away from the direction of falling or using the arms to cushion a fall probably depends on his or her confidence that a fall can be avoided. In all age groups, the direction of initial arm movements was determined by the initial (stimulus-induced) trunk motion. Thus, in all age groups, initial arm movements were directed toward the side of impending trunk displacement. For the young this meant that the arms were already used as a counterweight to compensate for the displaced center of gravity. In contrast, the elderly's initial arm movements placed the arms more in the direction of tilt. The next stage in the arm movement involves a rapid activation of arm muscles to create a counterrotating reaction movement on the trunk. For example, for a leftward support-surface tilt, rapidly abducting the arm (outward rotation away from the trunk and downhill) rotates the trunk more uphill. For the young, these movements can be larger and therefore more effective because the arms are already rotated uphill. However, for the elderly with their arms already downhill, this motion must be smaller as otherwise the final position of the arms at the end of such a movement would be even more destabilizing. The delayed arm muscle responses that we observed in the deltoid muscles of the elderly may have arisen because of their having to decide, albeit subconsciously, between continuing to stretch the arms out in the direction of a fall to grasp support (e.g., a handrail) or cushion possible contact with the floor or rapidly activating the arms to help move the trunk uphill. Presumably, this decision is connected with fear of falling in the elderly. Alternatively, the responses could simply be delayed as part of a CNS processing delay in the elderly (discussed later). The strategy that we observed in the elderly of placing the arms in the direction of a fall does not aid their stability because the arms further displace the center of gravity and thus increase the likelihood of a fall.

## Central Processing Delays in the Elderly

The latency changes we observed in muscle responses could indicate either a general reduction in sensory thresholds or slower processing time for balance corrections with age. The latter is the most parsimonious explanation for our results, although we also observed evidence of reduced stretch reflex gains in ankle and trunk muscles. In most muscles, balance-correcting responses in the young had an onset latency around 100 ms. This value was observed for arm, hip, and ankle muscle responses, suggesting that the balance corrections must be centrally timed to occur in all muscles more or less simultaneously. Invariably, these onsets were delayed in the elderly at these three locations by some 20 ms. The simultaneous activation of balance corrections across many segments has been noted before (Allum et al., 1993; Carpenter et al., 1999; Keshner et al., 1988). We can now extend this finding to arm muscles and hypothesize that the simultaneous activation arises from the constraint to have righting torques at each of the major joints precisely coordinated. This aspect of the timing differs from those compensatory trunk and leg responses that occur prior to voluntary arm movements (Cordo and Nashner, 1982; Friedli et al., 1984; Hodges et al., 2000).

Changes in sensory thresholds with age with concomitant increases in onset times of stretch reflexes were not found in this study. Thus, the concept of central processing delays in the elderly is supported by the lack of any obvious shifts in onset delays in stretch reflexes and unloading responses of the order of 20 ms (as found for balance corrections). Rather, only reductions in the amplitudes of early stretch reflexes in soleus and paraspinal muscles were observed, which appeared to be related to reduced muscle stretch caused by increased joint stiffness. The joint stiffness may have been caused by changes in intrinsic muscle stiffness, as the mean levels of background activity in the soleus and paraspinal muscles increased with age (see figure 8.4). The increased stiffness, especially at the trunk, caused the head to accelerate initially more for the elderly than for the young, and this increased acceleration could possibly overcome any age-related reductions in vestibular thresholds. Nonetheless, the apparently earlier vestibular input in the elderly compared with possibly later proprioceptive input might require increased processing time in order to generate appropriate balance corrections.

## Outlook for Preventive Treatment

The pathophysiology underlying age-related falls and injuries remains incompletely understood. We used two approaches to bridge this gap. First, we used unpredictable balance perturbations to provide information on how the CNS corrects falls in different directions. Second, we studied whether analysis of trunk and arm movements might clarify the mechanisms underlying hip or wrist fractures.

We observed three types of age-related changes in balance corrections. First, lower-leg responses adapted well to the effects of aging. For all perturbation directions, onsets of balance-correcting responses in these ankle muscles were delayed by 20 to 30 ms and had smaller amplitudes (between 120 and 220 ms) in the elderly compared with the young. This delayed and reduced early activity was compensated by increased lower-leg activity after 240 ms in elderly compared with young subjects. These EMG changes were paralleled by comparable differences in ankle torque responses, which were also initially smaller in the elderly but subsequently greater. Findings in the middle-aged group were generally midway between those in the young and the elderly.

Second, age-related changes occurred in trunk responses. Stimulus-induced trunk roll, but not trunk pitch, changed dramatically with age. Young subjects responded with early and large roll movements of the trunk in the opposite direction to platform roll. A similarly directed but reduced amplitude of trunk roll occurred in the middle-aged. The elderly had very little initial trunk roll modulation and also smaller stretch reflexes in paraspinal muscles. Balance-correcting responses (at 120-220 ms) in gluteus medius and paraspinal muscles were normally roll sensitive in the elderly but were reduced in amplitude. Onset latencies increased with age in gluteus medius muscles. Following the onset of balance corrections, trunk roll was in the same direction as support-surface motion for all groups but resulted in overall trunk roll toward the fall side in the elderly but not in the young. Response asymmetries between left- and right-side muscles tended to change with age, consistent with an attempt to achieve greater trunk stability in the elderly.

Finally, protective arm movements changed with age. Initial arm roll movements were largest in the young, smaller in the middle-aged, and smallest in the elderly. Initial arm roll movements were in the same direction as initial trunk motion in the young and middle-aged but in the opposite direction in the elderly. Initial pitch motion of the arms was similar across age groups. Subsequent arm movements depended on the amplitude of deltoid muscle responses, which commenced at 100 ms in the young and 20 to 30 ms later in the elderly. Deltoid responses were largest in all age groups for backward platform rotations. These deltoid muscle responses led to additional arm roll motion, which left the arms directed downhill (in the direction of the fall) in the elderly but uphill (to counterbalance motion of the pelvis) in the young.

## Conclusions

We conclude that decreased trunk roll flexibility is a key biomechanical change with age. This interferes with early compensatory trunk movements and leads to trunk displacements in the direction of the impending fall. This may contribute to the genesis of hip fractures. The reversal of protective arm movements in the elderly may reflect an adaptive strategy to cushion the fall, but arm extension in the fall direction can also cause wrist fractures. The uniform delay and amplitude reduction of balance-correcting responses across many segments (legs, hips, and arms) suggests a neurally based alteration in processing times and response modulation with age. Interestingly, the elderly compensated for reductions in early compensatory trunk movements with enlarged later responses in the legs, but no similar adaptation was noted in the arms or trunk. One possible explanation is that trunk stiffness and reversed arm movements are themselves compensatory strategies that, although perhaps self-perceived to be beneficial, in fact aggravate the falling risk when stance is perturbed.

These results help us to understand the mechanisms underlying fall-related injuries in the elderly and offer possible approaches for their prevention. Corrective balance responses in the arms and trunk of the elderly seem to be maladjusted to achieving overall stability of the body. By placing the arms more downhill than the young, the elderly place a greater mass downhill and thus increase the likelihood of a fall. The young adopt a more stable strategy by keeping the downhill arm uphill, in the direction of overall trunk movement. In contrast to the trunk, subsequent arm movements after balance corrections appear to be larger than those of the trunk, indicating the ease with which the arms can be moved compared with the trunk (see figure 8.7). In this respect, these results have a major significance for understanding the mechanisms underlying falls in the elderly and their possible prevention. If the young can plan different arm movement control when falling as part of martial arts training or learn to point their arms downhill to enhance dynamic continuous downhill falling while skiing, we should ask why the middle-aged do not acquire trunk and arm responses that decrease rather than increase the likelihood of a fall once tipped.

## Acknowledgments

This work was supported by a grant from the Swiss National Science Foundation (31-59319.99) to J.H.J. Allum. B.R. Bloem was supported by a grant from the Dutch Parkinson's Association. We thank Mrs. E. Clarke for typographical assistance.

## References

Alexander, N.B., Shepard N., Gu, M.J., and Schultz, A.B. (1992) Postural control in young and elderly adults when stance is perturbed: Kinematics. *J Gerontol* 47: M79-M87.

Allum, J.H.J., Honegger, F., and Schicks, H. (1993) Vestibular and proprioceptive modulation of postural synergies in normal subjects. *J Vestib Res* 3: 59-85.

Baloh, R.W., Corona, S., Jacobson, K.M., Enrietto, J.A., and Bell, T. (1998) A prospective study of posturography in normal older people. *J Am Geriatr Soc* 46: 438-443.

Baloh, R.W., Spain, S., Socotch, T.M., Jacobson, K.M., and Bell, T. (1995) Posturography and balance problems in older people. *J Am Geriatr Soc* 43: 638-644.

Bartlett, S.A., Maki, B.E., Fernie, G.R., Holliday, P.J., and Gryfe, C.I. (1986) On the classification of a geriatric subject as a faller or nonfaller. *Med Biol Eng Comput* 24: 219-222.

Bloem, B.R., Allum, J.H.J., Carpenter, M.G., Verschuuren, J.J.G.M., and Honegger, F. (2002) Triggering of balance corrections and compensatory strategies in a patient with total leg proprioceptive loss. *Exp Brain Res* 142: 91-107.

Bloem, B.R., van Dijk, J.G., Beckley, D.J., Zwinderman, A.H., Remler, M.P., and Roos, R.A. (1993) Correction for the influence of background muscle activity on stretch reflex amplitudes. *J Neurosci Meth* 46: 167-174.

Brocklehurst, J.C., Robertson, D., and James-Groom, P. (1982) Clinical correlates of sway in old age: Sensory modalities. *Age Aging* 11: 1-10.

Campbell, A.J., Borrie, M.J., and Spears, G.F. (1989) Risk factors for falls in a community-based prospective study of people 70 years and older. *J Gerontol* 44: M112-M117.

Carpenter, M.G., Allum, J.H.J., and Honegger, F. (1999) Directional sensitivity of stretch reflexes and balance corrections for normal subjects in the roll and pitch planes. *Exp Brain Res* 129: 93-113.

Carpenter, M.G., Allum, J.H., and Honegger, F. (2001) Vestibular influences on human postural control in combinations of pitch and roll planes reveal differences in spatiotemporal processing. *Exp Brain Res* 140: 95-111.

Chiu, J., and Robinovitch, S.N. (1998) Prediction of upper extremity impact forces during falls on the outstretched hand. *J Biomech* 31: 1169-1176.

Cordo, P.J., and Nashner, L.M. (1982) Properties of postural adjustments associated with rapid arm movements. *J Neurophysiol* 47: 287-302.

Fernie, G.R., Gryfe, C.I., Holliday, P.J., and Llewellyn, A. (1982) The relationship of postural sway in standing to the incidence of falls in geriatric subjects. *Age Aging* 11: 11-16.

Fife, T.D., and Baloh, R.W. (1993) Disequilibrium of unknown cause in older people. *Ann Neurol* 34: 694-702.

Friedli, W.G., Hallett, M., and Simon, S.R. (1984) Postural adjustments associated with rapid voluntary arm movements: 1. Electromyographic data. *J Neurol Neurosurg Psychiatry* 47: 611-622.

Furman, J.M.R., Baloh, R.W., Barin, K., Hain, T.C., Herdman, S.J., Konrad, H.R., and Parker, S.W. (1993) Assessment: Posturography. Report of the therapeutics and technology assessment sub-committee of the American Academy of Neurology. *Neurology* 43: 1261-1264.

Gill, J., Allum, J.H.J., Carpenter, M.G., Held-Ziolkowska, M., Honegger, F., and Pierchala, K. (2001) Trunk sway measures of postural stability during clinical balance tests: Effects of age. *J Gerontol* 56A: M438-M447.

Greenspan, S.L., Myers, E.R., Maitland, L.A., Resnick, N.M., and Hayes, W.C. (1994) Fall severity and bone mineral density as risk factors for hip fracture in ambulatory elderly. *JAMA* 271: 128-133.

Hodges, P.W., Cresswell, A.G., Daggfeldt, K., and Thorstensson, A. (2000) Three dimensional prepara-tory trunk motion precedes asymmetrical upper limb movement. *Gait Posture* 11: 92-101.

Imms, F.J., and Endhold, O.G. (1981) Studies of gait and mobility in the elderly. *Age Ageing* 10: 147-156.

Keshner, E.A., Allum, J.H.J., and Honegger, F. (1993) Predictors of less stable postural responses to support surface rotations in healthy human elderly. *J Vestib Res* 3 (4): 419-429.

Keshner, E.A., Woollacott, M.H., and Debu, B. (1988) Neck and trunk muscle responses during postural perturbations in humans. *Exp Brain Res* 71: 455-466.

Lichtenstein, M.J., Burger, M.C. , Shields, S.L., and Shiavi, R.G. (1990) Comparison of biomechanics platform measures of balance and videotaped measures of gait with a clinical mobility scale in elderly women. *J Gerontol* 45: M49-M54.

Lichtenstein, M.J., Shields, S.L., Shiavi, R.G., and Burger, M.C. (1988) Clinical determinants of bio-mechanics platform measures of balance in aged women. *J Am Geriatr Soc* 36: 996-1002.

Lord, S.R., Clark, R.D., and Webster, I.W. (1991) Postural stability and associated physiological factors in a population of aged persons. *J Gerontol* 46: M69.

Lord, S.R., Rogers, M.W., Howland, A., and Fitzpatrick, R. (1999) Lateral stability, sensorimotor func-tion and falls in older people. *J Am Geriatr Soc* 47: 1077-1081.

Maki, B.E. (1993) Biomechanical approach to quantifying anticipatory postural adjustments in the elderly. *Med Biol Eng Comput* 31: 355-362.

Maki, B.E., Holliday, P.J., and Fernie, G.R. (1990) Aging and postural control: A comparison of spon-taneous- and induced-sway balance tests. *J Am Geriatr Soc* 38: 1-9.

Maki, B.E., Holliday, P.J., and Topper, A.K. (1991) Fear of falling and postural performance in the elderly. *J Gerontol* 45: M123-M131.

Maki, B.E., Holliday, P.J., and Topper, A.K. (1994) A prospective study of postural balance and risk of falling in an ambulatory and independent elderly population. *J Gerontol* 49: M72-M84.

Maki, B.E., and McIlroy, W.E. (1998) Control of compensatory stepping reactions: Age-related impair-ment and the potential for remedial intervention. *Physiother Theory Pract* 15: 69-90.

Maki, B.E., McIlroy, W.E., and Perry, S.D. (1996) Influence of lateral destabilization on compensatory stepping responses. *J Biomech* 29: 343-353.

McIlroy, W.E., and Maki, B.E. (1994) Compensatory arm movements evoked by transient perturbations of upright stance. In Taguchi, K., Igarashi, M., and Mori, S., eds., *Vestibular and neural front.* Amsterdam: Elsevier. 489-492.

Melton, L.J., Chao, E.Y.S., and Lane, J. (1988) Biomechanical aspects of fractures. In Riggs, B.L., and Melton, L.J., eds., *Osteoporosis: Etiology, diagnosis and management.* New York: Raven Press. 111-131.

Murray, M.P., Seireg, A.A., and Sepic, S.B. (1975) Normal postural stability and steadiness: Quantita-tive assessment. *J Bone Joint Surg Am* 57: 510-516.

Nevitt, M.C., and Cummings, S.R. (1993) Type of fall and risk of hip and wrist fractures: The study of osteoporotic fractures. The Study of Osteoporotic Fractures Research Group. *J Am Geriatr Soc* 41: 1226-1234.

O'Neill, T.W., Varlow, J., Silman, A.J., Reeve, J., Reid, D.M., Todd, C., and Woolf, A.D. (1994) Age and sex influences on fall characteristics. *Ann Rheum Dis* 53: 773-775.

Overstall, P.W., Exton-Smith, A.N., Imms, F.J., and Johnson, A.L. (1977) Falls in the elderly related to postural imbalance. *Br Med J* 1: 261-264.

Rivner, M.H., Swift, T.R., and Malik, K. (2001) Influence of age and height on nerve conduction. *Muscle Nerve* 24: 1134-1141.

Shepard, N.T., Schultz, A.B., Alexander, N.B., Gu, M.J., and Boismier, T. (1993) Postural control in young and elderly adults when stance is challenged: Clinical versus laboratory measurements. *Ann Otol Rhinol Laryngol* 102: 508-517.

Stelmach, G.E., Phillips, J., Di Fabio, R.P., and Teasdale, N. (1989) Age, functional postural reflexes, and voluntary sway. *J Gerontol* 44: B100-B106.

Stelmach, G.E., Teasdale, N., Di Fabio, R.P., and Phillips, J. (1989) Age related decline in postural control mechanisms. *Int J Aging Hum Dev* 29: 205-223.

Williams, H.G., McClenaghan, B.A., and Dickerson, J. (1997) Spectral characteristics of postural control in elderly individuals. *Arch Phys Med Rehabil* 78: 737-744.

Woollacott, M.H. (1986) Gait and postural control in the aging adult. In Bles, W., and Brandt, T., eds., *Disorders of posture and gait*. Amsterdam: Elsevier Science (Medical Division). 325-314.

# 9

# Signs of Long-Term Adaptation to Permanent Brain Damage As Revealed by Prehension Studies of Children With Spastic Hemiparesis

*Bert Steenbergen and Ruud G.J. Meulenbroek*
University of Nijmegen

One of the most intriguing capacities of living creatures is adaptation. Organisms are remarkably capable of adapting to changes in the environment or their own makeup. Across species, adaptations occur on a phylogenetic time scale. Within a member of a species, adaptations can occur during a life span or even on a smaller time scale, as is the case with learning. An example of immediate adaptation can be found in the instant compensation for an unexpected perturbation during an unfolding action. A prerequisite common to all kinds of adaptation is redundancy. Without redundancy adaptation would be impossible. This is most clearly illustrated by the first generation of robots. Even though these machines were capable of performing actions with utmost precision and speed over and over again, they lacked any capacity to cope with novel situations.

In this chapter we review a series of studies on the planning and coordination of unrestricted grasping movements in children with hemiparetic cerebral palsy. The aim of our review is to try to find signs of adaptation to the brain damage that these children sustained at birth. In our view, looking for signs of long-term adaptation in this group of children may contribute to the study of motor disorders in general since this domain has traditionally overemphasized negative symptoms. When signs of adaptation to permanent brain damage become better known, diagnostics and treatment may change in character. Rather than focusing on restrictions and limitations, interventions could then focus on conditions under which the remaining potential can be exploited in a constructive way.

We expect to be able to pinpoint signs of adaptation in the group of children under study because, due to the problems they are confronted with on a daily basis, these children have learned to deal with suboptimal movement conditions for many years. Indeed, the majority of children with cerebral palsy sustained brain damage at or around birth, mostly due to lack of oxygen to the immature brain. As a consequence some cortical motor areas have permanently lost their function. It is apparent in this group of children that the unaffected brain areas have not fully taken over this functionality because, when we observe an adolescent with spastic hemiparesis performing a motor task, his or her postural changes still seem very awkward. Such awkward postures, however, can also be observed in people who have not sustained any brain damage. An example is the excessively cramped writing postures that young children frequently display during the initial stages of mastering the complex skill of handwriting. Surprisingly, the quality of the output of these children's' writing attempts is not affected by these strange postures (Sassoon et al., 1986). Likewise, children with spastic hemiparesis are also surprisingly successful in performing most daily tasks despite their deviant motor behavior. An important question here is how these children managed to adapt to the damage to their brain to the extent that they are able to perform the tasks as efficiently as they do. Another relevant question is why some tasks remain impossible for them to perform and others not. We keep these questions in mind as we review a series of studies on prehension movements.

Having formulated the main goal of our review, that is, looking for signs of adaptation in grasping movements performed by children with spastic hemiparesis, we first discuss ways in which our search can profit from insights obtained in the study of adaptation on an evolutionary time scale.

## Signs of Adaptation at Different Time Scales: Evolution

On the phylogenetic time scale, Darwin showed that evolution is guided by a process of random variation and guided selection. Only those species survive that are best fitted to the prevailing environmental contingencies, hence the well-known principle of "survival of the fittest" of which many explanations (e.g., Gould, 1992), implications (the most notorious being social Darwinism), and variations (e.g., neural Darwinism; Edelman, 1987) have been formulated. Some of the important claims and caveats of Darwin's theory are relevant to our search for signs of long-term adaptation to permanent brain damage.

The basic tenet of the theory is that of random variation. For a species to evolve, and thus survive, it has to produce random variations in its design or makeup. The way in which these variations are instigated is still heavily debated within the scientific community concerned with evolution (Gould, 1992). What is clear, however, is that without variation a new species cannot evolve, or, to put it bluntly, evolution would come to a dead end. The capacity for variation is the driving force behind evolution and provides a playground where new solutions can be tried out. This is one of the main differences between machines and organisms, as the former do not have redundancy and therefore will always have difficulties adapting to environmental contingencies. Consequently, in the context of the present search for signs of long-term adaptation to permanent brain damage, the first sign, or rather prerequisite, of adaptation we need to look for is redundancy in the neuromotor system or in the particular ways the tasks under study are performed.

A potential caveat in Darwin's theory is relevant to mention here. If only the best-fitted organisms survive, then the danger of overspecialization lurks. Surely, bacteria cannot be said to have altered their basic makeup to a large extent over their many years of survival. Still, they are among the organisms with the longest evolutionary history. The danger of overspecialization becomes painfully clear nowadays, when many species (e.g., panda bears) are endangered because their natural habitat (bamboo forest) is taken over by other species (humans mostly). Species that are flexible enough to alter their makeup or habits (i.e., that remain capable of producing random variation) will survive, but others will become extinct. An example of this is coyotes, which developed a way of living alongside humans, whereas their close relatives, the wolves, remain shy and consequently see their natural habitat shrinking.

It is outside the scope of this chapter to explore evolutionary theories further, but for the present purposes two things should be noted. First, to be successful in adapting to alterations in the environment, a species should have some redundancy in its makeup or habits. Second, overadaptation leads to rigidity, eventually leading to extinction.

## Ontogeny

The signs of adaptation that we are particularly interested in here are those that occur during the course of a life span. Later we present examples of such signs derived from studies on unrestricted reaching and grasping movements in children with cerebral palsy. We focus on "deviant" characteristics of these movements. The recurring and difficult question to be answered is whether the deviations are due to organismic limitations or, alternatively, should be seen as efficient adaptation to these constraints. The studies we discuss were conducted mainly in our own lab, but other studies are mentioned as well. For reading convenience, we do not include details of the experimental procedures. These are mentioned only when vital for understanding the studies.

Studies of children with cerebral palsy who are diagnosed with spastic hemiparesis can shed light on adaptation for two reasons. First, as indicated earlier, these children's brain damage dates back from birth, so they have had many years to adapt to their altered movement systems. In our attempt to discern signs of long-term adaptation processes, we studied *unrestricted* grasping movements so that the full adaptive capacity of the movement system could become visible. In our view, restricting movements in one way or another (e.g., by not allowing trunk movement)—although interesting from the point of view of studying adaptation under boundary conditions—may obscure the view of natural adaptation processes. Second, because of the lateralized nature of the disorder, comparisons between both body sides can be made within a child. Even though these within-subject analyses have methodological advantages, comparisons between the affected and unaffected body side need to be made with care since proximal movements are controlled bilaterally (e.g., Aglioti et al., 1993; Wiesendanger et al., 1994). The distal movements of the hand and fingers that are realized near grasp completion, however, are unilaterally controlled (e.g., Di Stefano et al., 1980). Consequently, signs of adaptation can most validly be discerned in movements of the hand and fingers contralateral to the damaged hemisphere.

The approach that we take here is rather straightforward. It consists of dividing the prehension act into a number of constituent parts and examining the performance deviations in each part separately. The deviations in movement coordination on the impaired side are compared with the performance of the unimpaired side or the performance of control subjects without neurological deficits. By scrutinizing the performance deviations on the impaired side, we try to capture possible optimization or efficiency principles that may guide the behavior. If such principles can be distinguished, we reason that the behavior under study shows signs of adaptation since these principles imply the presence of redundancy. If, however, such principles cannot be found, we conclude that the aspects we analyzed do not show any sign of adaptation. In the latter case, we conclude that the behavior is rigid and most likely reflects the impairment proper (see Mulder et al., 2001). Our expectations regarding deviant performance characteristics stem from existing knowledge on the cause and symptoms of hemiparetic cerebral palsy.

## Spastic Hemiparesis and Cerebral Palsy

All participants in the studies discussed in this chapter have spastic hemiparesis as a consequence of cerebral palsy. In general, spasticity is characterized by a velocity-dependent permanent increase in tonic reflexes that results in an excessive and awkward activation of skeletal muscles (cf. Barnes et al., 1994; Lance, 1980). Historically, it was assumed that the increase in resistance to passive movement was due to exaggerated stretch reflexes. Dietz et al. (1981), however, provided evidence that altered mechanical properties of muscles may also contribute to hypertonicity in spastic individuals. Therefore, the increased muscle tone (i.e., hypertonia) may stem from both neural and nonneural components (for a discussion, see O'Dwyer and Ada, 1996; O'Dwyer et al., 1996).

The nonneural components reflect the changes in muscle and connective tissue that in turn lead to an increased resistance to lengthening. Muscle contracture, a shortening of the muscle length as a consequence of a decrease in the number of sarcomeres, can be regarded as a major contributor to increased resistance to passive stretch. It is well known that the number of sarcomeres is not fixed but can change, even in adult muscle (Tabary et al., 1972; Williams and Goldspink, 1973). It is apparent that permanent loss of sarcomeres is accompanied by alterations in the length–tension curve. The reduced compliance (i.e., reduced flexibility of the muscle) can probably also be attributed to a remodeling of muscle connective tissue (Goldspink and Williams, 1990; O'Dwyer et al., 1989). The range of motion may therefore be reduced both by the shortening of the muscle fibers and by the loss of muscle compliance.

The neural basis of hypertonia, on the other hand, reflects deviant motor unit activity, in particular, stretch-reflex-generated muscle activity in reaction to muscle lengthening. In addition, decreased central inhibitory signals to the antagonist muscles further promote hypertonia.

Cerebral palsy, or "disease of the brain," most frequently occurs before, during, or immediately following birth as a consequence of lack of oxygen to the immature brain. It may, however, also result from (the removal of) a brain tumor. Cerebral palsy has been defined in a variety of different ways (e.g., Balf and Ingram, 1955; Bax, 1964; Ingram, 1966; Kurland, 1957; MacKeith et al., 1959). Bax (1964, p. 297), for example, defined it as "a non-progressive disorder of movement and posture due to a defect or lesion of the immature brain." In spite of the fact that the underlying disorder is nonprogressive, the classification of cerebral palsy is made difficult by the fact that the central nervous system develops very quickly during early childhood. As a consequence, the clinical expression of cerebral palsy in an individual child may not be stable but subject to alterations. This is particularly so in very young children. The subjects participating in the studies reviewed here, however, were between 14 and 20 years of age at the time that the studies were conducted, and their conditions were described at the time as relatively stable.

## Components of the Grasping Movement

The final issue that needs to be discussed before we turn to the prehension studies is a decomposition of the prehension act. Figure 9.1 shows such a tentative decomposition.

Suppose you want to pick up a cup of coffee. The first thing you need to do is to plan an appropriate grip with which to grasp the cup. The type of grip employed strongly depends on what you intend to do with the cup. Do you just want

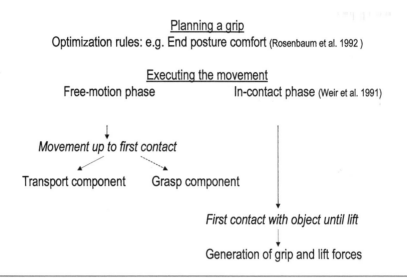

**Figure 9.1**    Tentative decomposition of the prehension movement into its elements.

to transport the cup, turn it over to empty it in the sink, or place it somewhere else with high precision? After establishing the goal, you need to transport one of your hands to the cup. During this transport the movements of the different components of the body (i.e., trunk, arm, and hand) need to be precisely coordinated, and the hand with which you chose to grasp the cup needs to be opened and closed in time so that the cup is grasped rather than missed or collided into. Once the finger and thumb make contact with the surface of the cup, the appropriate amount of grip and load forces need to be exerted so that the cup can be elevated without letting it slip away or crushing it between the fingers.

    Although the description of the prehension act just given is a simplified schema, it already demonstrates that the planning and coordination of this seemingly simple act is quite complex and involves many processes. In the remainder of this chapter we review similar analyses of prehension movements and highlight the deviations that we observed in different components of the grasping movements performed by children with spastic hemiparesis. Deviations in grip planning, interjoint coordination during the free-motion phase, and grip force control during the in-contact phase are discussed successively.

## Grip Planning

In the majority of grasping actions, we pick up objects for a certain purpose, and this purpose may already be partly unveiled in the type of grip that is employed at the start. Although it may appear to be an exercise in fortune telling, the following example may clarify this. Consider the acts of picking up a needle for sewing and a hammer for nailing: The first is a task with high precision demands, while the second demands quite some force. Each object, or tool, is picked up with a different grip. When high precision is demanded, as in the case of the needle, the object is picked up with a precision grip in which it is held between the fingers of one hand (cf. Napier, 1956). In contrast, for the forceful task, a power grip is used in which the tool is clamped firmly in the palm of the hand. Both grip types are well suited for the purpose of the tasks. Furthermore, the examples clarify that the end goal of the task to a large extent determines the grip type that is employed for picking up the object. This observation implies a process of planning that takes place before the movement is initiated but after the goals for the prehension task have been selected either consciously or unconsciously.

Rosenbaum and co-workers have taken this observation to the laboratory for systematic experimental research. In several studies they showed that individuals initially pick up objects in such a way that they can end a task with the arm and hand adopting a comfortable posture (Rosenbaum et al., 1990, 1993; Rosenbaum and Jorgensen, 1992). We discuss two tasks here in more detail, a bar transport task and a handle rotation task.

In the bar transport task, subjects had to pick up a bar that was placed horizontally on a cradle and subsequently place it vertically with one of the ends on a designated spot on the table (Rosenbaum and Jorgensen, 1992). Since the bar was on a cradle, subjects could grasp it with either an underhand grip (palm of the hand facing upward and forearm supinated) or an overhand grip (palm of the hand facing downward and forearm in a relatively neutral position). Both grips were rated differently in terms of awkwardness by the subjects, with the overhand grip as least awkward. From this it may be hypothesized that subjects would use only an overhand grip to pick up the bar, under the assumption that they plan only the start of the bar transport movement and not its end. However, the results showed that an underhand grip was also used to pick up the bar, and this use was not random. Rather, it was found that subjects consistently employed an underhand grip at the start when it assured them of attaining a comfortable posture of the arm and hand at the end of the task (a posture in which the thumb side of the hand points upward). According to Rosenbaum and co-workers, these results indicate that subjects plan end postures. Subjects sometimes sacrifice comfort at the start for the sake of ending comfortably.

In the second task, subjects had to rotate a pointer on a clock face to different positions from various starting positions (e.g., Rosenbaum et al., 1993). This setup allowed a more meticulous measurement of the effect of end-posture comfort. Again, planning for comfortable end postures was seen. A grip type was selected at the start that ensured that the arm–hand system was in a comfortable posture at the end of the task. Other studies followed up on these and also proved planning for comfortable end postures (e.g., Short and Cauraugh, 1997, 1999).

This raises the question of why people optimize the comfort of the end posture. Several explanations have been put forward, but the most promising one is that a comfortable posture allows more precision (the precision hypothesis; e.g. Rosenbaum et al., 1996; Short and Cauraugh, 1999), owing to a more optimal signal-to-noise ratio (e.g. Rossetti et al., 1994).

Do subjects with spastic hemiparesis employ the same so-called optimization rule (maximizing the comfort of the end posture) when they pick up objects, or is their optimization rule systematically different from subjects without neurological disorders? Stated differently, is the deviant movement behavior observed in this group of subjects a result of disorders in grip planning? Do they anticipate the end posture of the arm–hand system when they pick up objects? To answer these questions, we had subjects with spastic hemiparesis perform both a bar-handling task and a clock rotation task (Steenbergen, Hulstijn, and Dortmans, 2000). The bar-handling task was similar to the one used by Rosenbaum and Jorgensen (1992). Subjects had to pick up a bar that was placed horizontally on a cradle and subsequently had to put it vertically in a box on either one of the two ends. As an elaboration, the location of the boxes in the work space varied. Five boxes were placed in a semicircle around the subject, but always 30 cm distant from the cradle. This was well within the functional range of motion. Subjects used both their impaired as well as their unimpaired hand to pick up the bar. In addition to scoring the actual performance (grip used, overhand versus underhand at the start resulting in either thumb up or thumb down at the end), we also asked subjects to rate the awkwardness of the different postures at the start and end, from 1, "not awkward," to 5, "very awkward." A control group was also tested as a validation of the experimental setup.

Figure 9.2 shows the percentages of grips used that resulted in a comfortable end posture. Similar to the subjects of Rosenbaum and Jorgensen (1992), the control group adapted their starting grip so that they would end the task attaining a comfortable posture with the thumb pointing upward in the majority of trials (figure 9.2, right bar). This was not the case for the individuals with spastic hemiparesis. With their unimpaired hand these individuals appear to be indifferent with respect to their grip

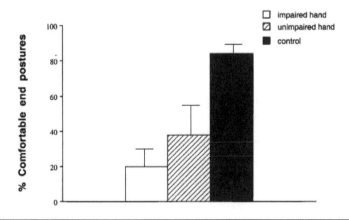

**Figure 9.2** Percentage of starting grips that led to a comfortable end posture used by a control group, the unimpaired side of subjects with spastic hemiparesis, and the impaired side of subjects with spastic hemiparesis.

choice. That is, they did not consistently employ a grip type that would enable them to end the task in a comfortable posture (figure 9.2, middle bar). Clearly, end-posture comfort was not used as an optimization rule for this hand. From the comfort ratings of this hand it became clear that subjects did not discriminate among the different postures in terms of awkwardness. All possible postures were rated as 1, "not awkward." Given this finding, it was not surprising to find no preference for a particular end posture, as comfort was not differentiated between postures. With the impaired hand, the percentage of grips employed that led to a comfortable ending was even smaller (figure 9.2, left bar; approximately 20%), pointing to the fact that end-posture comfort was not an optimization rule for this hand. Indeed, the overall difference between ratings for the thumbs-up and thumbs-down end posture was rather small (averages of 0.9 and 2.3, respectively), while the difference in ratings between overhand and underhand start posture were far more distinct (1.4 and 4.4, respectively). Nonetheless, it could not be concluded from the performance with the impaired hand that start posture comfort was optimized.

Given these results, we examined whether total posture comfort might be employed as an optimization rule for grip planning with the impaired hand. To that aim, two possible manners of task completion were distinguished. One starts with an underhand grip (supination of the forearm) and ends with a thumbs-up posture, while the other starts with an overhand grip and ends with a thumbs-down posture. The majority of subjects gave the movement combination starting with an overhand grip posture and ending with a thumbs-down posture a lower average awkwardness rating, and used this combination most often. This suggests that, rather than optimizing end-posture comfort, subjects with spastic hemiparesis optimized total posture comfort.

To test the assumption of optimization of total comfort, we asked the same subjects to perform a clock rotation task. Specifically, we examined whether optimization of total comfort, operationalized as the reduction of the total joint rotations, determined grip selection for the impaired hand. Subjects had to grasp a bar that was mounted on a clock face and turn one of the ends to the top position (i.e., 12 o'clock on an analog clock) without altering their grip during rotation. The clock face was divided into 15 positions that served as starting positions. Hand posture at the end was scored. Two end postures were possible, thumbs up (comfortable end) and thumbs down (uncomfortable end). For the test of optimization of total comfort, we determined the potential (theoretical) task solutions for each of the 15 starting positions separately and calculated the amount of joint rotation necessary for each task solution. For each starting position, at least two ways to complete the task were possible. The task solution that required the least joint rotation was compared with the actual performance of the subjects. The results showed that grips were employed with the impaired hand that ensured a minimal total amount of joint rotation. Again, subjects did not optimize comfort of the end posture, as they ended in a thumbs-down posture as well. In these instances, this end posture enabled them to minimize the total amount of joint rotation.

Taken together, the results suggest that grip planning for the impaired hand is adapted to the motion difficulties of the joints of this body side. Movements with this hand are difficult to perform, resulting in grips that decreased these movements. It has to be noted that both experiments were not very stringent with respect to the endpoint accuracy that had to be achieved. Therefore, we followed up on these experiments by manipulating endpoint accuracy, under the assumption that increased accuracy constraints at the end would force a comfortable ending, given the increased signal-to-noise ratio in this comfort range (the precision hypothesis; e.g. Rosenbaum et al., 1996; Rossetti et al., 1994; Short and Cauraugh, 1999).

In the follow-up experiment, a variation of the bar-handling task was used (Steenbergen et al., submitted). Subjects had to pick up a pencil from a cradle and use it to place a dot in a circle that was drawn on a sheet of paper. Endpoint accuracy was manipulated by varying the diameter of the target circle (0.6 cm and 3.5 cm). The results for the unimpaired hand showed that for both the large and small circle sizes, subjects optimized comfort of the end posture and ended with a thumbs-up posture. Concurrently, realized precision was high; most dots were placed inside the circles. To comply with the instruction to place the dots within the circle, subjects adapted their grips so that they ended in a comfortable posture. In this posture range, the signal-to-noise ratio is apparently optimal and allowed high precision to be attained. With the impaired hand, it was found that optimization of start comfort, and to a less degree total comfort, was a constraint on grip selection. These results suggest that grip planning per se is not disturbed in subjects with spastic hemiparesis. Rather, they point to a specific planning rule being employed that is closely adapted to the constraints of the moving organ.

With respect to the latter, we also showed that meaningfulness or significance of the task influenced grip selection of the unimpaired hand (Steenbergen et al., submitted) . If meaningfulness of the task increased (from just picking up a bar and turning it over to picking up a glass and turning it over to picking up a glass, turning it over, and filling it with water), the tendency to plan comfortable end postures increased, especially in individuals with right spastic hemiparesis.

Adaptation or impairment? Taken collectively, these results suggest that in the domain of grip planning, subjects with spastic hemiparesis are able to adapt their starting grip to both task constraints (unimpaired hand) and organismic constraints (impaired hand). Grip planning per se is not disturbed but appears to be closely adapted to the constraints imposed even though it leads to ostensibly deviant behavioral outcomes. The demonstration that the subjects applied optimization rules and were capable of selecting among alternative courses of action shows that their deviant ways of grasping objects reflect adaptation.

## *The Total Grasping Movement: From Start to Pick-Up*

As stated earlier, a methodological advantage of the study of spastic hemiparesis is the within-subject comparison of the impaired and unimpaired side. It is clear that the movement behavior of one body side is very different from the other. One of the most obvious differences is the total time that it takes to complete tasks. Total movement duration is one of the most frequently used assessment scores in the practical field (e.g., occupational therapy). Many dexterity tests measure the time it takes to complete a task (e.g. McPhee, 1987). In this context, total movement duration is even considered to be an index of the level of impairment. Although total movement duration may be a very useful measure for practical and assessment use, for intervention purposes it gives few clues about the processes that are disturbed. Moreover, it does not shed any light on the way in which movements are performed, which components are particularly impaired, or how subjects have adapted to their disorder. If an intervention program is to have any impact, manual control needs to be decomposed into its constituent parts (e.g. Wann et al., 1998). Establishing the processes that are involved in these components and measuring their duration may shed more light on the specific disorder.

A grasping movement can be decomposed into a free-motion phase, involving the transport of the hand to the object and the opening and closing of the hand, and an in-contact phase, in which grip and load forces are applied to the object. Measuring these components separately may clarify the cause of the slowness in grasping with the impaired hand. We had subjects with spastic hemiparesis grasp disks 50 mm in diameter and subsequently lift them to a height of approximately 2 cm (Steenbergen, Hulstijn, Lemmens, and Meulenbroek, 1998). At the start of each trial, subjects placed one hand on a start button. A switch underneath this start button permitted a consistent measurement of the start of the movement. Underneath the target disk a second switch was placed for consistent measurement of the end of the task. The time between the triggering of both switches was the measure of the total duration of the movement. A third landmark was the velocity profile of the hand. As the hand approached the target disk, its velocity decreased to nearly zero (we used 5% of peak velocity as the cutoff). At this point in time, the hand had reached the object and closed. The time between this moment and the disk lift was the measure of the duration of the in-contact phase. The duration between movement onset and zero velocity provided a measure of the duration of the free-motion phase.

In figure 9.3, the duration of the different phases is displayed. As expected, total movement duration of the impaired hand was longer than that of the unimpaired hand. The largest difference between the hands occurred during the in-contact phase rather than the free-motion phase. The duration of the in-contact phase for the unimpaired hand was rather small. Subjects approached the object, grasped it, and almost instantly lifted it. This was different for the impaired hand, for which a very large in-contact duration was found. This may indicate that subjects had difficulties grasping the object and generating the right amount of force with this hand, an aspect that we discuss later in this section.

Adaptation or impairment? This analysis of the decomposed grasping movement provides more insight into the components that are most affected. Although there were the differences in duration of the free-motion phase between both body sides, the largest proportional difference was in the in-contact phase. This result indicates that the largest movement difficulties for the spastic arm are distal, that

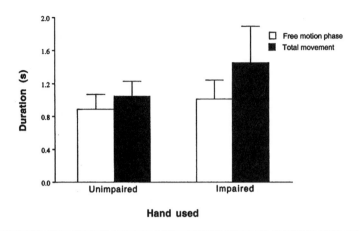

**Figure 9.3**    Duration of the free-motion phase and total movement for the unimpaired and impaired sides.

is, at the fingers. A step deeper into the deficiencies in both phases can be obtained by looking at (1) the coordination of the different elements during the free-motion phase and (2) force development during the in-contact phase.

## *The Free-Motion Phase*

The free-motion phase consists of two components: grasping and transport. This section also describes inter-segment and inter-joint coordination during transport.

### Grasp Component

In the free-motion phase, the hand is brought to the object, and during this transport the hand is typically opened larger than the diameter of the target object. The closing of the hand around the object is a landmark that signifies the end of the free-motion phase. Shown in figure 9.4 are the aperture profiles of both the impaired and unimpaired hand when grasping a 6-cm object. Note the flat tails at the end of the profiles of the impaired hand. Because the profiles show the hand opening from start to object lift, the flat tails represent the time that the hand is in contact with the object before it is lifted. It may also be noted from these profiles that hand opening and closing proceeds more smoothly in the unimpaired hand. Profiles of the impaired hand show a very undulating pattern, suggesting pronounced feedback-controlled regulation of the finger movements during hand opening and closing.

To gain insight into the question of whether hemiparesis is merely a peripheral muscular co-contraction disorder or also a more central parameterization problem, we examined peak aperture as a function of object size. Peak aperture is linearly related to object size in healthy individuals (e.g., Marteniuk et al., 1990). We had subjects with spastic hemiparesis grasp disks either 4, 6, or 8 cm in diameter, and we examined

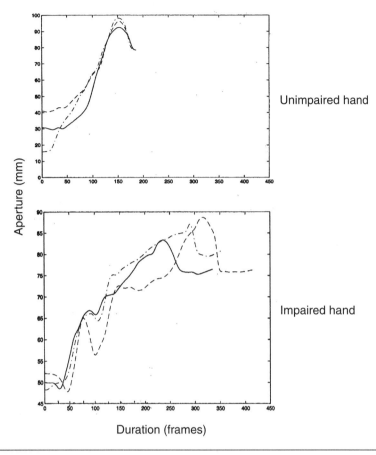

**Figure 9.4**    Hand aperture profiles for the unimpaired and impaired hands.

peak aperture as a function of disk size (Steenbergen and Van der Kamp, submitted). Aperture was defined as the absolute distance between the marker placed on the index finger and the marker placed on the thumb. Figure 9.5 shows peak aperture as a function of object size for both the impaired and unimpaired hand.

Both hands show a similar pattern of results. With an increase in object size, peak aperture increased accordingly. However, despite this similarity, there was a difference between the two hands. Closer inspection of figure 9.5 reveals that the peak aperture for the impaired hand was consistently larger. To examine this in more detail, we analyzed the overshoot in peak aperture as a function of hand used and object size. Overshoot was defined as the absolute distance between the thumb marker and index finger marker at peak aperture minus this distance at the moment of contact with the object. Note that this calculation corrects for differences among subjects in marker placement on the thumb and index finger. The results are displayed in figure 9.6.

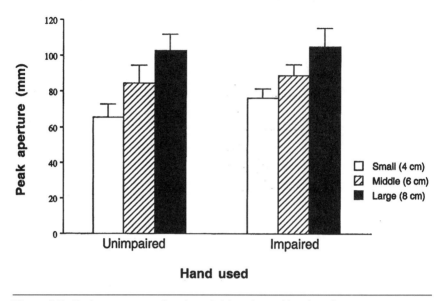

**Figure 9.5** Peak aperture as a function of object size and hand used.

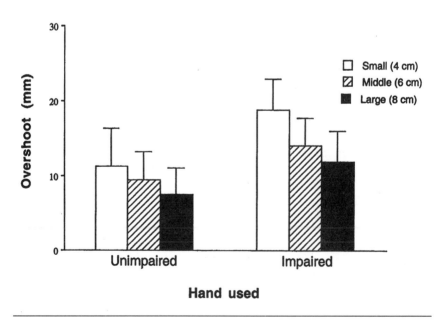

**Figure 9.6** Overshoot of hand aperture as a function of object size and hand used. See text for details on the calculation of overshoot.

It is clear from figure 9.6 that overshoot for the impaired hand was larger than for the unimpaired hand. This may signify that subjects increased the safety margin for grasping. By opening the hand more widely, they were less liable to bump into or push over the object. In addition, overshoot varied inversely with object size. With smaller objects, a larger overshoot was observed for both hands. This effect may point to a precision effect, as smaller objects demand more precision.

Adaptation or impairment? Taken collectively, the studies on grip aperture indicate that, although hand opening and closing do not proceed as smoothly in the impaired hand as in the unimpaired hand, adaptation to object size is still possible, albeit with a larger safety margin. These results suggest that central parameterization of hand opening to object size is still intact but that the more peripheral impairment disturbs smooth aperture formation.

## Transport Component

Besides hand opening and closing, the hand needs to be transported to the object in the free-motion phase by movements of the trunk, shoulder, elbow, and wrist joints. In this section we examine the contribution of the different segments to the transport of the hand. We then discuss the timing between shoulder and wrist displacement at movement onset and at peak velocity, and the coordination between shoulder and elbow in joint-angle space.

*Contribution of Different Segments to Wrist Transport*    In general, the transport of the wrist in grasping movements is brought about mainly by angular changes in the shoulder and elbow joints. As stated earlier, in subjects with spastic hemiparesis the functional range of motion in the elbow joint is reduced as a consequence of increased antagonistic activity. While there is ample evidence for this so-called hypertonia from neurophysiological studies, we sought to find out how it affects the coordination in functional movements. More specifically, how does the system solve the degrees-of-freedom problem when the characteristics of some of these degrees of freedom are altered or limited? Is the system capable of drawing upon other degrees of freedom for the successful completion of the task? In addition, what can the deployment of extra (formerly "silent") degrees of freedom tell us about central control processes?

Figure 9.7 shows typical examples of velocity profiles of the end effector—namely, the wrist—when approaching an object. The velocity profiles of the unimpaired wrist are very similar to the profiles frequently observed for grasping movements in subjects without movement disorders. That is, the profiles are smooth and bell shaped, with one clear velocity peak. The profiles of the impaired hand differ greatly from this. The profiles are multipeaked and undulating. Smooth transport to the object, as observed for the unimpaired hand, is not seen for the impaired hand. Furthermore, the profiles are positively skewed, indicating that subjects need additional time to home in on the object. The deceleration phase of the movement is considerably prolonged. Can we find clues in the angular changes of, and coordination between, segments that underlie these typical kinematic profiles of the impaired hand?

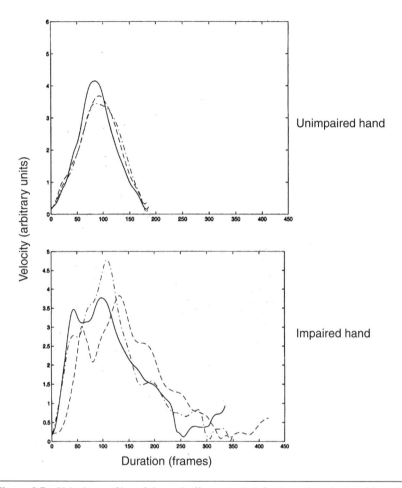

**Figure 9.7**    Velocity profiles of the end effector (wrist) for the unimpaired and impaired hands.

The first step for discovering such clues is to examine the contribution of the different joints and trunk to the transport of the hand to the object (see also Steenbergen, Van Thiel, Hulstijn, and Meulenbroek, 2000). As the elbow has only one degree of freedom (flexion and extension), calculation of this angle is straightforward. This angle was calculated as the angle formed by the line segment of the wrist and elbow marker and the line segment of the shoulder and elbow marker. Calculating the shoulder angle was less straightforward, since this joint has more than one degree of freedom. For this joint we calculated two angles. The first angle represents a 2D projection on the horizontal plane, and we called this angle shoulder flexion. The second angle represents the 2D projection on the sagittal plane and was denoted shoulder elevation. Figure 9.8 shows the changes of the three angles during movement execution for both the unimpaired and impaired side.

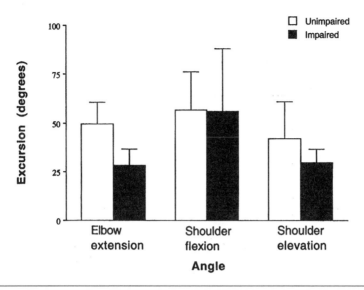

**Figure 9.8**    Contribution of elbow extension, shoulder flexion, and shoulder elevation to the grasping movement for the unimpaired and impaired sides.

As expected, the angular change in the elbow joint of the impaired side was substantially smaller (28.1°) than that of the unimpaired side (49.5°). Hence, the contribution of the elbow joint to the transport of the impaired hand was significantly decreased. A similar reduction was observed for shoulder elevation. Whereas angular change in shoulder elevation for the unimpaired side was quite substantial (41.9°), it was decreased on the impaired side (29.5°). Conversely, the amount of shoulder flexion was similar for both body sides, 56.5° for the unimpaired side and 55.8° for the impaired side.

Given this reduction in angular motion at the shoulder and elbow joints, it is interesting to examine how the object was reached. Since most of the transport movement is generally brought about by angular changes in these joints, the reductions on the impaired side beg the question of how the object was actually reached. To examine this, we looked at the displacement of both the ipsilateral and contralateral shoulder in the y direction, which was the main axis of movement. The displacement of both shoulders informs us about the contribution of the trunk to movement completion. Differentiating between both shoulders discriminates trunk translation (which involves both shoulders by an even amount) from trunk rotation (one of the two shoulders moves to a larger extent). Figure 9.9 displays the results of this analysis.

For both the impaired and unimpaired sides, most of the displacement was brought about by movement of the ipsilateral shoulder. However, when grasping with the impaired hand, the displacement of the ipsilateral (hence, impaired) shoulder was almost twice the displacement of the unimpaired shoulder when moving the unimpaired hand (see figure 9.9). To get a clearer picture of the type of trunk

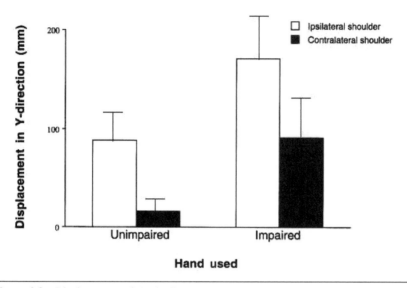

**Figure 9.9**   Displacement of the ipsilateral shoulder and contralateral shoulder for the unimpaired and impaired sides.

involvement, namely, rotation or translation, we also considered the displacement of the contralateral shoulder. Again, the displacement of this shoulder was larger when moving the impaired hand. However, the extent of this displacement was as much as the displacement of the ipsilateral shoulder when moving the unimpaired hand (compare the fourth with the first bar in figure 9.9). The difference between ipsilateral and contralateral shoulder displacement, a measure that indicates trunk rotation, was similar for both body sides (see figure 9.9). Stated differently, the trunk rotation component was constant irrespective of the hand with which the movement was performed. In combination with the increased displacement of both the contra- and ipsilateral shoulder during movements with the impaired hand, this result indicates that the displacement of the impaired hand was brought about by an increased translation of the trunk on top of its "basic" rotation.

Adaptation or impairment? Taken collectively, the results of our study of the contribution of the different effector segments show that both elbow extension and shoulder elevation are decreased on the impaired side, possibly due to decreased muscle compliance and contractures. Subjects adapt to this decrease by increasing the amount of trunk translation in order to be able to reach the target.

*Sequencing Between Shoulder and Wrist Displacement*   As a further test of the coordination between the proximal shoulder displacement and distal wrist displacement, we examined the sequencing of both segments at two discrete temporal landmarks in effector space. First, we determined a measure of onset asynchrony by subtracting movement onset of the shoulder from the movement onset of the wrist. Second, a measure of peak-velocity asynchrony was assessed by subtracting the moment of peak velocity of the shoulder from that of the wrist (see also Van Thiel and Steenbergen, 2001). The results showed that for both the unimpaired and impaired hand, the shoulder started to move before the wrist, yielding positive values. This onset asynchrony was larger on the unimpaired side. At peak velocity the asynchrony was reversed. For both the impaired as well as the unimpaired side, peak velocity of the hand was reached prior to peak velocity of the shoulder. Still, the time between both peaks was significantly larger on the impaired side. Peak-velocity asynchrony was small on the unimpaired side, signifying that both body segments reached peak velocity at virtually the same points in time.

Adaptation or impairment? These findings suggest that, on the impaired side, both arm segments move in isolation and that their relative contributions are reversed as the movement unfolds. On the unimpaired side, apart from an initial asynchrony at the start of movement, both segments appear to become synchronized during the course of the movement. To obtain a clearer view of this matter, we examined the relationship between shoulder-joint and elbow-joint rotations.

*Coordination in Joint-Angle Space*    In joint-angle space we looked at the coordination between two joint-angle pairs, shoulder flexion/elbow extension and shoulder elevation/elbow extension. Coordination between shoulder and elbow on the unimpaired side is smooth. Increases in shoulder elevation and flexion parallel an increase in elbow extension, signifying a tight coupling between both joint pairs on the unimpaired side. Again, this was different on the impaired side. The results showed that the shoulder joint was flexed first, with only a small angular change in the elbow joint. As shoulder flexion reached approximately 140°, the elbow joint started to extend. For the elbow extension/shoulder elevation coupling, a similar phenomenon was found. Movements started with elevation in the shoulder joint and little elbow extension, followed by an increase in elbow extension and a concurrent decrease in shoulder elevation. This pattern points to segmentation of the movement in joint-angle space.

Adaptation or impairment? Summing up the findings of coordination in joint-angle space, we can conclude that movements on the impaired side were clearly segmented. Rotations of the joints were performed more serially than simultaneously. This segmentation points to independent control of the joints on this side. It can be presumed that segmentation of the movement is a manner in which the total set of degrees of freedom of the altered action system is compressed to render control possible (cf. Bernstein, 1967). Segmentation of the movement, that is, moving the shoulder and elbow in relative isolation, may obviate the increased stretch reflexes that might occur if both segments move simultaneously. For the unimpaired side, the angle–angle plots result in a fairly straight line, indicating strict dependence of the movement from one joint on movement from the other joint, hence a tight coupling between both joints.

## In-Contact Phase: Generation of Grip and Load Forces

Earlier we showed that the duration of the in-contact phase especially was lengthened on the impaired side. What is the possible cause of this extended contact with the object before it is lifted? During the in-contact phase, forces have to be applied to the object in order to lift it. Two types of forces can be distinguished in this respect, a grip force, which is applied perpendicularly to the surface of the object by the thumb and index finger and serves to hold the object, and a load force, which serves to lift the object. In a number of experiments, Johansson and Westling (1984, 1988a, 1988b, 1990) examined the application of these forces in a healthy subject population. They found a parallel generation of grip and load forces. In addition, they found that heavier objects elicited a faster increase in grip and load forces, but over an extended period of time, resulting in an increased duration before the object started to move (Johansson and Westling, 1988a).

Weir et al. (1991) examined the duration of the free-motion and in-contact phase when objects differing in weight (20, 55, 150, and 410 g) were picked up. Their findings corresponded with those of Johansson and Westling and indicated that the time needed for the application of the appropriate force level is reflected in the duration of the in-contact phase. Hence, the in-contact phase forms a kinematic representation of the sum of the preload phase (when the grip is established and grip force increases until a positive increase in load force occurs) and the load phase (when grip and load forces increase in parallel until they overcome gravity and the object starts to move), as distinguished by Johansson and Westling (1984).

The application of grip and load forces by children with cerebral palsy was the focus of a number of studies by Eliasson et al. (1991, 1992, 1995). They showed that children with cerebral palsy needed additional time in the preload phase because the increase in grip force was accompanied by a negative load force at first and the onset of a positive load force was delayed in comparison with healthy subjects. In a group of subjects with hemiparetic cerebral palsy, we examined the effect of object weight on the timing of the grasping movement by dividing the total action into a free-motion phase and an in-contact phase (Steenbergen et al., 1998). Two object weights were used (20 g and 200 g). In addition to determining the duration of the in-contact phase for these weights, we also examined whether subjects with hemiparetic cerebral palsy were able to control and modify the force output in advance on the basis of weight information from a previous lift. For healthy subjects, Johansson and Westling (1988a) showed that the necessary grip and load forces are planned in advance based on a weight that was lifted previously. Weir et al. (1991) showed that this anticipatory timing could also be revealed in the kinematic features of the movement (the duration of the in-contact phase). In children with cerebral palsy, Eliasson et al. (1992) showed impaired anticipatory programming of isometric force output before liftoff. In a separate study, however, Eliasson et al. (1995) showed that, when allowed enough lifts with an object of a given texture, children with cerebral palsy were able to scale the amount of isometric grip force to the frictional conditions of the object.

Assuming a correspondence between force application and contact duration, we examined whether subjects with hemiparetic cerebral palsy were able to modify force output in advance on the basis of information about weight picked up in preceding lifts. Objects were presented in both randomized and blocked (same weight within a condition) order. Two experiments were performed. In the first experiment, no speed demands were imposed, whereas in the second experiment, speed of response was stressed. The results of the first study confirmed the difficulties present in the in-contact phase. The duration of this phase was prolonged to a large degree in the impaired hand as compared with the unimpaired hand. Overall, the duration of the in-contact phase amounted to 470 ms for the impaired hand but 139 ms for the unimpaired hand. Furthermore, the results showed that the initial lift with the light weight that was preceded by a lift of the heavier weight displayed a longer time in contact, suggesting that force programming for the light weight was based on the heavier weight. Interestingly, this effect decreased after only two consecutive lifts with the light weight, indicating adaptation of force generation to the actual weight. Still, the increased duration of the in-contact phase in the impaired hand compared with the unimpaired hand remained. In a second experiment, we examined whether this contact lengthening by the impaired side was a higher-order movement strategy adapted to the disorder, that is, a strategy to ensure that the established grip is accurate before lifting the object. One possible way to circumvent such a strategy is to instruct subjects to move as quickly as possible, thereby ensuring quick force development. This was done in the second experiment with the same object weights. The results of this experiment showed that the typical duration of the free-motion phase relative to the in-contact phase remained intact on the impaired side. That is, the increased duration of the in-contact phase for the impaired hand remained unaltered. It can be concluded from this result that the disproportionate prolongation of the in-contact phase represents a pathological constant in subjects with hemiparetic cerebral palsy, not a side effect of a higher-order movement strategy.

Adaptation or impairment? Taken collectively, the results of the in-contact phase experiments suggest that subjects with cerebral palsy have difficulties controlling the distal musculature of the impaired hand and fingers. They need additional time during this phase to build up the necessary forces. Despite this impairment, they were able to adapt the force level to the different object weights.

## Conclusions

In this chapter we provided an overview of behavioral phenomena that reflect either adaptive planning and coordination or rigidity in grasping movements by subjects with spastic hemiparesis. We examined deviations in the different components of the grasping movement in the impaired hand for signs of long-term adaptation to permanent damage to the brain. In this section we summarize the deviant patterns that we observed in the different components of the movement and

<u>Grip planning</u>

*Optimization of total comfort*


<u>Executing the movement</u>
**Free-motion phase    &    In-contact phase**
*Slowness of responding predominantly due to increased in-contact duration*

**Grasp component**
*Undulating hand opening and closing profiles*
*Scaling of peak aperture to object diameter*

*No parallel generation of grip and lift force*
*Increased duration between contact and liftoff,*
*even under speeded conditions*

**Transport component**
*Undulating velocity profiles of the wrist*
*Contribution of elbow flexion and shoulder*
*elevation decreased*
*Increased contribution of trunk translation*
*Segmentation of shoulder and elbow movements*

**Figure 9.10**   Tentative decomposition of the prehension movement into its elements and the deviations that were found for the spastic hemiparesis group.

point out the various adaptive processes that can be discerned in these patterns. Then, we try to establish the extent to which the adaptive processes can be regarded as long term.

Figure 9.10, like figure 9.1, outlines the different components of the grasping movement. We list the deviations that were observed for the impaired hand in these components. A ubiquitous feature found in all studies is that movements of the impaired limb were slower than those of the unimpaired counterpart. This slowness was caused largely by increased time spent in contact with the object before lifting it, owing to impaired force control at the level of the fingers. Despite this, the subjects were shown to be able to adaptively plan forces in advance on the basis of weight information from a previous lift. Besides increased contact time, we also observed a consistent lengthening of the free-motion phase on the impaired side. We further observed that the relative contribution of the different segments to movement completion was altered in an adaptive way. Trunk involvement (mainly forward translation) increased, while angular changes in the elbow and shoulder elevation decreased. In addition, movements of the shoulder and elbow were systematically performed serially instead of in parallel, pointing to a segmentation of the movement. This was further confirmed by the time between the shoulder and wrist movements. At the start, asynchrony between shoulder and wrist was in favor of the shoulder, but this was reversed at peak velocity. Probably due to this segmented movement coordination, we observed dysfluent velocity profiles of the transport of the wrist; the trajectories undulated. For hand opening and closing over time, the kinematic profiles were also undulating and dysfluent. Nonetheless, subjects were able to adaptively scale peak aperture to the width of the object, albeit with a larger safety margin than that observed for the unimpaired hand. With respect to movement planning, optimization of end-posture comfort was not observed on the impaired side. Rather, for this hand an initial grip was selected that would ensure a decrease in the total amount of joint rotation. Thus, total comfort was optimized. In sum, irrespective of the typical symptoms associated with spasticity, the participants in our studies proved to be able to use alternative strategies and hence adapt their movement performance to the task demands to a surprisingly large extent.

Remember that all the studies we reported here were concerned with unrestricted grasping movements so that the full potential of adaptation would become visible. Additionally, the subjects who performed the experiments had gone through elaborate rehabilitation programs, and it is therefore likely that they already had established a new coordination pattern well adapted to their altered neural and motor structures. Two important questions need be asked. First, do the deviations observed really represent adaptive processes, or are these merely a reflection of the disorder? Second, when adaptation has been established, are the deviations observed long-term adaptations, or do they reflect short-term, instantaneous adaptive processes?

Apart from its more fundamental theoretical relevance, the disorder–adaptation issue has important implications for the practical field of therapy because therapists need to know what aspect of the deviant movement performance needs to be treated (cf. Latash and Anson, 1996; Steenbergen and Hulstijn, 2001). Still, how can a distinction be made between disorder and adaptation? According to Latash and Anson (1996, p. 68), the distinction cannot yet be made because "Our present lack of understanding of the basic principles of motor control prevents us from making recommendations about how to distinguish between primary and adaptive changes in motor patterns. Obviously, one needs to know the original basic priorities of the CNS in order to be able to study deviations from these priorities." We have taken a rather straightforward route in the present chapter by comparing the movement performance of both body sides in spastic hemiparesis, under the assumption that the unimpaired side represents the "basic priorities" of the CNS. It has to be noted that this comparison is at an epistemological level rather than an ontological one. Due to the diffuse nature of the brain damage and interhemispheric transfer, the unimpaired body side probably does not really represent the basic priorities of the CNS. Indeed, previous research showed that this side is not unimpaired if compared with a control group of subjects without neurological disorders (e.g., Brown et al., 1989).

Probably merely comparing both body sides is not enough to gain insight into the disorder–adaptation issue. Therefore, we looked for principles of efficiency or optimization that were adaptive in the sense that they substitute for the "original basic priorities." Related to this is the concept of redundancy. If no redundancy is left to perform the task in any alternative way, then adaptation is impossible and the resulting behavioral outcome is rigid. In these cases we concluded that the deviations observed are a representation of the impairment proper. We discuss two findings that illustrate these phenomena. First, at the level of coordination, joint excursions in the shoulder and elbow were decreased, probably due to contractures, increased antagonistic activity, and hyperactive stretch reflexes. The decrease in angular change that was found for the impaired limb may be a direct consequence of the increased antagonistic muscle activity, a feature characteristic of spasticity. Subjects adapted to this impairment in two ways. In order to reach the target, they increased the level of trunk involvement. In addition, shoulder and elbow angular changes were not performed simultaneously but in a segmented manner. Hence, subjects employed an alternative strategy to perform the task. Second, with respect to the impairment proper, the extended in-contact phase may be illustrative. It was shown that this phase was lengthened on the impaired side. Even when speed of movement was stressed, subjects were not able to adapt to this instruction and remained in contact with the object before lifting it for sustained periods of time. Stated differently, subjects could not adapt to this task requirement by using an alternative strategy that would allow the in-contact phase to be decreased.

There may be a potential caveat here. As Mulder et al. (2001) pointed out, requesting individuals with chronic (lifelong) disease to perform familiar tasks with the aim of establishing momentary performance levels may be problematic as these tasks have been performed so many times that subjects exploit all possible control routes. Clearly, for the in-contact phase, no alternative control routes were possible. For coordination there were alternatives, such as the segmentation of the movement and the increased contribution of the trunk. Can we conclude on the basis of these findings that segmentation was adaptive and not a consequence of the impairment proper? Again, we have to examine whether it is a pathological constant. Testing the movement system under boundary conditions (e.g., increasing speed of responding, as was done in the second experiment of the in-contact phase study, Steenbergen et al., 1998) may be a logical next step for this. As an example, Levin (1996) had subjects with spastic hemiparesis resulting from stroke make planar arm movements. Trunk movement of the subjects was limited but not completely blocked by strapping both shoulder girdles to the high back of the chair. It was shown that segmentation was quite severe, especially for movements made to a contralateral target. We can speculate from these findings that the segmentation of shoulder and elbow movements is adaptive. If trunk involvement is impossible, then, owing to the redundancy of the movement system, segmentation is increased; without this segmentation, movements would probably not have been possible as a consequence of the increase in stretch reflexes.

This brings us to another problem of defining adaptation, which may be clarified by the grip planning study and the coordination study. The adaptation observed in grip planning is quite categorical. Subjects either optimize end-posture comfort or total comfort. Hence, a clear distinction can be made. For the coordination study, this is more difficult, as possible adaptations appear more gradual. When do we denote trunk involvement as adaptive? How much (relative) contribution does the trunk need to make to be called an adaptive strategy? Additionally, might this then be denoted a long-term adaptive strategy or merely an instantaneous, short-term adaptation?

A way of examining short-term adaptation processes can be derived from studies focusing on the phenomenon of flexibility of movement performance. A direct test of flexibility of the movement pattern of the impaired limb can be performed, for instance, by introducing a task-switch paradigm (e.g., Paulignan et al., 1991). This may also reveal why spastic subjects, despite their apparently stable behavior, encounter difficulties with activities of daily living. Most manual dexterity tests used in clinical settings do not measure task-switching behavior but present tasks that are highly predictable. Recently, however, Van Thiel et al. (2002) showed that subjects with spastic hemiparesis displayed a remarkable ability to adjust movements quickly. Subjects had to quickly hit a target projected on a frontoparallel screen. Targets were either stationary or started to move after hand movement onset. Kinematic analysis of the movements revealed no between-arm differences in latency, that is, the time until visual information on target displacement becomes apparent in the lateral hand displacement. Furthermore, although latency was longer for the spastic hemiparetic group than for a control group, it was only longer by 25 ms. This study therefore shows that, even on a very short time scale, subjects with spastic hemiparesis display remarkable flexibility in responding.

In conclusion, the present chapter described various patterns of adaptation. In all cases where movement characteristics of the impaired side deviated from those of the unimpaired side and were accompanied by alternative courses of action guided by efficiency principles, the deviant behavior was considered to represent optimization principles based on adaptation to organismic or task constraints. In cases where rigidity was established, there was no reason to conclude that the findings reflected adaptation. On the contrary, in those cases the deviant planning, coordination, and execution aspects were considered to reflect the neuromotor impairment proper. It may be clear that patterns of impairment and adaptation differ strongly among individuals. As stated earlier, the severity of spasticity varies among individuals and largely determines the degree to which adaptation can be observed. Average data across individuals were reviewed in this chapter, but individual differences should not be underestimated. Also note that individuals with relatively mild spastic hemiparesis participated in our studies as they had to meet the baseline requirement of at least being able to grasp an object. Future research should therefore also include severity of the disorder as a factor in the analyses discussed here. In sum, several issues need to be tackled, and in the long run it has to be established whether the disorder–adaptation issue can really be solved or will turn out to be a spurious one.

# References

Aglioti, S., Berlucchi, G., Pallini, R., Rossi, G.F., and Tassinari, G. (1993) Hemispheric control of unilateral and bilateral responses to lateralized light stimuli after callosotomy and in callosal agenesis. *Exp Brain Res* 95: 151-165.

Balf, C.L., and Ingram, T.T.S. (1955) Problems in the classification of cerebral palsy. *Br Med J* 2: 163-166.

Barnes, M., McLellan, L., and Sutton, R. (1994) Spasticity. In Greenwood, R.J., Barnes, M.P., McMillan, T.M., and Ward, C.D. (Eds.), *Neurological rehabilitation,* pp. 161-172. Edinburgh: Churchill Livingstone.

Bax, M.C.O. (1964) Terminology and classification of cerebral palsy. *Dev Med Child Neurol* 6: 295-297.

Bernstein, N.A. (1967) *The co-ordination and regulation of movements.* Oxford: Pergmon Press.

Brown, J.V., Schumacher, U., Rohlmann, A., Ettlinger, G., Schmidt, R.C., and Skreczek, W. (1989) Aimed movements to visual target in hemiplegic and normal children: Is the "good" hand of children with infantile hemiplegia also normal? *Neuropsychologia* 27: 283-302.

Dietz, V., Quintern, J., and Berger, W. (1981) Electrophysiological studies of gait in spasticity and rigidity: Evidence that altered mechanical properties of muscle contribute to hypertonia. *Brain* 104: 431-449.

Di Stefano, M., Morelli, M., Marzi, C.A., and Berlucchi, G. (1980) Hemispheric control of unilateral and bilateral movements of proximal and distal parts of the arm as inferred from simple reaction time to lateralized light stimuli in man. *Exp Brain Res* 38: 197-204.

Edelman, G.M. (1987) *Neural Darwinism.* New York: Basic Books.

Eliasson, A.C., Gordon, A.M., and Forssberg, H. (1991) Basic co-ordination of manipulative forces of children with cerebral palsy. *Dev Med Child Neurol* 33: 661-670.

Eliasson, A.C., Gordon, A.M., and Forssberg, H. (1992) Impaired anticipatory control of isometric forces during grasping by children with cerebral palsy. *Dev Med Child Neurol* 34: 216-225.

Eliasson, A.C., Gordon, A.M., and Forssberg, H. (1995) Tactile control of isometric finger forces during grasping in children with cerebral palsy. *Dev Med Child Neurol* 37: 56-71.

Goldspink, G., and Williams, P.E. (1990) Muscle fibre and connective tissue changes associated with use and disuse. In Ada, L., and Canning, C. (Eds.), *Foundations for practice: Topics in neurological physiotherapy,* pp. 197-218. London: Heinemann.

Gould, S.J. (1992) *Ever since Darwin.* London: Penguin Books.

Ingram, T.T.S. (1966) The neurology of cerebral palsy. *Arch Dis Child* 41: 337-357.

Johansson, R.S., and Westling, G. (1984) Roles of glabrous skin receptors and sensorimotor memory in automatic control of precision grip when lifting rougher or more slippery objects. *Exp Brain Res* 56: 550-564.

Johansson, R.S., and Westling, G. (1988a) Coordinated isometric muscle command adequately and erroneously programmed for the weight during lifting tasks with precision grip. *Exp Brain Res* 71: 59-71.

Johansson, R.S., and Westling, G. (1988b) Programmed and triggered actions to rapid load changes during precision grip. *Exp Brain Res* 71: 72-86.

Johansson, R.S., and Westling, G. (1990) Tactile afferent signals in the control of precision grip. In Jeannerod, M. (Ed.), *Attention and performance XIII,* pp. 677-736. Hillsdale, NJ: Erlbaum.

Kurland, L.T. (1957) Definitions of cerebral palsy and their role in epidemiologic research. *Neurology* 7: 641-654.

Lance, J.W. (1980) Symposium synopsis. In Feldman, R.G., Young, R.R., and Koella, W.P. (Eds.), *Spasticity: Disordered motor control,* pp. 485-494. Miami, FL: Symposia Specialists.

Latash, M.L., and Anson, G. (1996) What are "normal" movements in atypical populations? *Behav Brain Sci* 19: 55-106.

Levin, M.F. (1996) Interjoint coordination during pointing movements is disrupted in spastic hemiparesis. *Brain* 119: 281-293.

MacKeith, R.C., MacKenzie, I.C.K., and Polani, P.E. (1959) Memorandum on terminology and classification of "cerebral palsy." *Cereb Palsy Bull* 1: 27-35.

Marteniuk, R.G., Leavitt, J.L., MacKenzie, C.L., and Athenes, S. (1990) Functional relationships between grasp and transport components in a prehension task. *Hum Mov Sci* 9: 149-176.

McPhee, S.D. (1987) Functional hand evaluations: A review. *Am J Occup Ther* 41: 158-163.

Mulder, T., Den Otter, R., and Van Engelen, B. (2001) The regulation of fine movements in patients with Charcot-Marie-Tooth, type Ia: Some ideas about continuous adaption. *Motor Control* 2: 200-214.

Napier, J.R. (1956) The prehensile movements of the human hand. *J Bone Joint Surg* 38B: 902-913.

O'Dwyer, N.J., and Ada, L. (1996) Reflex hyperexcitability and muscle contracture in relation to spastic hypertonia. *Curr Opin Neurol* 9: 451-455.

O'Dwyer, N.J., Ada, L., and Neilson, P.D. (1996) Spasticity and muscle contracture following stroke. *Brain* 119: 1737-1749.

O'Dwyer, N.J., Neilson, P.D., and Nash, J. (1989) Mechanisms of muscle growth related to muscle contracture in cerebral palsy. *Dev Med Child Neurol* 31: 543-547.

Paulignan, Y., Mackenzie, C., Marteniuk, R., Jeannerod, M. (1991) Selective perturbation of visual input during prehension movements I. The effects of changing object position. *Exp Brain Res* 83: 502-512.

Rosenbaum, D.A., and Jorgensen, M.J. (1992) Planning macroscopic aspects of manual control. *Hum Mov Sci* 11: 61-69.

Rosenbaum, D.A., Marchak, F., Barnes, H.J., Vaughan, J., Slotta, J.D., and Jorgensen, M.J. (1990) Constraints for action selection: Overhand versus underhand grips. In Jeannerod, M. (Ed.), *Attention and performance XIII,* pp. 321-342. Hillsdale, NJ: Erlbaum.

Rosenbaum, D.A., Van Heugten, C.M., and Caldwell, G.E. (1996) From cognition to biomechanics and back: The end-state comfort effect and the middle-is-faster effect. *Acta Psychol* 94: 59-85.

Rosenbaum, D.A., Vaughan, J., Barnes, H.J., & M.J. Jorgensen (1992). Time course of movement planning: Selection of handgrips for object manipulation. *Journal of Experimental Psychology: Learning, Memory, and Cognition, 18,* 1058-1073.

Rosenbaum, D.A., Vaughan, J., Jorgensen, M.J., Barnes, H.J., and Stewart, E. (1993) Plans for object manipulation. In Meyer, D.E., and Kornblum, S. (Eds.), *Attention and performance XIV: Synergies in experimental psychology, artificial intelligence, and cognitive neuroscience,* pp. 803-820. Cambridge, MA: MIT Press.

Rossetti, Y., Meckler, C., and Prablanc, C. (1994) Is there an optimal arm posture? Deterioration of finger localization precision and comfort sensation in extreme arm-joint postures. *Exp Brain Res* 99: 131-136.

Sassoon, R., Nimmo-Smith, I., and Wann, A.M. (1986) An analysis of children's penholds. In Kao, H.S.R., van Galen, G.P., and Hoosain, R. (Eds.), *Graphonomics: Contemporary research in handwriting,* pp. 93-106. Amsterdam: North-Holland.

Short, M.W., and Cauraugh, J.H. (1997) Planning macroscopic aspects of manual control: End-state comfort and point-of-change effects. *Acta Psychol* 96: 133-147.

Short, M.W., and Cauraugh, J.H. (1999) Precision hypothesis and the end-state comfort effect. *Acta Psychol* 100: 243-252.

Steenbergen, B., and Hulstijn, W. (2001) Themes in movement disorder research. *Motor Control* 2: 95-98.

Steenbergen, B., Hulstijn, W., and Dortmans, S. (2000) Constraints on grip selection in cerebral palsy: Minimising discomfort. *Exp Brain Res* 134: 385-397.

Steenbergen, B., Hulstijn, W., Lemmens, I.H.L., and Meulenbroek, R.G.J. (1998) The timing of prehension movements in subjects with cerebral palsy. *Dev Med Child Neurol* 40: 108-114.

Steenbergen, B., Meulenbroek, R.G.J., and Rosenbaum, D.A. (submitted) Constraints on grip selection in hemiparetic cerebral palsy: Effects of lesional side, end-point accuracy and context.

Steenbergen, B. and Van der Kamp, J. (submitted) Planning and execution of prehension at the unimpaired and impaired side of spastic hemiparetic adolescents.

Steenbergen, B., Van Thiel, E., Hulstijn, W., and Meulenbroek, R.G.J. (2000) The coordination of reaching and grasping in spastic hemiparesis. *Hum Mov Sci* 19: 75-105.

Tabary, J.C., Tabary, C., Tardieu, C., Tardieu, G., and Goldspink, G. (1972) Physiological and structural changes in the cat's soleus muscle due to immobilization at different lengths by plaster casts. *J Physiol* 224: 231-244.

Van Thiel, E., Meulenbroek, R.G.J., Smeets, J.B.J., and Hulstijn, W. (2002) Fast adjustments of ongoing movements in hemiparetic cerebral palsy. *Neuropsychologia* 40 (1): 16-27.

Van Thiel, E., and Steenbergen, B. (2001) Shoulder and hand displacements during hitting, reaching, and grasping movements in hemiparetic cerebral palsy. *Motor Control* 2: 166-182.

Wann, J.P., Mon-Williams, M., and Carson, R.G. (1998) Assessment of manual control in children with coordination difficulties. In Connolly, K. (Ed.), *The psychobiology of the hand,* pp. 213-229. London: Mac Keith Press.

Weir, P.L., MacKenzie, C.L., Marteniuk, R.G., Cargoe, S.L., and Frazer, M.B. (1991) The effects of object weight on the kinematics of prehension. *J Mot Behav* 23: 192-204.

Wiesendanger, M., Wicki, U., and Rouiller, E. (1994) Are there unifying structures in the brain responsible for interlimb coordination? In Swinnen, S., Heuer, H., Massion, J., and Casaer, P. (Eds.), *Interlimb coordination: Neural, dynamical, and cognitive constraints,* pp. 179-207. San Diego: Academic Press.

Williams, P.E., and Goldspink, G. (1973) The effect of immobilization on the longitudinal growth of striated muscle fibres. *J Anat* 116: 45-55.

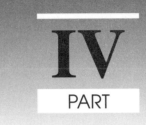

**PART IV**

# Motor Rehabilitation After Stroke or Spinal Cord Injuiry

# 10

# Optimizing Locomotor Function With Body Weight Support Training and Functional Electrical Stimulation

*Hugues Barbeau and Anouk Lamontagne*
McGill University and Jewish Rehabilitation Hospital,
Laval, Quebec, Canada

*Michel Ladouceur*
Brock University
Ontario, Canada

*Isabelle Mercier*
Jewish Rehabilitation Hospital,
Laval, Quebec, Canada

*Joyce Fung*
McGill University and Jewish Rehabilitation Hospital,
Laval, Quebec, Canada

The purpose of this chapter is to review some of the basic concepts developed in the last decade regarding enhanced recovery of locomotor function. The specific objectives are to determine (1) how two forms of locomotor training, one using body weight support and the other using functional electrical stimulation, can improve locomotion in clients with spinal cord injuries and stroke; (2) whether the gain in gait speed achieved on the treadmill can be transferred to overground locomotion; and (3) how locomotor and postural training can be more challenging to achieve a better functional recovery.

## Important Basic Concepts in Developing Locomotor Training Approaches

It is well known that the modulation of many reflexes is task and phase dependent and contributes to the control of locomotion. Many different sensory inputs have been studied in relation to their capacity to control important parameters in gait. For example, the angular position of the hip plays an important role, as demonstrated by the result that hip extension facilitates the initiation of the swing phase in locomotion (Pearson and Rossignol, 1991). Other proprioceptive inputs, such as the proprioceptive receptors that detect the load on the ankle extensors, also play an important role in the initiation of the swing (Duysen and Pearson, 1980) or in modulating the amount of electromyographic activity (Capaday and Stein, 1986). Sensory afferents, such as cutaneous inputs, are modulated quite differently during different phases of locomotion (stance versus swing). Their roles are especially important in the recovery of locomotion after complete transection (see Rossignol, 1996, for a review).

Numerous plastic changes have also been studied to understand the control and recovery of locomotion in spinalized animals. For example, it is now known that, after a complete spinal transection, the animal can learn specific tasks following locomotor or standing training. When two groups of spinal cats were trained differently to stand or to walk, their performances at the end of the training were quite different. The ones that were trained to stand perform very well in standing but walk poorly, whereas the ones that were trained to walk did so at a faster speed than the standing-trained group (Lovely et al., 1986). Pharmacological intervention can elicit locomotion in the early stage and modulate the walking pattern when patterns have been well established following spinal cord transection. Furthermore, the combination of pharmacology and locomotor training can further accelerate the locomotor recovery process to within a week compared with the two to three weeks it normally takes to recover with locomotor training alone.

Bouyer and collaborators (2001) performed a unilateral section of the lateral gastrocnemius-soleus nerve in chronic spinal cats, which caused a marked yield at the ankle joint during walking. Within a week following the lesion, a substantial recovery of the walking pattern was observed, suggesting that plastic changes had occurred within the spinal cord without the influence of supraspinal pathways. These results and others suggest strongly that several plastic changes occur within the spinal cord even in the absence of supraspinal descending pathways. From these studies, some principles that can enhance plastic changes have emerged for the enhancement of functional recovery in patients with neurological insults. These include (1) task-specific training, (2) stimulating appropriate sensory inputs, (3) challenging both posture and locomotor adaptation while training, (4) timing the initiation of training appropriately, and (5) minimizing compensation (see Barbeau et al., 1998; Barbeau and Fung, 2001, for comprehensive reviews).

# Gait Training With Body Weight Support as a Training Strategy

The use of locomotor training with body weight support (BWS) systems, first proposed by Finch and Barbeau (1986), has now been extended to human beings. Several studies of BWS or unloading have reported favorable effects on the gait pattern of patients with neurological conditions. In subjects with both stroke and spinal cord injury (SCI), unloading a percentage of a person's weight during treadmill walking has been shown to improve gait and balance immediately and to increase walking speed. Several open clinical trials have yielded positive results (see Barbeau et al., 1998 for a review), including investigations of the effect of locomotor training with BWS for subjects with SCI (Barbeau et al., 1987; Barbeau and Blunt 1991; Behrman and Harkema, 2000; Wernig and Müller, 1992; Wernig et al., 1995, 1998), stroke (Hesse et al., 1995, 1997, 2001; Kosak and Reding, 2000), Parkinson's disease (Miyai et al., 2000), and cerebral palsy (McNevin et al., 2000; Schindl et al., 2000). Clinical studies conducted in the past 10 years have demonstrated that locomotor training using BWS has a greater effect than conventional or locomotor training with full weight bearing (FWB).

Figure 10.1 summarizes some of the key results from a recent randomized clinical trial (Visintin et al., 1998). Briefly, this clinical trial, involving 79 subjects with stroke, reported better mobility outcomes for the experimental group that was trained with BWS during treadmill walking than for the control group that was trained to walk on the treadmill with FWB. This study differed from other studies in that both groups received the same type and amount of gait training during a 6-week period. The only difference was that the experimental group was provided with up to 40% BWS, and the amount of weight support was progressively decreased as the gait pattern improved (Visintin et al., 1998).

After 6 weeks of locomotor training, a significant improvement in mobility outcomes could be observed in both groups as compared with pretraining scores. However, the BWS group scored significantly higher for overground walking speed (compare the first columns in figure 10.1, a and b), balance, lower-limb motor recovery, and overground walking endurance. A 3-month follow-up revealed that patients trained with BWS continued to have significantly higher scores for overground walking speed and lower-limb motor recovery ($p < 0.01$).

## Locomotor Training Using Body Weight Support

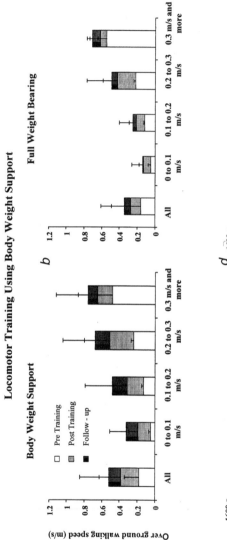

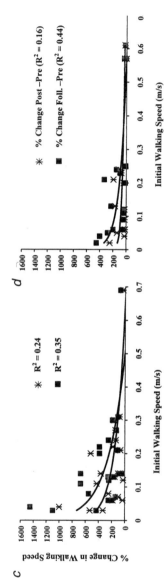

**Figure 10.1** *(a)* The effect of locomotor training using body weight support compared with *(b)* locomotor training using full weight bearing in the subacute stage of recovery after stroke (*n* = 79). The overall effect before and after intervention as well as the effects in subgroups of different initial gait speeds are shown. (Modified from Visintin et al., 1998). (*c* and *d*) Scatter plots of individual data showing the relationship of change in walking speed (as a percentage) to the initial walking speed using the best-fitting curve for the BWS (*c*) and FWB (*d*) groups.

Adapted from Visintin et al., (1998).

When the subjects were stratified according to their initial walking speed, significant main effects due to time (6 weeks post training vs. 3-month follow-up, $p$ < 0.001) and group (BWS vs. FWB, $p$ < 0.01) were seen. Stroke clients with an initial walking speed of 0.3 m/s or less increased their speed significantly more when trained with BWS at both the end of the training period (6 weeks) and at follow-up (3 months; compare figure 10.1a with 10.1b for other speeds). For patients walking at initial speed above 0.3 m/s, both the BWS and FWB groups improved significantly with time ($p$ < 0.001), but only a small difference could be observed between those two groups (compare the last columns in figure 10.1, a and b). Whether using BWS or FWB, treadmill training has a greater effect than conventional overground gait training (Hesse et al., 2001). Furthermore, the more severely impaired showed more improvement than the less severely impaired, and this difference was more pronounced in the BWS group than in the FWB group (compare figure 10.1, c and d). Similarly, Kosak and Reding (2000) compared treadmill training with BWS versus aggressive bracing-assisted walking (ABAW) in a randomized clinical trial ($n$ = 56) and observed significant improvement in walking speed (from 0.08 to 0.20 m/s) and endurance (from 44 to 90 m) in a subgroup of severe stroke subjects. These studies were done in the subacute stage of recovery, when a strong association has been found between acuteness of the lesion and the functional gain in outcome in subjects with stroke (Paolucci et al., 2001) and SCI (Sumida et al., 2001). Locomotor training with BWS was also demonstrated to be successful in the early postlesion stage in SCI subjects. Nymark et al. (1998) found a marked enhancement in both treadmill and overground speeds in higher-functioning SCI patients (classified as C and D on the ASIA scale), while the lower-functioning patients (ASIA B) who needed manual assistance during training with BWS showed minimal improvement. Behrman and Harkema (2000) observed a similar magnitude of change in ASIA scale C and D patients but not in ASIA scale A patients. However, this therapeutic modality (locomotor training using BWS) is extremely labor intensive, and the use of a mechanized gait trainer or robot-aided sensorimotor stimulation could be useful to restore some gait function in the nonambulatory SCI and stroke subjects (Hesse et al., 2001, Volpe et al., 2000). The success of these clinical trial studies has now led to a multicenter randomized clinical trial to evaluate the effectiveness of locomotor training using BWS as compared with conventional rehabilitation in 237 SCI subjects (Dobkin, 1999). An interim analysis was planned for the June of 2003.

# Gait Training With Functional Electrical Stimulation

The use of locomotor training combined with functional electrical stimulation (FES) has also demonstrated great potential to enhance walking recovery, even though the efficacy had not been established yet. Figure 10.2 summarizes the results of a recent Canadian multicenter trial ($n$ = 40) on the effect of FES during locomotion in clients with both chronic SCI and stroke (Wieler et al., 1999) and the effect of locomotor training combined with FES ($n = 14$, Ladouceur and Barbeau, 2000a, 2000b). The patients were fitted with functional electrical stimulators and tested before and after 1 year of use. There was a small gain in overground gait speed (0.11 m/s) in these patients (figure 10.2b, first column). Ladouceur and Barbeau (2000a) demonstrated in a longitudinal study ($n = 14$) that the combination of a simple FES system with locomotor training was effective for improving walking in chronic SCI subjects (figure 10.2a, first column). The average gain in speed was 0.26 m/s after 1 year of locomotor training with FES. Thus, the gain was more than double when comparing locomotor training with FES to the FES alone (figure 10.2, a and b, first columns, $p < 0.003$).

Furthermore, the gain was significant across all levels of initial gait speed (compare different speeds in figure 10.2, a and b). The gain in gait speed was retained in both groups even when the stimulator was turned off (not shown). Finally, the subjects with the most severe SCI and stroke impairments, as measured by the overground walking speed, showed marked relative changes in gait speed (as a percentage), but the linear regression lines were quite low ($R^2 = 0.13$ to $0.17$), showing that there is no correlation between the initial walking speed and relative improvement in walking speed. In patients with the most chronic SCI (more than one year post-injury) who underwent locomotor training with FES, changes in their use of assistive ambulatory devices from crutches to canes to no walking aids and an increase in the ergonomic efficiency of their walking behavior were also observed (Ladouceur and Barbeau, 2000b). The researchers concluded that an increase in maximal walking speed during training with FES was due mostly to a therapeutic effect, indicating that some plastic changes occurred, even when SCI subjects were trained in the later stage of recovery.

## Task Specificity of Training and Transfer From Treadmill to Overground Locomotion

Although treadmill training with BWS has been shown to have a greater effect on gait recovery than conventional gait training (Hesse et al., 1995), the magnitude of its effects is limited. In the study of Visintin et al. (1998), the BWS group reached an average overground walking speed of 0.52 m/s at the 3-month follow-up, which is important but still much slower than age-matched healthy subjects (1.0 to 1.3 m/s; Bohannon, 1997). In a post hoc analysis, we also found that people with an initial overground walking speed of 0.5m/s or faster did not seem to benefit as much from BWS during treadmill training (figure 10.1). Furthermore, the transfer of speed gain from treadmill to overground walking was incomplete after training in the BWS group (see figure 10.3a). In fact, the transfer was important but incomplete for about half the subjects in the BWS group and for most of the patients in the FWB group (figure 10.3a). This result contrasts with the results for subjects who were trained over ground with FES, illustrated in figure 10.3b. Most of the points were situated near the diagonal line (slope indicating a 1:1 ratio), suggesting that

# Locomotor Training Using Functional Electrical Stimulation (FES)

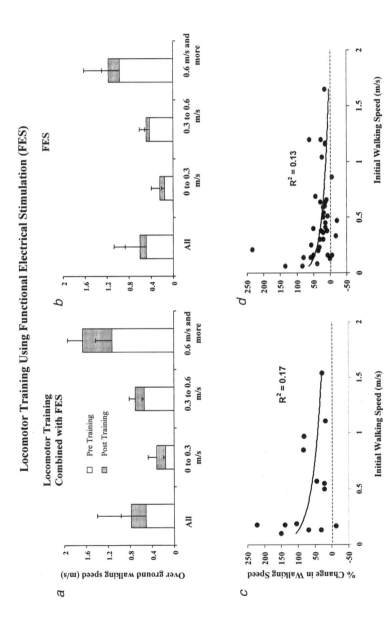

**Figure 10.2** (*a* and *b*) The effect of FES with locomotor training (*n* = 14) and of FES alone (*n* = 40). The overall effect before and after intervention as well as the effects in subgroups of different initial gait speeds are shown (modified from Wieler et al., 1999, and Ladouceur and Barbeau, 2000a). (*c* and *d*) Scatter plots of individual data showing the relationship of change in walking speed (as a percentage) to the initial walking speed using the best-fitting curve for FES with locomotor training (*c*) and FES groups (*d*).

Adapted from Visintin et al. (1998).

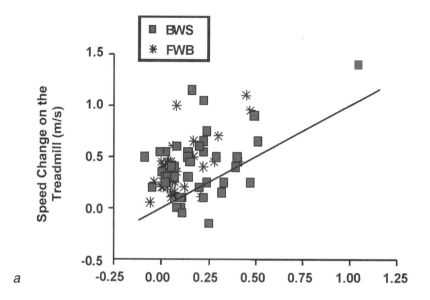

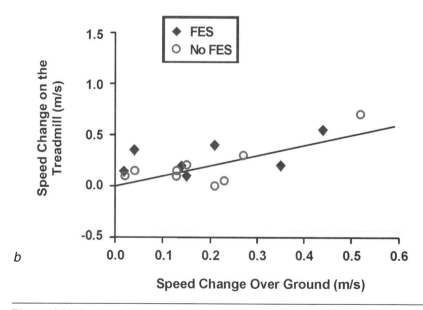

**Figure 10.3** Scatter plots of the walking speed change on the treadmill in relation to the walking speed change over ground *(a)* with locomotor training at FWB and with BWS and *(b)* with locomotor training using FES and when the stimulator was turned off.

the transfer in gait speed improvements from overground to treadmill locomotion was nearly complete.

# Rationale for the Development of an Overground Locomotor Training System

One of the new advances in gait retraining is the development of an overground BWS strategy. Indeed, some differences between overground and treadmill gait parameters have been demonstrated in cats (Wetzel et al., 1975) and in nondisabled individuals (Arsenault et al., 1986; Murray et al., 1985; Savelberg et al., 1998; Stolze et al., 1997; Strathy et al., 1983; Van Gheluwe et al., 1994; White et al., 1998). During walking over ground, the environment as seen by the individual is changing (open field), which is not generally the case on a treadmill. Speed is also internally driven during overground walking instead of externally driven as on a treadmill. The rationale behind overground gait retraining is that the transfer of the acquired walking skills to functional ambulation could be more challenging for both posture and locomotion. Thus the skill transfer will be more complete (or maybe *easier*) because overground training challenges posture and locomotion in the same way as functional ambulation. In fact, figure 10.3b illustrates that the transfer is almost complete when the patients have been trained over ground. However, the speed of treadmill and overground walking is relatively similar, suggesting an important transfer from overground to treadmill walking (figure 10.3b).

There is minimal information in the literature about the center-of-mass displacement during walking with FWB or with BWS in spinal cord and in hemiplegic subjects. In normal subjects, the center of mass moves through a vertical sinusoidal pathway during the gait cycle. The center of mass goes up when the leg is propelled into swing and then goes down until midstance. It actually undergoes a vertical displacement of around 7 cm and reaches its maximum at middle swing and its minimum at the end of load acceptance (see figure 10.4b; Simon et al., 1977). The BWS systems used to date do not allow this complete natural displacement (Barbeau et al., 1987; Gazzani et al., 1996; He et al., 1991; Norman et al., 1995; Siddiqi et al., 1997). Indeed, the patient is lifted while in quiet standing in order to provide the desired level of BWS. The patient then remains lifted at this height for the entire trial. Therefore, BWS limits the normal center of mass (COM) in the downward direction compared with normal walking (a decrease in the lower part of the sinusoidal pathway). On the other hand, the center of mass can go up,

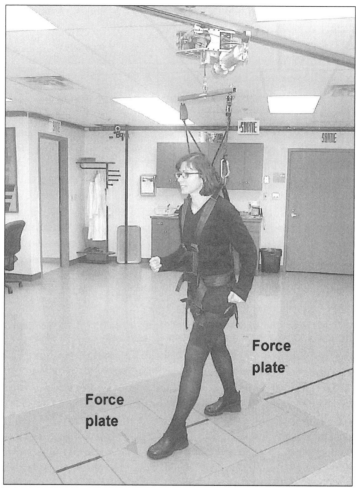

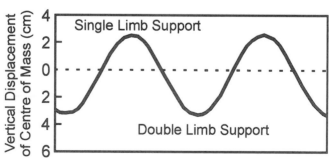

**Figure 10.4** *(a)* The subject is mechanically supported in a harness while walking on two force plates to determine the amount of BWS provided. *(b)* The center of mass goes up during single limb support and then down until double limb support period while walking in the harness in *(a)*.

and this elevation results in a lower level of body weight support. This means that not only was the vertical displacement of the center of mass disrupted, but also a constant BWS was not maintained during the gait cycle.

One question is whether constant BWS is important to retrain gait more effectively. The very essence of the BWS strategy is to symmetrically unload the lower extremities in order to decrease the need for compensation on the unaffected side and discourage the asymmetrical gait pattern of hemiplegics. Thus, one great advantage of BWS is that it forces the use of the most severely affected lower limb and thus minimizes the compensation pattern. Indeed, another form of partial weight support, such as handrails or parallel bars, can also be used during gait training but encourages compensation by the upper extremities and the less-affected lower limb (Barbeau and Blunt, 1991).

# Novel Overground Training System for Locomotor Training

A new BWS system (patent pending) that provides a constant level of load removal during bidirectional walking over ground has been built at the Jewish Rehabilitation Hospital in Canada (figure 10.4a). A pilot study was recently carried out to investigate the feasibility of using this new device during overground locomotion in patients with different levels of locomotor disability. Subjects were instructed to walk at comfortable speed with FWB and while 30% of their weight was supported. This weight removal was determined during quiet standing. Figure 10.5 illustrates how gait speed changed with BWS as compared with FWB. Absolute gait speed values are shown in figure 10.5a, whereas relative changes in gait speed are represented in figure 10.5b. Overall, BWS caused gait speed to increase by an average of 52% as compared with walking with FWB. It should be noted that these increases in gait speed were instantaneous changes and that the patients were not trained with the BWS system. This is the first report of instantaneous changes in gait speed with the use of BWS in stroke patients, since previous studies were carried out during locomotion on a treadmill at a controlled speed (Hesse et al., 1997). A closer examination of individual data, however, reveals that some patients may benefit more from BWS than others. First, patients whose preferred gait speed with FWB was less than 0.45 m/s experienced a mean absolute increase in gait speed of 0.15 m/s with BWS (figure 10.5a). The two patients who initially walked at 0.45m/s, however, showed minimal changes (+0.06 m/s) in gait speed with BWS. Second, relative changes in gait speed (figure 10.5b) also showed that the more severely disabled the patients, the larger the percent changes in gait speed with BWS. For instance, although patients 1 and 4 show absolute increases in gait speed of 0.15 m/s, this represents a 143% increase for patient 1 and a 48% increase for patient 4. From a functional perspective, improving gait speed by 0.15 m/s in a severely disabled patient has much more impact on locomotor capability than in a less disabled patient. Altogether, these findings show not only that BWS

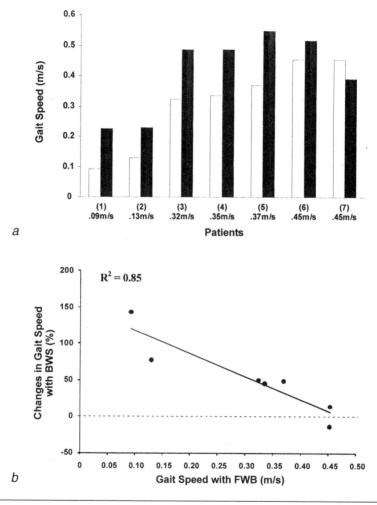

**Figure 10.5** *(a)* Gait speed at FWB (white bars) and at 30% BWS (black bars) in seven stroke subjects. Each bar represents one patient. *(b)* Gait speed changes as a percentage of FWB speed.

during overground walking can be used for severely disabled stroke patients, but also that these patients can benefit more from such intervention than less severely disabled patients.

Increases in gait speed with BWS were associated with improvements in both temporal and distance factors, as indicated by shorter cycle and stance duration and longer stride and step length for both the paretic and nonparetic limbs. In contrast to results reported for treadmill walking with BWS (Hassid et al., 1997), symmetry in spatiotemporal factors between the paretic and nonparetic sides was not significantly improved. When walking with BWS, patients also spent a larger proportion of time in single-limb support on both the paretic and nonparetic side as compared with walking with FWB. These spatiotemporal changes, especially the increased proportion of time spent in single-limb support, suggest an improvement in gait-related balance (Lamontagne et al., 2001). Patients also subjectively reported that their paretic limb felt "lighter" and "easier to swing forward" with BWS. Part of these preliminary findings have been reported previously (Lamontagne et al., 2001; Fung et al., 1999).

# Conclusions

Both spinal-cord-injured and stroke patients have the potential for functional recovery. This recovery process is also possible at the chronic stage, suggesting that some plastic changes can also occur during this late period. In recent years, several concepts for rehabilitation have emerged (see Barbeau and Fung 2001). It has been very well demonstrated from animal studies that the help of locomotor training is very specific (Lovely et al., 1986) and could not be replaced by other tasks. The present study examines the feasibility of overground locomotor training using BWS as the first step before a clinical trial comparing treadmill versus overground locomotor training using BWS. Challenging posture and walking adaptation force use of the lower extremities. Appropriate sensory inputs and timing of the intervention have also emerged as important concepts from our previous studies. These concepts should be integrated when we introduce the next phase of validation of this overground training approach. We should be able to facilitate and challenge both posture and locomotion as the patients progress. Finally, this rehabilitation approach should be combined with functional electrical stimulation and pharmacological therapy to maximize recovery of both balance and locomotion (Barbeau 2003).

# References

Arsenault, A.B., Winter, D.A., and Marteniuk, R.G. (1986) Treadmill versus walkway locomotion in humans: An EMG study. *Ergonomics* 29: 665-676.

Barbeau, H. (2003) Locomotor training in neurorehabilitation: Emerging rehabilitation concepts. *Neurorehabil Neurol Repair* 12: 3-11.

Barbeau, H., and Blunt, R. (1991) A novel interactive locomotor approach using body weight support to retrain gait in spastic paretic subjects. In Wernig, A. (Ed.), *Plasticity of motoneuronal connections,* pp. 461-474. Amsterdam: Elsevier Science.

Barbeau, H., and Fung, J. (2001) The role of rehabilitation in the recovery of walking in the neurological population. *Curr Opin Neurol* 14: 735-740.

Barbeau, H., Norman, K., Fung, J., Visintin, M., and Ladouceur, M. (1998) Does neurorehabilitation play a role in the recovery of walking in neurological populations? In Kiehn, D., Harris-Warrick, R., Jordan, L., Hultborn, H., and Kudo, N. (Eds.), *Neuronal mechanisms for generating locomotor activity,* pp. 377-392. New York: New York Academy of Sciences.

Barbeau, H., Wainberg, M., and Finch, L. (1987) Description and application of a system for locomotor rehabilitation. *Med Biol Eng Comput* 25: 341-344.

Behrman, A.L., and Harkema S.J. (2000) Locomotor training after human spinal cord injury: A series of case studies. *Phys Ther* 80: 688-700.

Bohannon, R.W. (1997) Comfortable and maximum walking speed of adults aged 20-79 years: Reference values and determinants. *Age Ageing* 26: 15-19.

Bouyer, L., Whelan, P.J., Pearson, K.G., and Rossignol, S. (2001) Adaptive locomotor plasticity in chronic spinal cats after ankle extensors neurectomy. *J Neurosci* 21: 3531-3541.

Capaday, C., and Stein, R.B. (1986) Amplitude modulation of the soleus H-reflex in the human during walking and standing. *J Neurosci* 6(5): 1308-1313.

Dobkin, B.H. (1999) An overview of treadmill locomotor training with partial body weight support: A neurologicially sound approach whose time has come for randomized clinical trials. *Neurorehabil Neural Repair* 13: 157-165.

Duysen, J., and Pearson, K.G. (1980) Inhibition of flexor burst generation by loading ankle extensor muscles in walking cats. *Brain Res* 187: 321-332.

Finch, L., and Barbeau, H. (1986) Hemiplegic gait: New treatment strategies. *Physiother Can* 38: 36-41.

Fung, J., Barbeau, H., and Roopchand, S. (1999) Partial weight support improves force generation and postural alignment during overground locomotion following stroke. *Soc Neurosci Abstr* 25: 907.

Gazzani, F., Macellari, V., Torre, M., Castellano, V., and Coratella, D. (1996) WARD: A pneumatic system for body weight relief in gait rehabilitation. In *Proceedings of the annual international conference of the IEEE*, p. 861. Engineering in Medicine and Biology Society. Piscataway, NJ: IEEE.

Hassid, E., Rose, D., Commisarow, J., Guttry, M., and Dobkin, B.H. (1997) Improved gait symmetry in hemiparetic stroke patients induced during body weight–supported treadmill stepping. *J Neurol Rehab* 11: 21-26.

He, J.P., Kram, R., and McMahon, T.A. (1991) Mechanics of running under simulated low gravity. *J Appl Physiol* 71: 863-870.

Hesse, S., Bertelt, C., Jahnke, M.T., Schaffrin, A., Baake, P., Malezic, M., and Mauritz, K.H. (1995) Treadmill training with partial body weight support compared with physiotherapy in nonambulatory hemiparetic patients. *Stroke* 26: 976-981.

Hesse, S., Helm, B., Krajnik, J., Gregoric, M., and Mauritz, K.H. (1997) Treadmill training with partial body weight support: Influence of body weight release on the gait of hemiparetic patients. *J Neurol Rehab* 11: 15-20.

Hesse, S., Werner, C., Bardeleben, A., and Barbeau, H. (2001) Body weight support treadmill training after stroke. *Curr Atheroscol Rep* 3: 287-294.

Kosak, M.C., and Reding, M.J. (2000) Comparison of partial body weight–supported treadmill gait training versus aggressive bracing assisted walking post stroke. *Neurorehabil Neural Repair* 14: 13-19.

Ladouceur, M., and Barbeau, H. (2000a) Functional electrical stimulation–assisted walking for persons with incomplete spinal cord injury: Longitudinal changes in maximal overground walking speed. *Scand J Rehabil Med* 32: 28-36.

Ladouceur, M., and Barbeau, H. (2000b) Functional electrical stimulation–assisted walking for persons with incomplete spinal injuries: Changes in the kinematics and physiological cost of overground walking. *Scand J Rehabil Med* 32: 72-79.

Lamontagne, A., Brosseau, L., and Fung, J. (2001). Changes in muscle activation and spatiotemporal profiles due to partial unloading and fast walking in subjects with hemiparesis. In *Proceedings of progress in motor control III: From basic science to applications,* p. 76. Montreal.

Lovely, R.G., Gregor, R.J., Roy, R.R., and Edgerton, V.R. (1986) Effect of training on the recovery of full weight bearing stepping in the adult spinal cat. *Exp Neurol* 92: 421-435.

McNevin, N.H., Coraci, L., and Schafer, J. (2000) Gait in adolescent cerebral palsy: The effect of partial unweighting. *Arch Phys Med Rehabil* 81: 525-528.

Miyai, I., Fujimoto, Y., Veda, Y., Yamamoto, H., Nuzaki, S., Saito, T., and Kang, J. (2000) Treadmill training with body weight support: Its effect on Parkinson's disease. *Arch Phys Med Rehabil* 81: 849-852.

Murray, M.P., Spurr, G.B., Sepic, S.B., and Gardner, G.M. (1985) Treadmill vs. floor walking: Kinematics, electromyogram, and heart rate. *J Appl Physiol* 59: 87-91.

Norman, K.E., Pepin, A., Ladouceur, M., and Barbeau, H. (1995) A treadmill apparatus and harness support for evaluation and rehabilitation of gait. *Arch Phys Med Rehabil* 76: 772-778.

Nymark, J., DeForge, D., Barbeau, H., Badour, M., Bercovitch, S., Tomas, J., Goudreau, L., and Mac-Donald, J. (1998) Body weight support treadmill gait training in the subacute recovery phase of incomplete spinal cord injury. *J Neurol Rehab* 12: 119-138.

Paolucci, S., Antonucci, G., Grasso, M.G., Bragoni, M., Troisi, E., Morelli, D., Coiro, P., De Angelis, D., and Rizzi, F. (2001) Early versus delayed inpatient stroke rehabilitation: A matched comparison conducted in Italy. *Arch Phys Med Rehabil* 81: 695-700.

Pearson, K.G., and Rossignol, S. (1991) Fictive motor patterns in chronic signal cats. *Neurophysiology* S66: 1874-1887.

Rossignol, S. (1996) Neural control of stereotypic limb movements. In Rowell, L.B., and Sheppard, J.T. (Eds.), *Handbook of physiology, Section 12,* pp. 173-216. American Physiological Society, Bethesda, MD.

Savelberg, H.H., Vorstenbosch, M.A., Kamman, E.H., van de Weijer, J.G, and Schambardt, H.C. (1998) Intra-stride belt-speed variation affects treadmill locomotion. *Gait Posture* 7: 26-34.

Schindl, M.R., Forstner, C., and Hesse, S. (2000) Treadmill training with partial body weight support in nonambulatory patients with cerebral palsy. *Arch Phys Med Rehabil* 81: 301-306.

Siddiqi, N., Gazzani, F., DesJardins, J., and Chao, E.Y. (1997) The use of a robotic device for gait training and rehabilitation. *Stud Health Technol Inform* 39: 440-449.

Simon, S.R., Knirk, J.K., Mansour, J.M., and Koskinen, M.F. (1977) The dynamics of the center of mass during walking and its clinical applicability. *Bull Hosp Joint Dis* 38: 112-116.

Stolze, H., Kuhtz-Buschbeck, J.P., Mondwurf, C., Boczek-Funcke, A., John, K., Deuschl, G., and Illert, M. (1997) Gait analysis during treadmill and underground locomotion in children and adults. *Electroencephalogr Clin Neurophysiol* 105: 490-497.

Strathy, G.M., Chao, E.Y., and Laughman, R.K. (1983) Changes in knee function associated with treadmill ambulation. *J Biomech* 16: 517-522.

Sumida, M., Fujimoto, M., Tokuhiro, A., Tominaga, T., Magara, A., and Uchida, R. (2001) Early rehabilitation effect for traumatic spinal cord injury. *Arch Phys Med Rehabil* 82: 391-395.

Van Gheluwe, B., Smekens, J., and Roosen, P. (1994) Electrodynographic evaluation of the foot during treadmill versus overground locomotion. *J Am Podiatr Med Assoc* 84: 598-606.

Visintin, M., Barbeau, H., Korner-Bitensky, N., and Mayo, N.E. (1998) A new approach to retrain gait in stroke patients through body weight support and treadmill stimulation. *Stroke* 29: 1122-1128.

Volpe, B.T., Krebs, H.I., Hogan, N., Edelstein, O.L., Diels, C., and Aisen, M. (2000) A novel approach to stroke rehabilitation: Robot-aided sensorimotor stimulation. *Neurology* 54: 1938-1944.

Wernig, A., and Müller, S. (1992) Laufband locomotion with body weight support improved walking in persons with severe spinal cord injuries. *Paraplegia* 30: 229-238.

Wernig, A., Müller, S., Nanassy, A., and Cagol, E. (1995) Laufband therapy based on "rules of spinal locomotion" is effective in spinal cord injured persons. *Eur J Neurosci* 7: 823-829.

Wernig, A., Nanassy, A., and Müller, S. (1998) Laufband (treadmill) therapy in incomplete paraplegia and tetraplegia. *J Neurotrauma* 16: 719-726.

Wetzel, M.C., Atwater, A.E., Wait, J.V., and Stuart, D.C. (1975) Neural implications of different profiles between treadmill and overground locomotion timings in cats. *J Neurophysiol* 38: 492-501.

White, S.C., Yack, H.J., Tucker, C.A., and Lin, H.Y. (1998) Comparison of vertical ground reaction forces during overground and treadmill walking. *Med Sci Sports Exerc* 30: 1537-1542.

Wieler, M., Stein, R.B., Ladouceur, M., Whittaker, M., Smith, A.W., Nieman, S., Barbeau, H., Bugarest, J., Aimone, E., and Biemann, I. (1999) Multi-center evaluation of electrical stimulating systems for walking. *Arch Phys Med Rehabil* 80: 495-500.

# Spinal Locomotor Capability Revealed by Electrical Stimulation of the Lumbar Enlargement in Paraplegic Patients

*Elena Yu. Shapkova*

Children's Surgery Clinic,
Institute of Phthisiopulmonology, St. Petersburg

Spinal cord electrical stimulation (SCES) induced steplike movements and was used for locomotor training in 23 completely and 6 incompletely paralyzed patients. Besides running-like and walking-like SCES-induced movements, other types of stereotypical leg activity were observed. The purpose of this chapter is to present in a systematic way our observations of SCES-induced motor activity in paraplegic patients, to discuss the data with respect to the possible central organization of a spinal locomotor generator (SLG) in humans, and to analyze the results of treatment with stimulation-evoked spinal locomotor activity in both completely and incompletely paralyzed patients.

An optimal level of SCES application for evoking locomotor-like movements (a "locomotor zone") was found at the midlumbar enlargement (about L3-L5, vertebrae T12-L1). The motor patterns induced by SCES in the locomotor zone could be typical or atypical of locomotion patterns. A transition from one pattern to another could occur with or without changes in SCES parameters. The frequency of stepping was often independent of the SCES frequency. After the end of the stimulation, rhythmic movements could continue for many cycles. Based on these observations, the induced activity was considered to be centrally generated.

The possibility of evoking well-coordinated, alternating, steplike movements by SCES in functionally completely paralyzed patients suggests the existence of a spinal locomotor generator in the human midlumbar enlargement (about L3-L5). Cases of atypical coordination between the two legs suggest the existence of separate spinal generators for each leg. Clinical results (an improved ability to walk in all incompletely paralyzed patients and different degrees of progress in locomotor ability in about 70% of originally completely paralyzed patients) show the high effectiveness of locomotor training with SCES for paralyzed patients, especially for those with functionally complete paralysis.

## The Evidence for Spinal Locomotor Generators

SLGs are well-established in animals (Grillner, 1973, 1981; Grillner and Zangger, 1975; Lundberg, 1981; Mori, 1987; Orlovsky and Shik, 1976; Pearson, 1993, 2000; Rossignol, 1996; Rossignol et al., 2000; Schomburg, 1995). The spinal cord of higher vertebrates deprived of all descending and peripheral signals is capable of generating rhythmic motor activity that partly resembles the main characteristics of normal locomotion, including coordination between the four limbs and between limb and trunk muscles (Edgerton et al., 1992; Koehler et al., 1984). It has been long questioned whether SLGs exist in primates and humans (Illis, 1995; Vilensky et al., 1992; Vilensky and O'Connor, 1997, 1999). Recent studies have provided evidence of SLGs in primates (Federichuk et al., 1998; Hultborn et al., 1993). There has also been indirect evidence of the existence of similar neuronal structures in humans. Most studies of human spinal locomotor activity are based on clinical findings such as the presence of myoclonus (Bussel et al., 1988, 1996), long-latency flexor reflexes (Bussel et al., 1989; Roby-Brami and Bussel, 1987, 1990, 1992), and involuntary steplike movements in patients with chronic, incomplete paralysis (Calancie et al., 1994). The existence of SLGs may also be inferred from the effects of training on the stepping abilities in patients with incomplete spinal lesions (Barbeau and Blunt, 1991; Barbeau and Rossignol, 1994; Dietz et al., 1994; Wernig and Müller, 1992; Wernig et al., 1995) and on EMG patterns in completely paralyzed patients (Dietz et al., 1995; Dobkin et al., 1995). Alternating locomotor-like activity in both completely and incompletely paraplegic patients has been demonstrated with epidural SCES (Dimitrijevic et al., 1996, 1998; Gerasimenko et al., 1996; Shapkov et al., 1995; Shapkova et al., 1997a, 1997b) and surface electrical stimulation of the lumbar enlargement (Shapkova et al., 1997a). A detailed comparison of voluntary stepping and steplike activity evoked with SCES in an incompletely paraplegic patient as well as the analysis of EMG patterns underlying human stepping evoked by SCES have supported the view that SCES-evoked stepping may be produced by an SLG (Shapkova and Schomburg, 1999a, 1999b, 2001). In healthy subjects, the possibility of evoking steplike movements with vibration of leg muscles has also been shown by Gurfinkel and colleagues (1998, 1999).

The loss of locomotor capability is a major disabling factor in various disorders. In particular, it is commonly seen in patients with cerebral palsy, spinal cord injury, and paraplegia secondary to disorders of the spine such as spondylitis, kyphosis, and kyphoscoliosis. Restoration of locomotion is a major problem, especially for functionally completely paralyzed patients. It has been shown by Barbeau et al. (1998, 1999) that an effective way to enhance locomotor capability in spinal-cord-injured (SCI) patients with partial paralysis is treadmill training with body weight support (BWS), an effect that can be increased with pharmacological agents (Fung et al., 1990). Despite the significant recent success in recovery of locomotion in incompletely paralyzed patients, this treatment has had no effect on patients with complete paralysis.

The findings obtained by different research groups suggest the existence of an SLG in humans, but it is still unknown how such neuronal structures are organized and how they interact with descending and peripheral signals. Both ethical and technical considerations limit this type of research in humans. The organization of the SLG can be studied indirectly in patients with complete and incomplete SCI by analyzing the characteristics of locomotor activity evoked by SCES applied for therapeutic purposes.

# Method

The observations were made over a 7-year period of treating paralyzed patients in the Children's Surgery Clinic with SCES-evoked spinal locomotor activity. In all patients, paralysis was secondary to a disease or damage of the spine. Etiology and neurological status before and after the SCES rehabilitation protocol are presented in table 11.1. The group of 29 patients included 23 patients with functionally complete paralysis (type A and B on the Frankel scale) and 6 patients with incomplete paralysis (type C, existence of minimal voluntary movements). Patients ranged from 2 to 19 years old. Eighteen patients received between two and five repeated courses of SCES at intervals of 6 to 9 months. In all cases, a surgical anterior decompression of the spinal cord and spine stabilization were done prior to the patients' entering the rehabilitation program. SCES began within 1 week to 1 month of decompression surgery in 7 cases, after 3 to 12 months in 10 cases, and after more than a year in 11 cases. The duration of the paralysis before the initiation of SCES treatment was more than a year in 10 cases, and SCES began in the acute phase in 4 cases.

The initial neurological status of the patients was estimated using the Frankel scale (types A-E; Ditunno et al., 1994; Frankel et al., 1969) on the basis of the clinical data, but this scale was not sensitive enough to estimate the results of rehabilitation.

**Table 11.1    Characteristics of Patients With Vertebrogenic Myelopathy Treated With SCES-Evoked Locomotor-Like Activity**

| Patient | Age (yr+mo) | Sex | Diagnosis | Level of damage | Duration of paralysis before SCES | Courses of SCES | Neurological status (on Frankel scale) +, – pelvic disorder Before rehab | | After rehab | |
|---|---|---|---|---|---|---|---|---|---|---|
| *Completely paralyzed (n = 23)* | | | | | | | | | | |
| P1 | 3 + 5 | M | Tuberculous spondylitis | T3-8 | 2 yr | 3 | A | + | A | – |
| P2 | 3 | M | Tuberculous spondylitis | T8-9 | > 1 yr | 3 | A | + | D | – |
| P3 | 3 + 5 | M | Tuberculous spondylitis | T11-L1 | 7 mo | 3 | A | + | D | – |
| P4 | 2 + 4 | F | Tuberculous spondylitis | T4-8 | 8 mo | 1 | A | + | E | – |
| P5 | 10 | M | Tuberculous spondylitis* | T12-L1 | 0 | 2 | A | – | D | – |
| P6 | 14 | F | Pathological fracture* | T5 | 0 | 3 | A | + | D | – |
| P7 | 10 | M | Trauma | T3-7 | 4 mo | 3 | A | + | C | + |
| P8 | 5 | M | Trauma | L1-2 | 4 mo | 2 | A | + | A | – |
| P9 | 14 | M | Fibrous dysplasia | T2-5 | 2 yr | 5 | A | + | AC | – |
| P10 | 16 | M | Tumor D3-D7 | T3-8 | 4 mo | 3 | A | + | AC | – |
| P11 | 9 | F | Abnormality of spine | T8-9 | 9 yr | 2 | A | + | A | + |
| P12 | 11 | F | Abnormality of spine | T6-8 | 1 yr | 2 | A | + | A | – |
| P13 | 9 | M | Trauma | C6 | 5 mo | 1 | A | + | A | + |
| P14 | 11 | M | Trauma | T6-8 | 6 mo | 1 | A | + | A | + |
| P15 | 3 | M | Tuberculous spondylitis | T5-7 | 1 yr | 2 | A | + | AC | + |

| Patient | | | Diagnosis | Level of damage | Duration of paralysis before SCES | Courses of SCES | Neurological status (on Frankel scale) +, – pelvic disorder | | | |
|---|---|---|---|---|---|---|---|---|---|---|
| | Age (yr+mo) | Sex | | | | | Before rehab | | After rehab | |
| P16 | 1 + 8 | F | Tuberculous spondylitis* | T7-10 | 0 | 1 | A | + | A | + |
| P17 | 15 | F | Trauma | T8-9 | 1 yr | 1 | A | + | BC | + |
| P18 | 16 | F | Tuberculous spondylitis | C7-T4 | 6 yr | 2 | B | – | C | – |
| P19 | 10 | F | Tuberculous spondylitis | T5-8 | 1 mo | 1 | B | + | C | – |
| P20 | 3 + 8 | M | Tuberculous spondylitis | T4 | 5 mo | 1 | B | + | E | – |
| P21 | 11 | M | Osteomyelitis | T1-5 | 7 yr | 2 | B | + | C | – |
| P22 | 11 | F | Tuberculous spondylitis | T5 | 1 yr | 2 | B | + | BC | – |
| P23 | 14 | F | Abnormality of spine* | T7-8 | 5 mo | 2 | B | + | BC | + |
| *Incompletely paralyzed (n = 6)* | | | | | | | | | | |
| P24 | 5 | F | Tuberculous spondylitis* | L1-3 | 0 | 1 | C | + | E | – |
| P25 | 16 | M | Tuberculous spondylitis | T7-8 | 5 mo | 1 | C | + | E | – |
| P26 | 3 + 1 | F | Tuberculous spondylitis | T2-6 | 8 mo | 1 | C | – | E | – |
| P27 | 15 | M | Trauma | L1-3 | 6 mo | 4 | C | + | D | – |
| P28 | 17 | F | Trauma | L1-3 | 6 mo | 1 | C | + | D | – |
| P29 | 14 | M | Trauma | T12 | 3 mo | 2 | C | + | D | – |

*Complication of surgery.

Therefore, two grades, AC and BC, were added to create categories of patients clinically estimated as types A and B (no movements or muscle contraction during neurological testing in the standard supine position) but capable of quadrupedal or supported bipedal walking. Six patients were estimated as type AC or BC on the basis of EMG recordings of leg muscle activity during quadrupedal walking.

The majority of patients (23 patients of 29) initially had various degrees of spasticity in the leg muscles (rectus femoris, biceps femoris, triceps surae, tibialis anterior) and clonic activity in distal leg muscles, 4 patients had leg muscle hypotonia, and only 2 patients initially had clinically normal muscle tone.

## *Determination of the Functional Completeness of the Spinal Lesion*

Anatomical damage to the spinal cord was visualized with MRI data of the spine and spinal cord in 18 patients. However, many patients with complete functional paralysis ($n = 22$) did not show anatomically complete lesions. On the other hand, a case (P17) of spinal cord gunshot damage with an MRI-confirmed diastasis of about 3.5 cm was functionally incomplete. Hence, we did not use MRI data as the only criterion of lesion completeness.

The absence of voluntary movements or muscle contractions tested clinically can be interpreted as a dysfunction of the corticospinal tract but not necessarily of other descending tracts. H-reflex amplitude modulation may reveal influences mediated by the reticulo-, rubro-, vestibulo-, and propriospinal descending tracts. Therefore, we paid particular attention to detailed neurophysiological testing, including the comparison of H reflexes on both sides of the body at rest and during and after certain tests such as the Jendrassik maneuver, auditory stimulation, passive head turning (vestibular stimulation), and fast alternating movements of the arms imitating running (propriospinal test). The integrity of the corticospinal tracts was tested by the presence of visible leg movements in response to transcranial magnetic stimulation over the primary motor cortical areas.

Standard H-reflex testing was performed by electrical stimulation of the tibial nerve and EMG recording of the activity of medial gastrocnemius with patients in supine position. The following procedure was used.

1. Repetitive 0.5-Hz stimulation of increasing intensity to determine an optimal strength for testing stimulation. The strength of the stimulation was adjusted to induce M and H responses of approximately equal magnitude. (M response was used for control.)

2. Control: Recording of 32 consecutive M and H responses.

3. Test: The same stimulation parameters were used as during the control test. The five initial stimuli were applied as in the control condition. During the next 20 s (10 stimuli) one of the following facilitatory or inhibitory procedures was performed: Jendrassik maneuver, auditory stimulation, vestibulospinal stimulation, or propriospinal stimulation. The last 17 stimuli were applied during recovery after the facilitatory procedure.

4. The amplitudes of M and H responses during the test procedure (step 3) were compared with the those during the control procedure (step 2).

An example of the comparisons between control and test procedures with propriospinal stimulation is presented in figure 11.1. The amplitudes of the control M and H responses were not significantly modulated. During the test procedure, five initial records were similar to the control. With the onset of fast alternating arm movements (running imitation), the H response was depressed with no modulation of the M response. After the arm movements were stopped, the magnitude of the H response increased and returned to the initial value. The data were interpreted as showing an inhibitory influence on the H response via descending long axonal propriospinal connections. Similar results following the Jendrassik maneuver, auditory stimulation, and vestibulospinal stimulation showed the presence or absence of influences by noncortical descending supraspinal pathways.

The state of ascending tracts was tested clinically and with cortical somatosensory evoked potentials (SSEP) in response to the electrical stimulation of the tibial nerve. For incompletely paralyzed patients, EMG records of the main leg muscles during standing and walking with additional support were done. All recordings were done on an 8-channel Nicolet Viking IV (USA) using standard or modified programs.

## SCES: Epidural Electrical Stimulation of the Cervical and Lumbar Enlargements

Iwahara et al. (1992) showed that epidural electrical stimulation of the dorsal surface of the cervical enlargement could induce stepping in all four limbs in cats, while similar stimulation of the lumbar enlargement could evoke hindlimb stepping even after acute midthoracic transection of the spinal cord. In line with these results, we

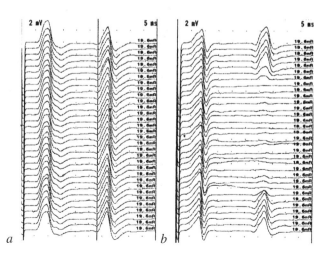

**Figure 11.1** Study of the descending influences on H-reflex amplitude. H-reflex during (a) control and (b) test with imitative arm movements. Thirty-two consecutive records, frequency of stimulation 0.5 Hz, patient P9.

hypothesized that electrical stimulation of both cervical and lumbar enlargements as well as the pathways between them can activate SLGs and induce locomotor-like activity. We used a similar stimulation technique in paralyzed patients to initiate steplike movements (Shapkova et al., 1997a, 1997b). SCES was applied at different spinal levels. During SCES, the patient was lying supine. The legs were suspended on elastic straps in a position such that the hip and knee joints were in semiflexion. In 5 patients, 6 wire electrodes were implanted transcutaneously at the level of the cervical enlargement (vertebrae C5-T1). In 6 patients 11 pairs of electrodes were implanted between the enlargements, above and below the spinal damage. In 11 patients 15 epidural electrodes were implanted at the lumbar enlargement level (vertebrae T11-L1), and in 2 patients electrodes were implanted below this level (vertebra L2; table 11.2). There were differences between the numbers of patients and implantations because some patients received repeated courses of epidural SCES.

Two different techniques evoking similar motor effects were used for this stimulation: (1) a pair of epidural electrodes implanted in the dorsal epidural space or (2) one active electrode implanted in the dorsal epidural space and a metal plate electrode (indifferent) placed on the abdomen. The implantations were done through a Touhe needle placed between L2 and L3. The electrodes were pushed up to the upper lumbar enlargement level or to a preenlargement level (vertebrae T10-11). Trial examinations were done at the initial electrode position and after consecutive displacement steps (pulling the electrode down by one to six steps of 5-10 mm per step). Electrodes were fixed at a level optimal for a bilateral alternating response

**Table 11.2   Levels of SCES Application in Paralyzed Patients**

| Method of SCES | Cervical enlargement (vertebrae C5-T1) | | Zone between cervical and lumbar enlargements (vertebrae T2-10) | | Lumbar enlargement (vertebrae T11-L1) | | Conus medullaris and cauda equina (vertebrae L2-3) | |
|---|---|---|---|---|---|---|---|---|
| | | Stepping-like activity induced (# patients) | | Stepping-like activity induced (# patients) | | Stepping-like activity induced (# patient) | | Stepping-like activity induced (# patients) |
| Epidural # patients # electrodes | 5 6 | 0 | 6 11 | 0 | 11 15 | 11 | 2 2 | 1 |
| Surface SCES | 3 | 0 | 7 | 0 | 29 | 29 | 18 | 1 |
| Total patients | 8 | 0 | 13 | 0 | 29 | 29 | 18 | 2 |

and used for therapeutic purposes. The optimal electrode position was documented with X-rays. The rate and amplitude of SCES were selected individually to induce alternating stepping and ranged from 0.5 to 100 Hz and 0.2 to 7 mA, respectively. Stimulus duration was 0.5 to 1 ms. The threshold (Th) for a bilateral response was defined as the amplitude of SCES that induced minimal bilateral movement. Visible, evoked, rhythmic, steplike activity was obtained after 1 to 30 sessions of SCES. Treatment lasted 1 to 7 months (on average, 2.5 mA) with five to six sessions per week, 40 to 180 min/day. The training load of the stimulation-evoked motor activity was assessed using pulse rate and blood pressure monitoring.

## Surface Percutaneous ES of the Lumbar Enlargement

Repeated courses of surface electrical stimulation applied at the same level, after previous courses of epidural SCES, have evoked similar steplike movements (Shapkova et al., 1997a). In some patients, we evoked steplike activity without an initial epidural stimulation. For surface SCES, metal plate electrodes were placed on the back (over the spinous processes) and the abdominal surface. The frequencies for SCES were the same as for epidural ES. SCES of the lumbar enlargement is noninvasive but requires a higher stimulation intensity. Initially, it could be as high as 70 to 85 mA, but after several sessions, a similar motor effect could be obtained with an intensity between 20 and 50 mA. This method can be painful for patients with intact sensation. The surface electrical stimulation can cause local cutaneous burns at the site of electrode application, particularly if the patient's sensitivity is impaired. The risk of burns can be decreased by the control of skin impedance during the stimulation and by ensuring good contact with the skin.

## Chronic Epidural ES of the Lumbar Enlargement
## With the Implanted Stimulator

We used the Neuroelect system, which includes epidural electrodes, an implanted receiver, and an external generator. The optimal electrode position was documented with X-rays. Evoked movements were documented with videotaped records and EMGs from rectus femoris (RF), biceps femoris (BF), soleus (Sol), and tibialis anterior (TA) and with knee displacement records for both legs.

# Results

Electrical stimulation was applied to the cervical and lumbar enlargements as well as to the pathways between them. The electrode position was documented with X-rays. Examples of spondilograms with implanted and surface electrodes are shown in figure 11.2.

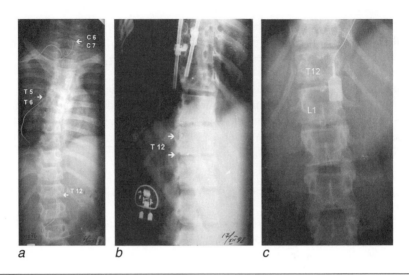

**Figure 11.2** X-rays of the spine with stimulating electrodes. *(a)* Epidural electrodes implanted at the cervical, midthoracic, and low-thoracic levels, patient P7. *(b)* Chronic epidural stimulation of the lumbar enlargement with an implanted system, patient P9. *(c)* Surface stimulation of the lumbar enlargement in patient P9.

Figure 11.2a is an X-ray of patient P7 showing epidural electrodes implanted at three levels, C6-7, T5-6, and T12. No coordinated rhythmic activity was obtained with SCES applied at either cervical or midthoracic levels. Stimulation at the T10 level evoked direct responses only, while stimulation at T11 evoked rhythmic in-phase but not alternating activity on both sides of the body. Alternating steplike movements were obtained only with T12 stimulation (indifferent electrode on the abdomen).

Figure 11.2b shows the implanted system for chronic epidural stimulation in patient P9. Epidural electrodes were implanted at T10 and T11, and after a few consecutive electrode displacements, an optimal zone was found at the T12 level. The X-ray image shows the implanted parts of the stimulation system (the receiver), but not the external generator. Figure 11.2c shows an X-ray image of the same patient during stimulation with surface electrodes (a year earlier). Comparison of the electrode positions in figure 11.2b and 11.2c suggests that similar zones were effective for inducing steplike movements by epidural and surface SCES. Displacement of the electrodes to the right or to the left from the midline was not critical for evoking symmetric alternating stepping. The zones of SCES application and methods of stimulation are presented in table 11.2.

All segments of the spinal cord were tested with electrical stimulation (table 11.2). Electrical stimulation of the cervical enlargement evoked synchronous direct responses in the muscles of both arms but no rhythmic activity in the arms or legs. No cases of rhythmic motor activity were found with stimulation of either the cervical enlargement (C5-T2; 8 patients) or the zone between the enlargements (T3-T10; 13 patients). In contrast, electrical stimulation of the lumbar enlargement

(T12-L1) evoked steplike movements in all patients. In two patients, stimulation of the lower zone (L2) was also effective.

We found that SCES at T11-L1 could evoke unilateral steplike movements as well as in-phase bilateral movements in most patients. In contrast, bilateral alternating stepping was induced only from a local zone that varied among individuals at a height about 15 to 20 mm. Alternating steplike movements could be lost as a result of a displacement of the electrode by a few millimeters from this optimal "locomotor zone."

The location of individual locomotor zones was constant with respect to the bone structures during the course of the stimulation. In most patients, no changes were found between the initial and subsequent courses. In only a few cases (P9, P21, and P28) this zone became wider after repeated courses of SCES, but the optimal zone with the lowest threshold for alternating response remained the same (figure 11.3).

Out of 29 patients, the locomotor zone was at the T12 level (including the T12-L1 disk) in 19 (66%), it was at L1 in 8 patients (28%), and it overlapped T12 and L1 in 2 patients. Two patients (6%) demonstrated alternating stepping with ES at both T12 and T11, and two others (6%) at both L1 and L2. Thus, in the majority of patients, the locomotor zone was within T12-L1, but it is necessary to note that the height of the locomotor zone was about 15 to 20 mm, and the height of vertebrae T12-L1 varied from 4 to 8 cm in patients of different ages.

To identify a locomotor zone within the lumbar enlargement, we compared X-ray images of the spine with the optimal position of the electrode using MRI or contrast myelography data. Such studies were done in only some patients, but the available observations show correspondence of the locomotor zone with the middle (wider) part of the lumbar enlargement.

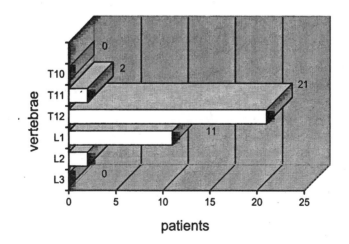

**Figure 11.3** Location of the effective zone for initiating alternating steplike movements with SCES in a group of paraplegic patients ($n = 29$).

The position of the stimulating electrode toward the spinal cord segments was controlled by low-frequency (0.5-Hz) stimulation of the spinal cord, resulting in EMG records of key muscles of the legs (Livenson and Ma, 1992). On the basis of these myotome studies, the location of the locomotor zone was estimated as the L3-L5 spinal cord segments.

## *Effective Parameters of SCES: Frequency and Amplitude*

For each patient, an effective frequency or a range of frequencies was found. The rate was considered effective if it evoked alternating stepping in the patient at least once. For two patients (P15 and P28), the range of effective rates was very wide, from 3 to 100 Hz, but more often it was between 3 and 5 Hz or between 7 and 12 Hz. These preferred frequencies were relatively unchanged during a course of stimulation but could change from one course to the next. For example, in patient P9, who was treated with SCES over 5 years, the optimal frequency during the initial course was 3 Hz; during the second and third courses the frequencies increased to 5 to 7 Hz and to 7 to 12 Hz respectively and then decreased to 7 Hz during the fourth course. A summary of results for the group ($n = 29$) are presented in figure 11.4.

As shown in figure 11.4, no cases of steplike activity were observed with stimulation rates below 2 Hz. A 2 Hz frequency was effective in only four patients. Frequencies between 3 and 12 Hz were effective in most patients, and a frequency of 3 Hz was effective in all patients. Among the higher frequencies, a range of 20 to 30 Hz was the most effective in 12 patients.

After an optimal zone and an optimal frequency of stimulation were defined, patterns of SCES-induced stepping were determined by the amplitude of the stimulation. The dependence between the amplitude and patterns of steplike movements was studied in 10 paralyzed patients (table 11.3).

A gradual increase in the SCES amplitude produced the following changes in the motor pattern: A low-amplitude (1.2-1.4 Th) stimulation evoked unstable movements for a few stepping cycles of one leg per cycle of the other leg or movements

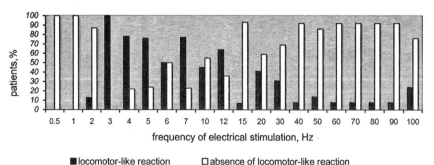

**Figure 11.4**   Probability of inducing locomotor-like responses with different frequencies of SCES in a group of paraplegic patients ($n = 29$).

From E. Shapkova et al. 1999.

Table 11.3    Amplitudes of SCES Evoking Different Kinds of Steplike Movements

| Patient | | Minimal bilateral response | | Alternating bilateral "stepping" | | | | In-phase "stepping" | |
|---|---|---|---|---|---|---|---|---|---|
| | | | | Unstable | | Stable | | | |
| | | mA | Th | mA | Th | mA | Th | mA | Th |
| 1 | P9 | 42.5 | 1 | 53 | 1.24 | 68-82 | 1.6-1.78 | 85-92 | 2-2.16 |
| 2 | P8 | 38 | 1 | 45-52 | 1.18-1.36 | 64 | 1.68 | 72-78 | 1.89-2.05 |
| 3 | P6 | 40 | 1 | 46 | 1.15 | 60-65 | 1.5-1.62 | 92 | 1.91 |
| 4 | P3 | 37.5 | 1 | 43 | 1.14 | 52-58 | 1.38-1.54 | 68 | 1.81 |
| 5 | P10 | 48 | 1 | 56 | 1.16 | 68-78 | 1.41-1.62 | 92 | 1.91 |
| 6 | P27 | 52 | 1 | — | — | 75 | 1.44 | 96-100 | 1.84-1.92 |
| 7 | P21 | 48 | 1 | — | — | 72 | 1.5 | 100 | 2.08 |
| 8 | P4* | 2.5 | 1 | 3 | 1.2 | 4.3 | 1.72 | 5-6 | 2-2.4 |
| 9 | P20* | 4.2 | 1 | 5 | 1.19 | 6.5 | 1.54 | 8.5 | 2.02 |
| 10 | P3* | 2.5 | 1 | 3.1 | 1.24 | 3.9 | 1.56 | 4.8-5 | 1.92-2 |
| | P3 | 31 | 1 | 38 | 1.22 | 50 | 1.6 | 58-60 | 1.87-1.93 |

*Epidural SCES

Th = threshold stimulation value

that stopped spontaneously. SCES between 1.4 and 1.8 Th evoked stable, bilateral, steplike movements that could continue for hours. Further amplitude increases led to synchronous leg stepping, and at amplitudes between 1.8 and 2.2 Th, only in-phase, bilateral, steplike movements could be evoked. Similar dependencies were obtained with epidural and surface SCES.

We classified motor reactions into four categories: (1) threshold for bilateral response, (2) unstable steplike movements, (3) alternating bilateral steplike movements, and (4) in-phase bilateral steplike movements (figure 11.5).

## Motor Reactions to SCES of Lumbar Enlargement

Electrical stimulation of the cervical enlargement and of the zone between the cervical and lumbar enlargements evoked short-latency responses in muscles on both sides of the body in exact correspondence with the spinal segments. Rhythmic, coordinated movements were not observed in the arms or legs. In contrast, SCES of the lumbar enlargement evoked a wide spectrum of motor reactions. The observed

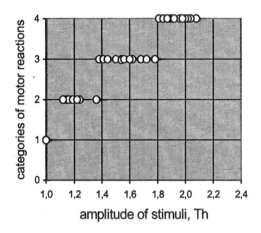

**Figure 11.5** Dependence between the amplitude of SCES and the pattern of induced steplike movements. Data are the means of 51 observations in 10 patients. The categories of motor responses induced with SCES are (1) threshold for bilateral response, (2) unstable steplike movements, (3) alternating bilateral steplike movements, (4) in-phase bilateral steplike movements.

rhythmic movements were classified into two general groups: *uncoordinated motor activity,* including synchronized muscle responses to each stimulus, tonic contraction, and clonic activity, and *coordinated stereotypical rhythmic motor activity,* including nonlocomotor movements and rhythmical movements comparable to locomotor activity. Our classification of types of SCES-evoked motor activity is presented in figure 11.6.

### Uncoordinated Motor Activity

Synchronous responses to every stimulus were observed in RF, BF, Sol, and TA muscles with low-rate (0.5-1 Hz) ES of the midlumbar enlargement. The latencies of the EMG responses (twitches) were about 3 to 7 ms in hip muscles and 14 to 17 ms in leg muscles. Applying SCES above the optimal zone (segments L2-L4) evoked responses in hip flexors, while SCES applied below the optimal zone (segments L4-S2) evoked responses in extensors corresponding to the segmental structure of the spinal cord. Uncoordinated simple responses to each stimulus could be also evoked with low-amplitude SCES between 2 and 12 Hz.

Tonic contraction could be evoked with ES at rates higher than 12 Hz. Even when the electrode was positioned in the body midline, tonic muscle contraction could be observed in one or both legs.

Clonic activity could be provoked by SCES of the lumbar enlargement at any rate. SCES-evoked clonic activity was rarely observed in patients with high levels of leg spasticity. When it occurred, clonic activity resembled rhythmic movement of the ankle at a frequency of 7 to 8 Hz with corresponding EMG bursts, mainly in muscles of the peroneal group, and did not stop immediately after the end of ES.

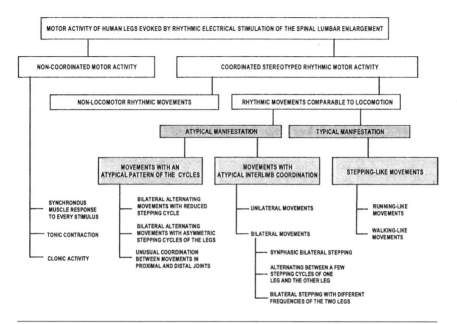

**Figure 11.6**   The classification of motor activity evoked with electrical stimulation of the lumbar enlargement, based on observations in paralyzed patients.

Rhythmic stereotypical movements evoked by the stimulation of the lumbar enlargement could have a nonlocomotor structure characterized by synchronous bilateral hip rotation or abduction. Such activity could take place prior to the beginning of steplike movements or as a stable reaction to SCES.

Locomotor leg movements in humans can be characterized by (1) the structure of a single cycle, (2) distinct bilateral alternating, and (3) repeated stereotypical rhythmic movements. SCES-induced movements fitting all these criteria were classified as typical locomotor-like activity. Besides rhythmical steplike movements that fit all the characteristics of human locomotion, many movements showed only some locomotor signs. These were classified as atypical manifestations of locomotor-like activity.

Well-coordinated steplike movements had the appearance of rhythmic leg flexions and extensions at the hip, knee, and ankle joints with a distinctive alternating pattern. The amplitude of movements varied from a few degrees to 75° at the hip, 85° at the knee, and 40° at the ankle. These ranges could be lower or higher than during natural locomotion (Vitenson, 1998). Either walking-like or running-like movements could be evoked in partially and completely paralyzed patients, though running-like movements were observed more often (figure 11.7).

Both running- and walking-like movements started 80 to 190 ms after the start of SCES (figure 11.8a) and continued for 10 to 27 cycles after the end of the stimulation (figure 11.8b). In a few cases, after the SCES was turned off, a transition from running-like to stepping-like movements was seen.

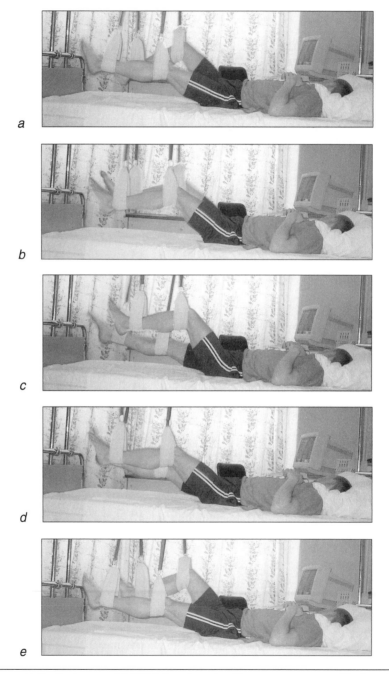

**Figure 11.7** Cyclogram of SCES-induced running-like movements. *(a–c)* Flexion of the left leg with extension of the right one; *(d–e)* extension of the left leg with flexion of the right one.

The frequency of SCES-induced alternating rhythmic movements varied from 1 to 7 Hz, and averaged 2.5 Hz. No clear relationship between the frequency of steplike movements and the rate of the stimulation was found. Fragments of EMG records during steplike activity evoked with different rates of SCES are shown in figure 11.8.

Records obtained with SCES rates of 20, 30, and 40 Hz (figure 11.9) show visible differences in the stimulus artifacts, while the EMG bursts and knee joint goniograms show similar rates. In other words, different rates of SCES could induce the same rate of stepping.

We also examined the step cycle duration as a function of SCES frequency in a patient (P28) who responded to a wide range of SCES frequencies. The duration of the step cycles obtained with each rate of SCES was calculated from video records. An increase in the SCES rate from 3 to 5 Hz shortened the step cycle while increasing the rate from 5 to 10 Hz stimulation frequency had no significant effects on the stepping cycle duration (see figure 11.9).

Note that a gradual decrease in the SCES rate had no effect on the rate of evoked stepping, even when the rates were 1 Hz and 0.5 Hz (figure 11.10). Stimulation at these frequencies was initially unable to evoke steplike movements. After the SCES was turned off, rhythmical movements continued with decreasing amplitude but relatively unchanged frequency for up to about 10 s. In contrast to the effects of gradual changes in SCES rates, an abrupt decrease in the frequency could turn a running-like movement into a walking-like pattern. In such cases, the running-like pattern continued for 3 cycles and then turned into a walking-like pattern at a slower rate and with lower amplitude EMG bursts. Similar observations have been obtained in animal experiments (Kniffki et al., 1981).

The comparison between SCES-induced and natural locomotion was done in a partially paralyzed patient (P28, type C on Frankel scale) who was initially able to imitate stepping in a supine position with suspended legs. Later, after a course of SCES-evoked locomotor training, this patient was able to ambulate over ground with support. We compared stimulation-induced steplike movements to both types of voluntary stepping. Walking-like and running-like activity are presented separately in figures 11.11 and 11.12 respectively.

SCES-evoked stepping and natural locomotor activity showed significantly different frequencies of stepping. A movement frequency of 3 Hz evoked by SCES resembled a fast running pattern with short steps. Our patient could not run but was able to imitate 1.5-Hz running movements in the air while supported by a parachute harness (body weight support 100%; figure 11.12c). Lying on her back with legs suspended, she easily developed a running-like activity of about 3 Hz (figure 11.12b). The maximal running-like movement rate for this patient was 3.85 Hz. The frequency of walking without support was under 1 Hz. After a course of SCES, the patient was able to perform six to eight steps without support, but the ability was limited with respect to both balance and locomotor capability.

Figures 11.11 and 11.12 show that during both running-like and walking-like movements, the EMG patterns were comparable to those obtained during voluntary

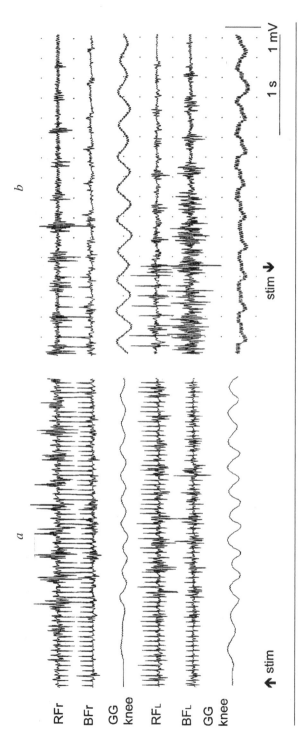

**Figure 11.8** (a) Running-like movements beginning with surface ES of 20 Hz applied at the level of vertebra L1. (b) Continuous rhythmic activity after the end of ES (15 Hz). ↑ beginning of ES; ↓ the end of ES. Patient P28.

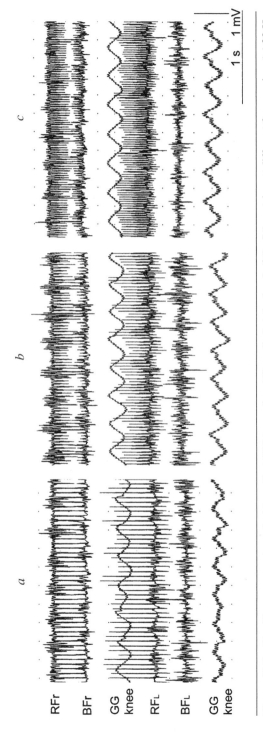

**Figure 11.9** Steplike movements evoked in patient P28 by surface ES applied at the level of the L1 vertebra at different frequencies: (a) 20 Hz, (b) 30 Hz, and (c) 40 Hz.

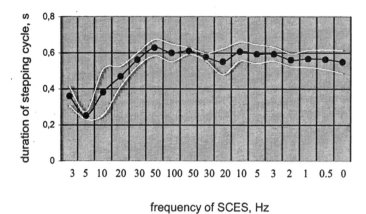

frequency of SCES, Hz

**Figure 11.10** Duration of stepping cycle in relationship to the frequency of SCES in patient P28. The frequency gradually increased from 3 to 100 Hz and then decreased from 100 to 0.5 Hz.

activity. During SCES-evoked "walking," EMGs of RF and BF within a leg showed different phases but partly overlapped. During the SCES-evoked "running" as well as during running imitation, this overlap was more significant. EMGs of the RF and BF of the other leg alternated in both SCES-evoked and voluntarily initiated stepping. In contrast to SCES-evoked "stepping," the end of voluntary stepping was never accompanied by repetitive, decreasing EMG bursts.

### Effects of Fatigue and Potentiation

ES-evoked and voluntary locomotor activities differed in that the former could last for more than 90 to 150 min with some potentiation during the stimulation period. Potentiation was characterized by an increase in the amplitude of steplike movements and in the recruitment of distal muscles, which are mostly silent at the beginning. Voluntary locomotor activity fatigued quickly and could not be sustained for more than 10 to 15 min (figure 11.13).

### Steplike Movements With Atypical Interlimb Coordination

Rhythmic movements with a typical single-step pattern but an atypical interlimb coordination, induced by SCES, were either *unilateral* or *bilateral.* During unilateral steplike movements, the contralateral leg could be relaxed or could show tonic contraction. Unilateral "stepping" could be caused by an off-midline electrode positioning or by SCES with low amplitude (unstable locomotion, see the section "Effective Parameters of SCES: Frequency and Amplitude"). In some cases, unilateral "stepping" as well as a transfer from unilateral "stepping" by one leg to "stepping" by the other leg was observed with SCES of the optimal zone with unchanged parameters. For example, in patient P6, repeated, stable, high-amplitude, left-leg stepping movements stopped for 2 to 3 cycles and then resumed in the right leg without any change in the stimulation.

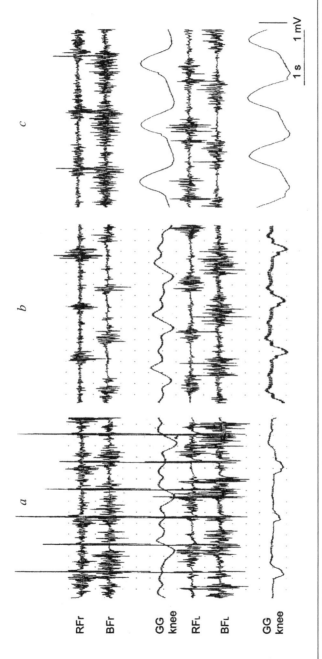

**Figure 11.11** Walking-like movements under different conditions (in patient P28): (*a*) Walking-like movements at 1 Hz evoked with 2-Hz SCES. (*b*) Voluntarily initiated imitative stepping in the same position. (*c*) Overground walking with additional support.

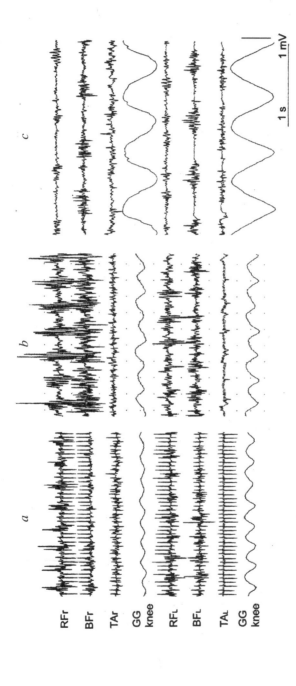

**Figure 11.12** Running-like movements under different conditions (in patient P28): (*a*) Running-like movements evoked with SCES. (*b*) Voluntarily initiated locomotor movements (while patient lay on her back). (*c*) Running-like stepping in the air while supported by a parachute system.

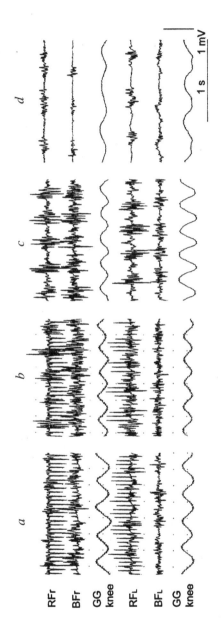

**Figure 11.13** Effects of fatigue and potentiation during voluntarily initiated and SCES-induced steplike activity (EMG records of RF and BF and knee goniograms, patient P28): (*a*) SCES-induced running-like movements at the beginning and (*b*) after 40 min of SCES; (*c*) voluntary imitation of stepping at the beginning and (*d*) after 10 min of activity.

In two patients (P13 and P22), unilateral steplike movements were regularly obtained because of the difference in the threshold rates of SCES that could initiate steplike movements in the right and left legs. In particular, in P22 (for whom the stimulating electrode was placed over the midline), stimulation at 3 to 5 Hz was optimal for the right leg but had no effect on the left leg. The left leg showed high-amplitude steplike movement with SCES at 12 Hz, but the right leg was in a state of tonic contraction. In this patient we trained the left and the right legs separately using the optimal parameters for each leg. Only after 3 weeks of daily training did it become possible to obtain alternating bilateral stepping with a compromise 6-Hz SCES, but the amplitude of the bilateral movements was lower than that during unilateral steplike movements at the optimal rates.

Atypical interactions between SLGs were manifested as in-phase bilateral movements as well as bilateral "stepping" with a constant phase shift between the legs and movements at different rates of the right and left legs. In-phase two-leg "stepping" was observed in all patients with electrical stimulation of the lumbar enlargement above or below the optimal locomotor zone. The same effect could be obtained during stimulation of the optimal zone but with a higher-amplitude SCES. Movements of the two other types were seldom observed and in only a few patients. During bilateral steplike movements with different right and left frequencies, the rates were commonly related in a 1:2 ratio and more rarely 1:3. Steplike movements with other rate ratios were unstable and stopped after a few cycles.

ES-induced movements with an atypical interlimb coordination revealed the possibility of different interactions between SLGs, including alternation, coactivation, and coupling of steplike movements with different rates.

Alternating bilateral movements with an atypical pattern were seen as alternating movements in one or two pairs of homonymous joints (incomplete locomotor pattern) or as movements with an unusual coordination between the proximal and distal joints. Rhythmical movements with an incomplete pattern were often observed at the beginning of SCES. During stimulation-evoked activity (after about 40 min), these movements could change into a typical locomotor cycle. However, in some cases movements with an incomplete pattern were stable and did not change during SCES. For example, alternating, rhythmical hip flexion and extension at 3 Hz with an amplitude of about 40° were observed in patient P12. The knee joints were not involved in these movements and remained in a flexed position. Similar alternating, rhythmical hip movements were observed in patient P19, but with a rate of about 1.5 Hz, an amplitude of 30°, and with the knee joints extended. Rhythmic movements with distinct alternation in the knee joints were recorded in patient P15, but more often such rhythmic activity was observed not in one but in two pairs of joints. Usually it was the hip and the knee or the knee and the ankle. No cases of rhythmic activity in the hip and the ankle joints in the absence of activity in the knee joints were observed. Average frequencies of these hip and knee movements varied from 1.5 to

3.5 Hz, whereas movements in distal joints could reach frequencies of 5 to 7 Hz.

Another kind of ES-induced atypical pattern was found in patient P9, in whom hip joint flexion was followed by extension in the knee and ankle joints. Such an unusual single-cycle pattern was observed during either alternating or in-phase bilateral movements. We also observed stereotypical rhythmic activity, which combined alternating movements in one pair of homonymous joints and synchronous movements in another pair. In patient P6, synchronous flexion in the hip joints was accompanied by flexion in the right and extension in the left knee joint. During the hip joint extension, the right knee extended and the left one flexed. Comparison of this unusual pattern to either alternating or in-phase bilateral "stepping" shows a different movement in one joint only (hip or knee joint).

# Clinical Implication of SCES With a Locomotor-like Effect

Locomotor recovery in paralyzed patients requires the restoration of ability for both rhythmic leg stepping and body weight support. Both these functions are controlled by descending commands. The absence or deficit of descending influences makes standing and walking extremely difficult for paraplegic patients, especially those with functionally complete lesions, despite the intact spinal locomotor structures. That is why we suggest that rehabilitative therapy has to include (1) activation and training of spinal locomotor activity, (2) activation of ascending and descending tracts, and (3) recovery and training of natural and adapted locomotion (quadrupedal walking and knee walking).

During the last 7 years, we have used SCES-evoked locomotor activity to facilitate motor recovery in paralyzed children as a part of their rehabilitation (Shapkova et al., 1999a). The aims and methods of rehabilitation depend on the neurological status and motor capability of the patients and are presented as a sequence of five stages (table 11.4).

For completely paralyzed patients (types A and B), training with locomotor-like activity evoked by SCES of the lumbar enlargement (invasive or noninvasive) was routinely used. Rhythmical SCES-induced motion was the main form of motor activity. Another method of activation of SLGs and of the long descending propriospinal connections was propriospinal stimulation, in which intensive arm movements imitating running produced an effect on rhythmic leg activity. Stimulation-induced locomotor training was complemented with physical exercises (passive movements assisted by a physiotherapist).

The appearance of the first elements of voluntary control, such as minimal muscle contractions or voluntary initiation of rhythmic leg activity (including initiation of spastic contractions) would bring the patient to the second stage. Patients were considered to be incompletely paralyzed, although some might have made no progress in the control of isolated muscles (types AC and BC). These patients might only have been able to initiate rhythmic activity, and there might have been no significant changes in neurological status. In the second stage, the SCES-evoked locomotor-like movements were also the main form of motor activity. Patients trained with both

**Table 11.4    Treatment Protocol for Restoration of Walking in Patients With Vertebrogenic Myelopathies as a Function of Neurological Status and Motor Capabilities**

| Neurological status, class on Frankel | The aims of rehabilitation | General forms of locomotor activity / Methods of physiotherapeutic treatment | Criteria for stage completion (restored motor capability) |
|---|---|---|---|
| Stage 1 A, B | 1. Activation and training of spinal locomotor activity 2. Activation of propriospinal connections between upper and lower extremities 3. Elements of motor control restoration | ES-evoked locomotor activit 1. Epidual or surface SCES 2. Propriospinal stimulation 3. Physical exercises (passive movements assisted by physiotherapists) | Initiation of voluntary movements or voluntarily induced spasticity |
| Stage 2 C, AC,* BC* | 1. Training of spinal locomotor activity 2. Training of propriospinal connections between upper and lower extremities 3. Available forms of posture and locomotion forming | Evoked locomotor activity 1. Epidural or surface SCES 2. Propriospinal stimulation 3. Treadmill training with BWS 4. Physical exercises (passive-active movements assisted by physiotherapists) | Quadrupedal standing, quadrupedal walking |
| Stage 3 C, AC,* BC* | 1. Training of spinal locomotor activity 2. Training of available forms of natural locomotor activity | Evoked and voluntary locomotor activity 1. Surface SCES 2. Treadmill training with BWS 3. Quadrupedal standing and walking 4. Physical exercises (active movements assisted by physiotherapists) | Walking on knees with additional support |

| Neuro-logical status, class on Frankel | The aims of rehabilitation | General forms of locomotor activity Methods of physiotherapeutic treatment | Criteria for stage completion (restored motor capability) |
|---|---|---|---|
| Stage 4 D, AC,* BC* | 1. Training of available forms of natural locomotor activity 2. Training of vertical posture 3. Forming of walk technique | Natural locomotor activity 1. Quadrupedal walking and kneeling 2. Treadmill training with BWS 3. Walk training with or without additional support 4. Walk training with or without visual or EMG control 5. Surface SCES (prewalk potentiating) | Vertical posture with additional support, walking with facilitation |
| Stage 5 D, AC,* BC* | 1. Training the muscle groups for limited walking 2. Walk training 3. Gait correction | Natural locomotor activity 1. Power- and endurance-oriented training programs (stepper, bicycle) 2. Treadmill training with or without limited BWS 3. Walk training with or without additional support 4. Walk training with or without visual or EMG feedback 5. Surface SCES (prewalk potentiating) | Standing and walking without time limits |

Reprinted from Shapkova, Mushkin, and Kovalenko (1999).
*Additional ranges. See "Method" on page 257.

SCES-evoked and treadmill stepping with body weight support. The third stage started when the patient was able to support himself or herself and ambulate in the quadrupedal position. At this stage, the training included both SCES-evoked and voluntary locomotion. With increasing motor capabilities, the training with SCES-evoked locomotion decreased, while that with voluntary locomotion increased. In stages 4 and 5, SCES-evoked stepping was no longer used for training patients who were able to walk, only for prewalking training, and voluntary locomotor activity became the main form of motor activity.

## Clinical Results of Treatment: Acute and Long-Term Effects

During consecutive sessions of SCES, an increase in the locomotor-like activity was observed in both completely and incompletely paralyzed patients. Despite this, contrary to our expectations, the completely paralyzed patients were unable to walk during the sessions of SCES because of instability in the vertical posture. In contrast, immediately after switching the stimulation off, standing and walking were facilitated for 30 to 60 min. For example, patient P9 (initially type A on the Frankel scale), after five annual ES courses (two epidural and three surface) had no voluntary isolated movements in the legs and could not stand without external fixation of the knees. He could, however, walk on hands and knees and on the knees. After 40 min of SCES-induced steplike activity, the patient was able to stand and walk with additional support during about 45 min (walking over 75 to 100 m). The dependence of the motor abilities of this patient on SCES and the absence of neurological improvement after a few courses of stimulation were the reason for implanting the system for chronic epidural stimulation. After the implantation, the same effects of evoked stepping with a limited poststimulation ability to stand and walk were managed by the patient.

After SCES, all patients who were able to walk increased walking distance by 150% to 200% of prestimulation distance. Muscle tone changed; it increased in patients with low muscle tone and decreased in those with high muscle tone and spasticity. Such effects lasted throughout the day.

A course of locomotor training with SCES improved the physical status of all patients, decreasing leg muscle atrophy and normalizing muscle tone. Most of the spastic patients (20 out of 23) were able to stop taking baclofen or other antispastic drugs. Most patients had improvements in control of bowel and bladder functions as well as in sensation. Clinical examination showed that, as a rule, changes in sensation preceded motor function. The results of motor function recovery are presented in table 11.5.

All incompletely paralyzed patients (6) recovered the ability to walk with (3) or without (3) assistance. Among the 23 initially completely paralyzed patients, 16

**Table 11.5   Results of Rehabilitation in Groups of Completely and Incompletely Paralyzed Patients**

| Effect of rehabilitation | Incompletely paralyzed patients | | Initially completely paralyzed patients | |
|---|---|---|---|---|
| Recovery of either muscle control or locomotion (different degrees) | 6 (100%) (3+ 3) | P24, P25, P26 P27, P28, P29 | 10 (43%) (2 + 4 + 4) | P4, P21 P2, P3, P5, P6 P7, P19, P20, P22 |
| Recovery of ability for quadrupedal and supported bipedal walk in absence of isolated leg muscle control | | | 6 (26%) | P9, P10, P15, P17, P18, P23 |
| No motor improvement | | | 7 (30%) | P1, P8, P11, P12, P13, P14, P16 |
| Total | 6 | | 23 | |

(about 70%) showed some improvement in motor abilities. We observed two types of motor improvement: (1) a steady progress in muscle strength and ability to ambulate and (2) an improvement in quadrupedal locomotion with poorly supported bipedal locomotion in the absence of any isolated leg movements or muscle contractions. We viewed only the first type of improvement as motor recovery. Recovery of either muscle control or locomotion was obtained in 10 patients (43%), including two cases of good recovery (unlimited walking and running) and four cases of muscle strength recovery and walking with support. Four patients had partial motor recovery and showed incomplete paraplegia with limited voluntary movements of the legs and some capability of walking with significant additional support.

Six patients had paradoxical effects. After a few courses of SCES, they had no isolated voluntary movements or muscle contractions in the legs but were able to walk on hands and knees or knees only. They later could perform limited bipedal walking with support. Seven completely paralyzed patients improved their general physical state with SCES-evoked locomotor training but made no progress in motor control.

Among patients treated with repeated courses of SCES, a group of seven completely paralyzed children did not show improvement in motor function despite the occurrence of pronounced SCES-evoked stepping. However, other benefits—such as a decrease in spasticity, improvements in sensation and in bladder and bowel control, and a decrease in muscle atrophy—were obtained during an 8- to 10-week course of SCES that persisted for 3 to 4 months.

Neurophysiological testing of patients with paradoxical walking showed an H-reflex modulation during both the Jendrassik maneuver and the propriospinal test (which was absent initially) but no responses in leg muscles to magnetic stimulation of the cortex. The data are interpreted as the existence of supraspinal and propriospinal influences on spinal motoneurons, which suggests that at least some descending spinal projections remained intact or were restored. In contrast, patients who made no progress in motor control showed no H-reflex modulation during these tests.

## Discussion

In recent studies, a group of patients (classes A and B on the Frankel scale) who had been trained to walk on a treadmill with body weight support showed a correlation between the amplitude of the EMG bursts in their tibialis anterior and gastrocnemius muscles during stepping and the level of their spinal cord lesion; that is, a "more normal" locomotor pattern was seen in patients with a larger section of the spinal cord separated from the brain (Dietz et al., 1999; Erni et al., 1999). This finding led those authors to suggest that the generation of EMG activity occurring during bipedal locomotion in humans is not localized in a specific part of the spinal cord. Our investigations do not support this suggestion. On the contrary, we observed different patterns of locomotor-like activity with SCES of the lumbar enlargement (at T11-L1), and the application of electrical stimulation above or below this level was ineffective in both completely and incompletely paraplegic patients. Moreover, a specific locomotor zone at which SCES could evoke alternating steplike activity was found within the lumbar enlargement. In all our patients, this zone was found at the level of the midlumbar enlargement. The absence of alternating steplike activity from SCES above and below the local locomotor zone suggests that some neuronal structures responsible for the reciprocal relations between the leg muscles, probably part of the SLG, are located at this level.

We did not find any dependence between either the SCES-induced locomotor pattern or the capacity for locomotion and the level of the spinal lesion except for cases of T12-L1 level trauma, in which steplike movements could not be evoked because of the destruction of the lumbar section of the spinal cord. In all patients with intact lumbar enlargement (damage at the level of vertebra T11 or above), steplike movements were obtained with SCES of the middle part of the enlargement. We view these observations as strong evidence for the existence of SLGs in the human lumbar enlargement.

## Effective Parameters for Stimulation

The wide range (2-100 Hz) of frequencies of SCES that could evoke steplike movements shows that electrical activation of SLGs cannot be viewed as resulting from activation of descending or peripheral excitatory inputs. Our results only partly corroborate the data of Dimitrijevic et al. (1996, 1998) and Gerasimenko et al. (1996), who obtained rhythmic leg movements in paraplegic patients with SCES of the L2 spinal segment (vertebra T11) at 20 to 30 Hz. We also found the range of 20 to 30 Hz to be effective, but for less than 40% of the patients, while the range of 3 to 12 Hz was effective for a majority of the patients, and 3 Hz was effective in all cases. The latter observation is similar to the data of Iwahara et al. (1992), who reported that rates of 0.5 to 10 Hz for SCES of the lumbar enlargement in spinalized cats were optimal for stepping initiation and that, moreover, rates of 3 to 5 Hz were effective in all experimental animals.

The dependence between the amplitude of SCES and the pattern of evoked steplike activity suggests relationships between the different manifestations of locomotor-like reactions, including those atypical of natural human locomotion. A similar dependence between the amplitude of electrical stimulation and the pattern of SCES-induced stepping has been described in decerebrated cats (Baev, 1991).

The unchanged site of SCES application and its unchanged frequency could suggest that similar neuronal structures were activated in cases of either atypical or typical locomotor-like activity. Moreover, a smooth transition from unstable motor patterns to a stable, alternating, bilateral "stepping" and then to an in-phase bilateral motion show that the intensity of SCES does not change the single-step pattern but does have an effect on interlimb coordination. On the basis of these amplitude-dependent changes in the motor behavior, we suggest that the in-phase bilateral movements are manifestations of locomotor-like activity.

## Reflexes or Centrally Generated Pattern?

Steplike activity induced by rhythmical electrical stimulation of the lumbar enlargement seems similar to rhythmically repeated reflexes or a centrally generated pattern. Two arguments refute the first and support the second suggestion. First, the frequencies of SCES and stimulation-evoked movements could be independent. Second, the rhythmic activity could last longer than the period of SCES. On the basis of these findings, we contend that SCES-induced steplike movements likely activate a centrally generated pattern.

## Comparison of SCES-Induced and Natural Locomotion

The locomotor activity that could be induced by SCES in an incompletely paraplegic patient had features similar to those of the stepping movements produced voluntarily by the patient under comparable conditions. The similarities included both the frequency of evoked responses and the performance of walking- and running-like movements.

The main frequency of stimulation-evoked stepping was 1.5 to 3.5 Hz. The latter frequency is quite high for human locomotion, particularly for paraplegic patients, but these rates are usual for sportlike cyclical movements that include locomotion: The stepping frequency in long-distance running is about 3.5 to 3.7 Hz, and in the sprint it is about 5 Hz, while the rate of rhythmic alternate cycling can reach 7.1 Hz (Bober, 1985). In comparison, the 3- to 3.5-Hz frequency of evoked stepping, which does not depend on the rate of SCES and which continued for hours without changes in the stepping rate, could be an optimal rate for running. The second point that needs explanation is the overlap of the EMG activity in antagonistic muscles. During walking, the EMGs of antagonistic muscles are typically out of phase or show some overlapping. It is known that overlapping increases with the rate of stepping. However, overlapping activity in antagonistic muscles also occurs in spasticity. The significant EMG overlapping observed in rectus femoris and biceps femoris muscles during SCES-evoked stepping was partly related to the rate of stepping. Keeping in mind that the SCES-evoked running-like movements were easily voluntarily reproduced at the same rates (and higher, up to 3.85 Hz) and showed similar EMG patterns, the SCES-evoked 3- to 3.5-Hz stepping might be regarded as an activation of a central pattern for running, that is, realization of a spinal running program.

The occurrence of both running-like and walking-like SCES-evoked movements with typical EMG patterns and sharp rather than gradual transitions from one type of locomotion to the other could indicate the existence of two central programs. The observations of both running-like or walking-like movements induced by SCES at the same rates suggest that the motor output may be determined by the state of the central rhythm generator.

The similarities in the frequency and patterns of walking- and running-like movements induced voluntarily and by SCES under comparable conditions may indicate that the same central structures were engaged in the performance of the movements. The observed differences between potentiation during SCES and fatigue during voluntarily initiated locomotor activity support the idea that spinal and supraspinal mechanisms are involved in the initiation of locomotor activity.

Summarizing the observations concerning the coordination of steplike movements induced by SCES, we conclude that they have (1) a centrally generated pattern, (2) similarities in frequency and pattern with walking- and running-like movements induced voluntarily under comparable conditions, and (3) specificity with respect to the level of stimulation. On the basis of these findings, we regard steplike movements evoked with SCES as spinal locomotor activity, and we suggest that the human lumbar enlargement contains SLGs similar to those described in vertebrate animals.

SCES with the same parameters at the optimal locomotor zone could also evoke stereotypical movements with an atypical cycle or atypical interlimb coordination. These "incorrect" coordination patterns are likely generated by the same neuronal structures as typical locomotor patterns. What could these movements say about the SLG organization?

The possibility of initiating unilateral "stepping" with SCES of the lumbar enlargement suggests the existence of an SLG for each leg and the possibility of activating them separately. Cases of bilateral movements at different stepping frequencies by the right and left legs also support this suggestion. Such activity as bilateral, alternating, rhythmic movements in one or two pairs of homonymous joints may indicate a centrally generated pattern for every pair of homonymous joints. A comparison between stereotyped bilateral movements with symmetric and asymmetric leg patterns shows differences between these centrally generated patterns concerning the movements in one joint. This could mean that the minimal unit of the centrally generated pattern is movement in one joint.

Summarizing our observations concerning SCES-induced activity with signs atypical for natural human locomotion, we suggest (1) the existence of an SLG for each leg, (2) a complex organization of interaction between SLGs, (3) the possibility of generating patterns for pairs of homonymous joints, and (4) movement in one joint as a minimal unit of a centrally generated pattern.

## *Diversity of Motor Reactions*

The wide diversity of motor reactions evoked by SCES of the lumbar enlargement could be induced by the activation of segmental short-latency reflexes and interneuronal networks that generate rhythmical activity, including clonus and stereotypical coordinated movements. Activation of these interneuronal structures in the lumbar enlargement by SCES could produce such stereotypical coordinated movements as atypical walking-like and running-like movements. Manifestations of SCES-evoked spinal activity seem to be much richer than the natural human locomotion manifested as the typical gaits of walking and running. The variety of SCES-induced movements can be explained in at least two ways. First, the artificial electrical stimulation of the lumbar enlargement, in addition to evoking the standard locomotor pattern, could activate some other patterns rarely or never used for natural locomotion. In fact, this could demonstrate not only the actual but also the potential abilities of the spinal cord. Second, the spinal cord could generate rhythmic movements of both a locomotor and nonlocomotor nature, probably using the same or partly overlapping interneuronal networks: The in-phase bilateral activity is an atypical pattern for human locomotion (although hopping is not atypical for children) but typical, for example, for spinal sexual behavior. Similar relationships between generators for locomotion and scratching are well described in decerebrated cats (Baev, 1991; Berkinblit et al., 1978; Gelfand et al., 1988).

The effectiveness of SCES-induced locomotor training in functionally completely paralyzed patients suggests that SCES has an effect not only at the spinal level. Such clinical results as the improvement in sensitivity and progress in locomotor ability in formerly functionally completely paralyzed patients indicates an effect of locomotor training with SCES not only on SLGs but also on ascending and descending spinal tracts. Similar effects were not observed with treadmill training, despite its being known as one of the most effective methods for locomotor recovery in patients with incomplete paralysis (Barbeau et al., 1998; Dietz et al., 1998; Edgerton et al., 1997, 2001). What are the main differences between these two methods?

First, SCES-induced locomotor-like activity can be applied for a longer period of time. Normal sessions of treadmill training last for about 30 to 40 min, while SCES-induced locomotor training can last up to 60 to 120 min or more without fatigue. Second, prolonged (longer than 40 min) sessions of SCES-evoked activity have a potentiating effect on locomotor activity. Third, SCES-evoked stepping occurs at higher (on average 1.5 to 3 Hz) frequencies than treadmill stepping (0.7 to 1 Hz), which makes training more intensive. Fourth, higher-intensity training not only affects locomotor pattern generation but also induces secondary sensory stimulation of the spinal cord via the afferents of the rhythmically activated muscles. Finally, during SCES the spinal cord (including its ascending and descending tracts) receives direct electrical stimulation at a high rate (often 3 to 12 Hz). It is not difficult to calculate that during every session of SCES-induced training the SLGs generate 2.25 to 16 times more motor and sensory patterns than during treadmill training.

Summarizing all these differences, we conclude that SCES-induced locomotor training is the most intensive method known for locomotor restoration, affecting both spinal locomotor generators as well as ascending and descending pathways. The method is effective in patients with both complete and incomplete paralysis, but its main mechanisms of action are different. In completely paralyzed patients, the main purpose is to compensate for the hypodynamia and achieve a state of incomplete paralysis. Locomotor training with SCES is the only form of motor activity for completely paralyzed patients (types A and B), and intensive training improves the fitness of the patient. If the patients show no progress in activation or recovery of descending tracts, they will stay completely paralyzed and will need periodic courses of stimulation-evoked locomotion or chronic epidural SCES to induce locomotion. Our experience with chronic epidural electrical stimulation of the lumbar enlargement with an implanted system is limited to two cases, but it offers a new possibility for chronically paralyzed patients. In incompletely paralyzed patients, locomotor training with SCES can be used in addition to treadmill training to facilitate the locomotor capability of the spinal cord as well as to intensify the training.

## Conclusions

1. The possibility to evoke well-coordinated alternating steplike movements by SCES in functionally completely paralyzed patients suggests the existence of an SLG in the human midlumbar enlargement.

2. A "locomotor zone," probably containing structures responsible for bilateral alternating movement, is likely located at about the L3-L5 spinal cord level.

3. The relative independence of the frequency of induced movements from SCES frequency and the continuing activity after the end of SCES indicate that these movements are centrally generated.

4. Cases of atypical coordination between the legs suggest the existence of separate generators for each leg with a complex interaction.

5. An improved ability to walk in all incompletely paralyzed patients and different degrees of progress in locomotor ability in about 70% of originally completely paralyzed patients show the effectiveness of locomotor training with SCES for paralyzed patients, especially for those with functionally complete paralysis.

6. Such clinical results as improvement in sensitivity and progress in locomotor ability in formerly functionally completely paralyzed patients indicate that locomotor training with SCES has an effect not only on SLGs but also on ascending and descending spinal tracts.

## Acknowledgments

I am very grateful to Eike D. Schomburg for his collaboration, to Mark L. Latash for many helpful discussions of the topics considered in this chapter, and to Mindy Levin for editing the manuscript.

## References

Baev, K.V. (1991) *Neurobiology of locomotion.* Nauka: Moscow (in Russian).
Barbeau, H., and Blunt, R. (1991) A novel interactive locomotor approach using body weight support to retrain gait in spastic paretic subjects. In Wernig, A. (Ed.), *Plasticity of motoneuronal connections,* pp. 461-474. Amsterdam: Elsevier.

Barbeau, H., McCrea, D.A., O'Donovan, M.J., Rossignol, S., Grill, W.M., and Lemay, M.A. (1999) Tapping into spinal circuits to restore motor function. *Brain Res Rev* 30: 27-51.

Barbeau, H., Norman, K., Fung, J., Visintin, M., and Ladouceur, M. (1998) Does neurorehabilitation play a role in the recovery of walking in neurological populations? *Ann NY Acad Sci* 860: 377-392.

Barbeau, H., and Rossignol, S. (1994) Enhancement of locomotor recovery following spinal cord injury. *Curr Opin Neurol* 7: 517-524.

Berkinblit, M.B., Deliagina, T.G., Feldman, A.G., Gelfand, J.M., and Orlovsky, G.N. (1978) Generation of scratching: 1. Activity of spinal interneurons during scratching. *J Neurophysiol* 41: 1040-1057.

Bober, T. (1985) Biomechaniczna charakterystika chodu i biegu. *Sport Wyczynowy* 5: 16-27.

Bussel, B., Roby-Brami, A., Azouvi, Ph., Biraben, A., Yakoleff, A., and Held, J.P. (1988) Myoclonus in a patient with spinal cord transection: Possible involvement of the spinal stepping generator. *Brain* 111: 1235-1245.

Bussel, B., Roby-Brami, A., Neris, O.R., and Yakovleff, A. (1996) Evidence for a spinal stepping generator in man. *Paraplegia* 34: 91-92.

Bussel, B., Roby-Brami, A., Yakovleff, A., and Bennis, N. (1989) Late-flexion reflex in paraplegic patients: Evidence for a spinal stepping generator. *Brain Res Bull* 22: 53-56.

Calancie, B., Needham-Shropshire, B., Jacobs, P., Willer, K., Zych, G., and Green, B.A. (1994) Involuntary stepping after chronic spinal cord injury: Evidence for a central rhythm generator for locomotion in man. *Brain* 117: 1143-1159.

Dietz, V., Colombo, G., and Jensen, L. (1994) Locomotor activity in spinal man. *Lancet* 344 (8932): 1260-1263.

Dietz, V., Colombo, G., Jensen, L., and Baumgartner, L. (1995) Locomotor capacity of spinal cord in paraplegic patients. *Ann Neurol* 37: 574-582.

Dietz, V., Nakazawa, K., Wirz, M., and Erni, Th. (1999) Level of spinal cord lesion determines locomotor activity in spinal man. *Exp Brain Res* 128: 405-409.

Dietz, V., Wirz, M., Curt, A., and Colombo, G. (1998) Locomotor pattern in paraplegic patients: Training effects and recovery of spinal cord function. *Spinal Cord* 36: 380-390.

Dimitrijevic, M.R., Gerasimenko, Y., and Pinter, M.M. (1998) Evidence for a spinal central pattern generator in humans. *Ann NY Acad Sci* 860: 360-377.

Dimitrijevic, M.R., Halter, J.A., Gerasimenko, Y., Sherwood, A.M., and McKay, W.B. (1996) Central pattern generator in humans: Motor responses evoked by and spinal cord evoked potentials recorded from epidural electrodes at different locations. *Soc Neurosci Abstr* 22: 543.8.

Ditunno, J.F., Young, W., Donovan, W.H., and Greasey, G. (1994) The international standards booklet for neurological and functional classification of spinal cord injury. *Paraplegia* 32: 70-80.

Dobkin, B., Harkema, S., Requejo, P.S., and Edgerton, V.R. (1995) Modulation of locomotor-like EMG activity in subjects with complete and incomplete spinal cord injury. *J Neurol Rehabil* 9: 183-190.

Edgerton, V.R., de Leon, R.D., Harkema, S.J., Hodgson, J.A., London, N., Reinkensmeyer, D.J., Roy, R.R., Talmadge, R.J., Tillakaratne, N., Timoszyk, W., and Tobin, A. (2001) Retraining the injured spinal cord. *J Physiol* 533 (1): 15-22.

Edgerton, V.R., de Leon, R.D., Tillakaratne, N.J., Recktenwald, N., Hodgson, J.A., and Roy, R.R. (1997) Use-dependent plasticity in spinal stepping and standing. In Seil, F.J. (Ed.), *Advances in neurology: Neuronal regeneration, reorganization and repair,* vol. 72, pp. 233-247. Philadelphia: Lippincott-Raven.

Edgerton, V.R., Roy, R.R., Hodgson, J.A., Prober, R.J., de-Guzman, C.P., and de-Leon, R. (1992) Potential of adult mammalian lumbosacral spinal cord to execute and acquire improved locomotion in the absence of supraspinal input. *J Neurotrauma* 9: 119-128.

Erni, Th., Nakazawa, K., Wirtz, M., and Dietz, V. (1999) The level of spinal cord lesion determines the locomotor activity in spinal man. In Gantchev, G., and Gantchev, N., *From basic motor to functional recovery: Concepts, theories and models,* pp. 257-263. Sofia: Professor Marius Drinov Academic Publishing House.

Federichuk, B., Jensen, J., Peterson, N., and Hultborn, H. (1998) Pharmacologically evoked fictive motor patterns in the acutely spinalized marmoset monkey *(Callithrix jacchus). Exp Brain Res* 122: 351-361.

Frankel, H.L., Hancock, D.O., Hyslop, G., Melzack, J., Michaelis, L.S., Ungar, G.H., Vernon, J.D.S., and Walsh, J.J. (1969) The value of postural reduction in the initial management of closed injuries of the spine with paraplegia and tetraplegia. *Paraplegia* 7: 179-192.

Fung, J., Stewart, J.E., and Barbeau, H. (1990) The combined effects of clonidine and cyproheptadine with interactive training on the modulation of locomotion in spinal cord injured subjects. *J Neurol Sci* 100: 85-93.

Gelfand, I.M., Orlovsky, G.N., and Shik, M.L. (1988) Locomotion and scratching in tetrapods. In Cohen, A.H., Rossignol, S., and Grillner, S. (Eds.), *Neural control of rhythmic movements in vertebrates*, pp. 167-199. New York: Wiley.

Gerasimenko, Y., McKay, W.B., Pollo, F.E., and Dimitrijevic, M.R. (1996) Stepping movements in paraplegic patients induced by epidural spinal cord stimulation. *Soc Neurosci Abstr* 22: 543.5

Grillner, S. (1973) Locomotion in the spinal cat. In Stein, R.B., Pearson, K.G., Smith, R.S., Redford, J.B. (Eds.), *Control of posture and locomotion*, pp. 513-535. New York: Plenum Press.

Grillner, S. (1981) Control of locomotion in bipeds, tetrapods and fish. In Brookhart, J.M., Mountcastle, V.B., and Geiger, S.R. (Eds.), *Handbook of physiology*, sect. 1, vol. II, part 2, *The nervous system: Motor control*. Oxford: American Physiological Society.

Grillner, S., Zangger, P. (1975) How detailed is the central pattern generation for locomotion? *Brain Res.* 88: 267-371.

Gurfinkel, V.S., Ivanenko, Y.P., Levik, Y.S., Kazennikov, O.V., and Selionov, V.A. (1999) The neural control of posture and locomotion: A lock with two keys. In Gantchev, G.N., Mori, S., and Massion, J. (Eds.), *Motor control, today and tomorrow*, pp. 111-121. Sofia: Professor Marius Drinov Academic Publishing House.

Gurfinkel, V.S., Levik, Y.S., Kazennikov, O.V., and Selionov, V.A. (1998) Locomotor-like movements evoked by leg muscle vibration in humans. *Eur J Neurosci* 10: 1608-1612.

Hultborn, H., Peterson, N., Brownstone, R., and Nielsen, J. (1993) Evidence of fictive spinal locomotion in the marmoset *(Callithrix jacchus). Soc Neurosci Abstr* 19: 225.1.

Illis, L.S. (1995) Is there a central pattern generator in man? *Paraplegia* 33: 239-240.

Iwahara, T., Atsuta, Y., Garcia-Rill, E., and Skinner, R.D. (1992) Spinal cord stimulation–induced locomotion in the adult cat. *Brain Res Bull* 28: 99-105.

Kniffki, K.D., Schomburg, E.D., and Steffens, H. (1981) Effects from fine muscle and cutaneous afferents on spinal locomotion in cats. *J Physiol* 319: 543-554.

Koehler, W.J., Schomburg, E.D., and Steffens, H. (1984) Phasic modulation of trunk muscle efferents during fictive spinal locomotion in cats. *J Physiol* 353: 187-197.

Livenson, J.A., and Ma, D.M. (1992) *Laboratory reference for clinical neurophysiology*. Philadelphia: Davis.

Lundberg, A. (1981) Half-centres revisited. In Szetagothai, J., Palkovits, M., and Hamori, J. (Eds.), Regulatory functions of the CNS: Principles of motion and organization. *Academiai Kiado*, vol. 1, pp. 155-167. Budapest: Pergamon Press.

Mori, S. (1987) Integration of posture and locomotion in acute decerebrate cats and in awake, freely moving cats. *Prog Neurobiol* 28: 164-195.

Orlovsky, G.N., and Shik, M.L. (1976) Control of locomotion: A neurophysiological analysis of the cat locomotor system. In Porter, R. (Ed.), *International review of physiology*. Neurophysiology II, vol. 10, pp. 281-317. Baltimore: University Park Press.

Pearson, K.G. (1993) Common principles of motor control in vertebrates and invertebrates. *Ann Rev Neurosci* 16: 265-297.

Pearson, K.G. (2000) Neural adaptation in the generation of rhythmic behavior. *Ann Rev Physiol* 62: 723-753.

Roby-Brami, A., and Bussel, B. (1987) Long-latency spinal reflex in man after flexor reflex afferent stimulation. *Brain* 110: 707-725.

Roby-Brami, A., and Bussel, B. (1990) Effects of flexor reflex afferent stimulation on the soleus H-reflex in patients with a complete spinal cord lesion: Evidence for presynaptic inhibition of Ia transmission. *Exp Brain Res* 81: 593-601.

Roby-Brami, A., and Bussel, B. (1992) Inhibitory effects on reflexes in patients with a complete spinal lesion. *Exp Brain Res* 90: 201-208.

Rossignol, S. (1996) Neural control of stereotypic limb movements. In Rowell, L.B., and Sheperd,

J.T. (Eds.), *Handbook of physiology,* sect. 12: *Exercise: Regulation and integration of multiple systems,* pp. 173-216. Oxford: American Physiological Society.

Rossignol, S., Bélanger, M., Chau, C., Giroux, N., Brustein, E., Bouyer, L., Grenier, C.-A., Drew, T., Barbeau, H., and Reader, T.A. (2000) The spinal cat. In Kalb, R.G., and Smittmatter, S.M. (Eds.), *Neurobiology of spinal cord injury,* pp. 57-87. Totowa, NJ: Humana Press.

Schomburg, E.D. (1995) Modes of rhythmic motor patterns generated by the spinal cord in the cat. In Taylor, A. (Ed.), *Alpha and gamma motor systems,* pp. 564-571. New York: Plenum Press.

Shapkov, Yu.T., Shapkova, H.Yu., and Mushkin, A.Yu. (1995) Spinal generators of human locomotor movements. In 4th IBRO World Congress of Neuroscience, Kyoto, Japan, p. 349.

Shapkova, E.Yu., and Schomburg, E.D. (2001) Two types of motor modulation underlying human stepping evoked by spinal cord electrical stimulation. *Acta Physiol Pharmacol Bulgarica* 26 (3): 155-159.

Shapkova, E., Mushkin, A., and Kovalenko, K. (1999) Motor rehabilitation for children with neurological complications of thuberculous spondylitis. *Problems of Tuberculosis* 3: 27-30.

Shapkova, H.Yu., and Schomburg, E.D. (1999a) Comparison of voluntary and stimulation-evoked locomotor activity in an incomplete paraplegic patient. *Progress in motor control II,* Aug 19-22, pp. 142-143. Pennsylvania State University.

Shapkova, H.Yu., and Schomburg, E.D. (1999b) Voluntary and stimulation-evoked locomotor activity in an incomplete paraplegic patient. In Gantchev, G.N., and Gantchev N. (Eds.), *From basic motor to functional recovery: Concepts, theories and models,* pp. 477-483. Sofia: Professor Marius Drinov Academic Publishing House.

Shapkova, H.Yu., Shapkov, Yu.T., and Mushkin, A.Yu. (1997a) Spinal cord stimulation–induced locomotion in human paraplegic. XXXIII International Congress of Physiological Sciences, June 30–July 5, St. Petersburg, P078.32.

Shapkova, H.Yu., Shapkov, Yu.T., and Mushkin, A.Yu. (1997b) Locomotor activity in paraplegic children induced by spinal cord stimulation. In Gurfinkel, V.S., and Levik, Yu. (Eds.), *Brain and movement,* pp. 170-171. Moscow: St-Petersburg-Moscow.

Vilensky, J.A., Eidelberg, E., Moore, A.M., and Walden, J.G. (1992) Recovery of locomotion in monkeys with spinal cord lesions. *J Mot Behav* 24: 288-296.

Vilensky, J.A., and O'Conner, B.L. (1997) Stepping in humans with complete spinal cord transection: A phylogenetic evaluation. *Motor Control* 1: 284-292.

Vilensky, J.A., and O'Conner, B.L. (1999) Stepping in nonhuman primates with a complete spinal cord transection: Old and new data, and implications for humans. *Ann NY Acad Sci* 860: 528-530.

Vitenson, A.S. (1998) *Regularities of normal and pathological human gait.* Moscow: Zerkalo-M (in Russian).

Wernig, A., and Müller, S. (1992) Laufband locomotion with body weight support improved walking in persons with severe spinal cord injuries. *Paraplegia* 30: 229-238.

Wernig, A., Müller, S., Nanassy, A., and Cagol, E. (1995) Laufband therapy based on "rules of spinal locomotion" is effective in spinal cord injured persons. *Eur J Neurosci* 7: 823-829.

# 12

# Motor Control and Learning After Stroke: A Review

## Mindy F. Levin
University of Montreal

In North America, 30% to 60% of all stroke survivors suffer from motor loss and the inability to use their affected arm in activities of daily living (Dombovy et al., 1987; DeLisa and Gans, 1998). This has an important impact on their level of independence and their return to active community life. In the first few months following stroke, therapy focuses on maximizing arm motor recovery. However, in the development of therapeutic techniques, little attention has been paid to concepts of motor learning derived from studies in healthy populations. In an attempt to bridge the gap between fundamental motor learning theory and therapeutic practice, this chapter reviews concepts of motor learning from the exercise and motor control literature and summarizes the evidence that this knowledge can be applied to the treatment of recovery of arm function in patients with neurological deficits following stroke-related brain damage.

Unilateral strokes resulting in hemiplegia are characterized by sensorimotor deficits such as spasticity (Lance, 1980) and pathological synergies in the limbs contralateral to the hemispheric lesion (Bobath, 1978). Sensorimotor deficits also influence the ability to activate appropriate muscles (Hammond, Kraft, and Fitts, 1988) and the coordination of movements between adjacent joints (Levin, 1996a). Impairments may be related to altered mechanical properties of motor units (Hufschmidt and Mauritz, 1985; Jakobsson et al., 1992; Petajan, 1983), abnormal agonist motor unit activation (Tang and Rymer, 1981; Gowland et al., 1992), deficits in segmental reflex organization such as antagonist inhibition (Hammond, Fitts, et al., 1988), reciprocal inhibition (Yanagisawa and Tanaka, 1978), and stretch reflex threshold regulation (Levin and Feldman, 1994; Levin et al., 2000). These impairments lead to muscle weakness (Colebatch et al., 1986) and improper spatial and temporal muscle recruitment, including inappropriate agonist–antagonist coactivation (Conrad et al., 1985; Dewald et al., 1995; Hammond, Kraft, and Fitts, 1988; Knutsson and Richards, 1979; Levin and Dimov, 1997).

Traditional physiotherapeutic stroke treatments (Bobath, 1978; Brunnstrom, 1970; Knott and Voss, 1968; Rood, 1956) are largely based on neurodevelopmental views of movement production and rely on the assumption of a hierarchical organization of the CNS for the control of movement (Gordon, 1987). This has led to the idea that recovery from brain damage follows a predictable sequence that mimics normal development and that movement recovery can be facilitated by specific sensory stimuli. Traditional therapies primarily use neurophysiological phenomena (i.e., reflexes) to enhance voluntary movement while placing less emphasis on behavioral and human ecology approaches. In contrast, some recent therapeutic approaches have broken away from traditional neurodevelopmental doctrine and have incorporated modern theories of motor control and learning. An example is the motor relearning approach (Carr and Shepherd, 1987) that focuses on elements of motor learning such as task analysis, practice of missing components, and transference of training. However, although based on sound theoretical considerations, to date there is little evidence that motor learning occurs in the same way in individuals with stroke as in healthy people.

An important consideration in the choice of therapeutic strategy is whether motor recovery results from the restoration of normal coordination patterns or from the substitution of new patterns (see Latash and Anson, 1996, and commentaries; Cirstea and Levin, 2000). To approach this fundamental problem, studies must identify which specific characteristics of reaching performance are altered following CNS lesions, whether these characteristics change with treatment, which treatments are the most effective, and whether changes may be related to measurable functional improvement.

This chapter begins by surveying the motor control principles underlying the production of voluntary movement and the principles of motor recovery and plasticity following stroke-related brain damage. Then, cognitive and sensorimotor processes related to motor learning are summarized. Finally, questions related to recovery of arm motor performance and motor learning in patients with stroke are discussed. Emphasis is placed on kinematic evidence of changes in reaching performance following different practice and feedback regimens. Analysis of this type of data may improve our understanding of the mechanisms underlying reaching deficits and lead to the development of more effective treatments for arm recovery based on objective movement analysis.

# The Production of Voluntary Movement

Since the time of Bernstein, motor control scientists have grappled with the problem of redundancy (see the chapters by Lestienne et al., Latash et al., and Bate and Thelen in this volume). It is now a well-accepted notion that the CNS takes advantage of the redundancy in the number of muscles and degrees of freedom (DFs) of the motor apparatus by selecting a desired trajectory and desired interjoint and intermuscle coordination from among many possible strategies to make a goal-directed movement. How the CNS uses this redundancy is fundamental to our understanding of motor control (Berkinblit et al., 1986; Bernstein, 1967; Feldman and Levin, 1995; Flash and Henis, 1991; Grossberg and Kuperstein, 1989; Kelso et al., 1993; Ma and Feldman, 1995; Mussa-Ivaldi et al., 1988; Reeke et al., 1990). For example, planar arm-reaching movements to a target can be produced by alterations in elbow and shoulder angles, leaving the trunk position and wrist angle unchanged (Flanagan et al., 1993). Thus, the CNS reduces the number of DFs in order to produce a unique arm configuration for each target position. This strategy can be changed, for example, by deliberately varying the wrist position during reaching (Koshland and Hasan, 1994). The CNS uses redundancy to produce topologically similar movement patterns while using different effectors (Gielen and Van Zuylen, 1986). In approaches to the redundancy problem, the concept of movement synergy has emerged (Bernstein, 1967), defined as the unit of coordination of many DFs fulfilling a specific functional goal. Recent studies have suggested that different synergies can be combined to meet several functional constraints simultaneously (Kaminski et al., 1995; Ma and Feldman, 1995; Saling et al., 1996; Pigeon et al., 2000; Adamovich et al., 2001).

Several hypotheses as to how the nervous system solves this "redundancy problem" have been proposed. Some authors have suggested that the CNS constructs coordinative structures or synergies linking together different DFs in a constantly varying task-specific way (Gelfand and Tsetlin, 1966; Turvey, 1990; Feldman and Levin, 1995). A new methodology for identifying the control laws by which the CNS might combine joint recruitment to reduce or contribute to redundancy, known as the uncontrolled manifold, has also been proposed (Schöner, 1995; Scholz and Schöner, 1999; Scholz et al., 2000; chapter 5 by Latash et al. in this volume).

A concept that has received increasing attention in motor control is the role of internal models in the learning, planning, and execution of movements (Wolpert et al., 1998; Shadmehr and Holcomb, 1997; Kawato, 1999). The internal model concept has its origin in control theory and robotics and was originally proposed as a model for cerebellar function (Ito, 1970). Kawato (1999) defines internal models as "neural mechanisms that can mimic the input/output characteristics, or their inverses, of the motor apparatus." Various forms of internal models have been proposed (Jordan and Rumelhart, 1992; Kawato, 1999; Wolpert et al., 1998). Forward models predict movement parameters from motor commands, and inverse models calculate appropriate motor commands from information about movement

parameters. Central to the concept of internal models is that motor skill acquisition may consist of the formation and refinement of an internal model of the limb
as a result of learning (e.g., Konczak et al., 1997). For the production of reaching
movements, it is proposed that already learned internal models function to produce
feedforward commands to motoneurons. It has also been suggested that movement
is represented by multiple internal models localized in different areas of the CNS,
most notably the cerebellum, and computational theories have been advanced in
which multiple internal models can be learned and combined adaptively (Wolpert
and Kawato, 1998; Haruno et al., 1999; Bastian et al., 1996).

Another approach to motor control suggests that active movements are produced
by resetting muscle activation thresholds via control variables. These determine
where, in spatial coordinates, muscles are active (Asatryan and Feldman, 1965).
EMG signals and forces emerge from this resetting and are therefore not directly
programmed by the CNS (Weeks et al., 1996; Feldman and Levin, 1995; Gribble
and Ostry, 2000). In this approach, task-specific control patterns (models or "en-
grams," according to Bernstein, 1967) rather than movement kinematics and forces
are stored in memory. Learning is associated with the ability of control systems
to recognize the appropriate external conditions, choose between different control
patterns stored in memory, and adjust the selected pattern according to changes in
task requirements (Feldman and Levin, 1995; Weeks et al., 1996).

Movement synergies and internal model formation may be further understood
by comparing motor behavior between healthy subjects and patients following a
stroke that results in movement planning or execution deficits. Neurophysiological studies in animals show that planning and sequencing of movement may be
distributed throughout different cortical and subcortical areas. The posterior parietal cortex is thought to play an important role in the integration of multimodal
sensory coordinate frames with emphasis on planning goal-directed movements
(Andersen et al., 1997; Posner et al., 1984). For example, in intact animals, the
activity of single cells in both parietal and premotor cortices is selectively tuned
to movement direction (Georgopoulos, 1990; Kalaska and Crammond, 1992).
The central control mechanism that codes target type and location and kinematic
parameters of limb movement may be partly localized in the parietal cortex
(Kalaska, 1991). Planning of coordinated arm and trunk movements may involve
both the parietal and premotor cortices, the latter playing a role in postural
adjustments through the control of axial musculature (Wise and Strick, 1984).
In addition, the supplementary motor area and the premotor cortex have been
implicated in movement control based on findings of disturbances in visually
guided reaching following lesion in monkeys (Haaxma and Kuypers, 1974;
LaMotte and Acuna, 1978; Lawrence and Kuypers, 1987). Distributed control
in humans is evidenced by a recent study of regional cerebral blood flow that
showed increased activity in the anterior cerebellum and the ventral premotor area during motor tasks requiring multijoint coordination and rapid reversals
(Winstein et al., 1997). Damage to any of those structures or their pathways likely
causes deficits in movement coordination or synchronization (Freund, 1987). Our

data suggests that, at a control level, motor "planning" may not be impaired in hemiparetic subjects with parietal or subcortical lesions. Nonapraxic patients are able to plan multijoint arm movements (Levin, 1996a) and more complex arm and trunk movements (Cirstea and Levin, 2000; Archambault et al., 1999; Esparza et al., 2003) into different parts of the workspace (figure 12.1). However, pointing movements of the affected arm are usually slower and more segmented than normal, suggesting deficits in interjoint coordination.

In conclusion, sensorimotor deficits in goal-directed movement may be associated with some disruption in premorbid internal models or may interfere with the production of new ones. The emergence of pathological movement synergies following stroke may be a manifestation of this disruption. The number of available synergies may be limited, and the ability of the control level to adapt existing synergies may be reduced. If redundancy in the motor system of stroke patients is constrained, then patients' ability to adapt motor output to different functional situations is reduced.

# Motor Recovery and Plasticity

The time course of recovery from stroke can vary from several weeks to years, with the most rapid recovery occurring within the first 3 months following the ictal event (Dombovy et al., 1987). Although mechanisms of recovery are not completely understood, evidence of recovery and reorganization suggests the presence of a notable amount of plasticity even in the adult CNS. Motor recovery following stroke depends on the location and the extent of the lesion (Heald et al., 1993) and cortical plasticity (Lee and van Donkelaar, 1995) associated with functional reorganization within areas of the cerebral cortex unaffected by the lesion (Brion et al., 1989; Chollet et al., 1991; Fries et al., 1990; 1993; Traversa et al., 1997; Weiller et al., 1992, 1993; for a review, see Hallett et al., 1998). This has been supported by direct studies of cortical reorganization in animals (Nudo and Milliken, 1996). The basis for reorganization may lie in the considerable functional overlap in cortical motor areas so that motor regions might be able to substitute for each other (Fries et al., 1993). Studies using transcranial magnetic stimulation (TMS) and neuroimaging with positron emission tomography (PET) have demonstrated activation in cortical areas not normally recruited with the type of movement studied. For example, using PET, Weiller et al. (1993) showed that movements of the recovered hand activated a large ventral extension of the hand field of the contralateral sensorimotor cortex in patients with lesions of the posterior limb of the internal capsule. They also found a greater activation than normal in supplementary motor areas, the insula, the frontal operculum, and the parietal cortex. Studies also suggest plastic reorganization of the ipsilateral hemisphere. For example, TMS of the damaged hemisphere can evoke motor responses not only in the contralateral but also in the ipsilateral hand. Substantial coactivation of ipsilateral motor cortex and contralateral nonprimary motor cortex was shown by cortical metabolic activity

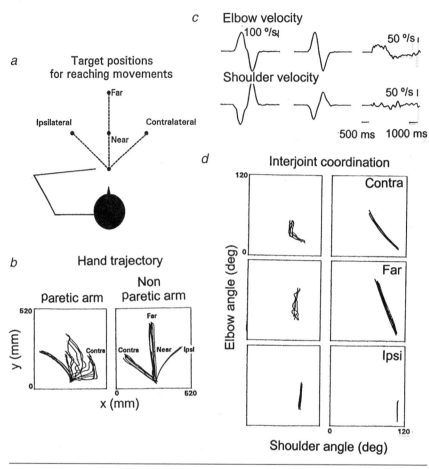

**Figure 12.1** *(a)* Schematic diagram of an experimental task in which patients with hemiparesis after stroke made movements with the paretic and nonparetic arms to different parts of a horizontally oriented work space. *(b)* Examples of 2D hand trajectories of both arms of a patient with moderate to severe paresis of the left arm *(left panel)*. Movements to far and contralateral (Contra) targets made by the paretic arm are possible but segmented. *(c)* The segmentation in trajectories is also evident in elbow and shoulder velocity profiles *(right panel)*. Joint velocity data is also shown for a healthy subject *(left panel)* and a patient with mild hemiparesis *(middle panel)* for comparison. *(d)* Comparison of movements of the paretic left arm *(left panels)* and the nonparetic right arm *(right panels)* of the same patient reveal disruption in interjoint coordination for contralateral (top panel) and far (middle panel) targets.

levels in stroke patients moving their formerly paretic hand (Chae et al., 1996). However, the presence of motor-evoked potentials of the ipsilateral sensorimotor cortex may be associated with poor motor recovery (e.g., Turton et al., 1996), whereas contralateral activity appears to be an indicator of good recovery (Turton et al., 1996; Rapisarda et al., 1996).

Overall, the evidence suggests that the damaged CNS retains the capacity for motor recovery through cortical reorganization. Identifying the optimal form of therapy to take advantage of this plasticity is the challenge in rehabilitation.

# Cognitive Processes Related to Motor Learning

The degree of poststroke motor recovery also depends on the ability of the damaged CNS to acquire new or recuperate lost skills through cognitive learning processes. After stroke, some or all components necessary for the acquisition of new movements may be impaired, depending on the site and severity of the CNS lesion (DeRenzi et al., 1977). This is particularly likely in light of recent evidence that different forms of motor memory are localized in different brain areas (Doyon et al., 1997). Of particular importance may be cognitive impairments, present in a large percentage of patients (Reding et al., 1993), that hinder the process of rehabilitation (Novack et al., 1987; Fong et al., 2001). For modification of the motor plan to occur, the CNS has to integrate sensory information emerging from the previous movement, store this information in short-term memory, and use it to adapt subsequent movements (Baddeley and Hitch, 1974). This strategy is similar to working memory tasks in which the individual has to keep track of previously presented material in order to successfully carry out a novel task (Petrides, 1994). Working memory is concerned with short-term retention, operating over seconds, and is used to maintain information online in order to carry out cognitive tasks such as comprehending, reasoning, and problem solving. In addition to working memory, executive functions of the frontal cortex as well as the striatum and cerebellum may be involved in visuospatial motor learning (Doyon et al., 1997; Owen et al., 1996, 1999). Posterior cortical areas implicated in the processing of visual, auditory, and somatosensory information can also influence the frontal cortex.

Stroke-related damage in sensorimotor cortical areas may affect both working memory and executive functions involved in motor learning (Halsband and Freund, 1993; Salmon and Butters, 1995). Most studies, however, have not found significant relationships between neuropsychological factors and motor learning deficits in stroke patients. However, recent evidence suggests that while healthy individuals can adapt their arm movements to changed load conditions after a single trial by reproducing motor commands stored in short-term memory (Weeks et al., 1996), this ability may not be preserved in all stroke patients (Dancause et al., 2002). In the study by Dancause et al. (2002), most patients who had mild to moderate strokes had a diminished ability to adapt their arm movements after a change in load (one-trial learning; figure 12.2). Similar conclusions can be drawn from studies in which patients had to learn new movement sequences (Pohl et al., 2001; Winstein et al., 1999). For patients with more severe strokes, however, there may be a relationship between motor performance and their decision-making ability based on previous information (executive function), a function related to the frontal lobe (Dancause et al., 2002). This suggests that more-sensitive testing is still needed to determine

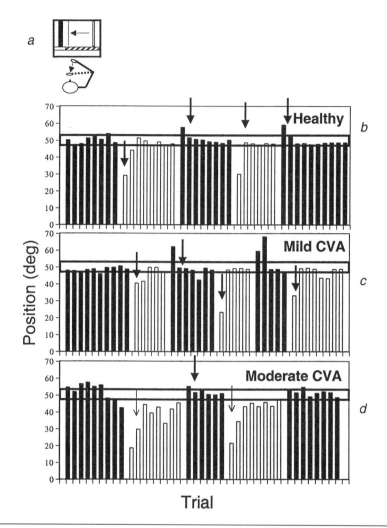

**Figure 12.2** Results of experiment in which healthy subjects and patients with hemiparesis made fast, 50° elbow flexion movements from one position *(white bar in a)* to another *(black bar in a)*. The arm and hand were supported by a splint attached to a manipulandum. Trials were either loaded (30% of subjects' maximal voluntary elbow flexor contraction, produced by a torque motor) or not loaded. A random number of loaded or nonloaded trials were presented in blocks. When load conditions changed from nonloaded *(black bars in b-d)* to loaded *(white bars in b-d)* conditions, the hand undershot the target position *(leftmost arrow in b),* and an error occurred. The subject could correct this error and in the next one or two trials in the same load condition, an accurate movement could be made *(bars ending in the zone outlined by the horizontal bar in each graph).* Such behavior was considered to be one-trial learning. *(b)* Healthy subjects and *(c)* patients with mild hemiparesis showed consistent one-trial learning *(thick arrows).* *(d)* Patients with moderate and severe hemiparesis required a larger number of trials in the same load conditions to adapt their movements to the change in load *(thin arrows).*

Adapted from Dancause et al. (2002).

the relationship between deficits in motor performance and motor learning for patients with CNS lesions.

# General Principles of Motor Learning

The previous section leads us to the conclusion that the understanding of motor recovery is related to the concepts of motor learning. This section reviews general principles of motor skill acquisition and relates them to movement reacquisition in stroke patients.

Much is known about motor skill acquisition in healthy subjects (Corcos et al., 1990; Newell, 1985; Salmoni et al., 1984; Schmidt, 1988; Winstein et al., 1997). For example, repeated practice of even very simple target-directed, rapid, single-joint elbow movements results in a decrease in movement time (Gottlieb et al., 1988). Learning a more complex multijoint task—characterized as the appearance of smooth, straight hand trajectories through a force field—occurs in healthy subjects after more prolonged practice (> 100 trials; Shadmehr and Mussa-Ivaldi, 1994). Learning has been defined as the set of internal processes related to practice or experience leading to a relatively permanent change in the capacity of the subject to respond (Schmidt, 1988). Among the many proposed theories of motor learning (Adams, 1971; Bernstein, 1967; Fitts and Posner, 1967; Newell, 1991), the most prevalent (Schmidt, 1975, 1988) suggests that, through practice, the CNS constructs generalized rules governing a number of movement elements that can be applied in a variety of contexts (Asanuma and Keller, 1991a, 1991b; Schmidt, 1975). After moving, information stored as a recall motor schema is used for the selection of a specific response, and a recognition sensory schema is used to evaluate the response. Support for this theory stems from animal studies in which sensory feedback induced by the movement may underlie the development of long-term potentiation in the sensorimotor cortex (Asanuma and Keller, 1991a, 1991b). Learning new movement elements may underlie the development of new interjoint coordinations (Bernstein, 1967; Gentile, 1972; Kugler et al., 1980; Thelen and Corbetta, 1994) and may be related to the formation of internal models.

Early research and theory in motor learning was based on the idea that improvements in motor performance should be reflected in the minimization or elimination of errors. This led to practice regimens stressing movement repetition with little rest between trials and a high frequency of feedback. The importance of precision as a motor goal was subsequently challenged. Another shift in thinking was that learning could be said to occur only if changes in behavior persisted beyond the period of training and if newly acquired skills could be generalized to other, related tasks (transfer of training; see Schmidt and Bjork, 1992). The essential principle is that instead of promoting errorless movement, practice should be designed to recruit the active participation of the individual in the solving of motor control problems. This would permit the individual to acquire the skills needed to adapt motor behavior to novel situations (Lee et al., 1994).

Different elements involved in learning have been studied, including the type and frequency of feedback; the use of demonstration and mental practice; and the amount, type, variability, and contextual dependency of practice (Christina, 1987; Corcos et al., 1990; for reviews, see Magill, 1989; Proteau et al., 1994; Schmidt, 1988). An essential variable in learning is feedback, which may be intrinsic (somatosensory information inherent in the task) or extrinsic (information not available in a task; Schmidt, 1988; Winstein, 1991). Extrinsic feedback may be provided through knowledge of results (KR) pertaining to augmented sensory information about task outcome and knowledge of performance (KP) pertaining to augmented information about how the task is performed.

The type of feedback (verbal or nonverbal) and also its frequency and time of delivery are critical in determining outcome (Salmoni et al., 1984). Continuous visual feedback about performance as well as feedback given right after every movement may improve performance immediately after training but may also have detrimental effects on retention (Lavery, 1962; Proteau and Marteniuk, 1993). Frequent guidance may inhibit performers from engaging the sensory encoding and retrieval processes necessary for learning. For example, studies in deafferented patients have shown that the visual system can almost completely compensate for the lack of proprioceptive feedback to produce accurate arm movements (Ghez et al., 1995; Levin et al., 1995). In addition, in conditions of continuous visual feedback, the CNS may have inadequate time to process and integrate augmented sensorimotor information into the new motor program for effective change to occur (Swinnen et al., 1990). Therefore, a condition for optimal learning is practice in the absence of continuous visual feedback. To summarize, it has been shown that the optimal form of KR for learning an arm movement is delayed summary KR, specifically, vision of the hand near the target with feedback given after a short delay following every few trials (Schmidt et al., 1989; Swinnen et al., 1990).

Finally, the type of practice (constant vs. variable) has been considered. Immediate improvement in task performance preferentially occurs when the same task (constant practice) is practiced in blocked fashion. However, the generalizability of learning is improved when different tasks, including the target task, are practiced in a random sequence (variable practice; Catalano and Kleiner, 1984; Schmidt, 1988; Shea and Morgan, 1979).

The optimal conditions for motor learning in healthy subjects occur when practice promotes the active involvement of the learner in the process of solving the motor problem (the use of variable blocked practice) and extrinsic feedback is provided in the form of summary KR or KP. It remains to be determined whether these principles apply equally to patients with poststroke brain injury.

# Motor Learning in Stroke

Movement repetition leads to motor improvements in healthy individuals. Assuming that this is the case for individuals with stroke-related brain damage, therapists encourage patients to practice different specific movements or combinations of movements. However, consideration of motor skill acquisition in neurological patients and how motor learning may differ in stroke patients compared with healthy individuals has begun only recently and has not been systematically studied (Platz et al., 1994; Winstein et al., 1999). Learning or adaptation depends on the constraints arising from the task, the environment, and the learner's body (Newell and McDonald, 1992), all of which may be modified by pathology. Patients with CNS lesions may adapt differently to the impairment according to optimization processes at different levels of motor control. These include the modification of the motor plan leading to different compensatory strategies, the modification of the motor program leading to new combinations of interjoint coordination patterns, and outright recovery of lost or impaired motor execution patterns.

The evidence that rehabilitation of the arm results in better arm motor function is equivocal. Studies of therapeutic approaches for recovery of arm motor function based on neurofacilitation techniques have not demonstrated that any one method is significantly better than any other (for reviews, see Duncan, 1997; Miller et al., 1998). Other studies analyzing the effects of specific treatments based on enhanced and repetitive training have shown more promising results, but methodologies are so different that it is difficult to draw conclusions from them. In rehabilitation, the paradigm most closely resembling KP is biofeedback, in which auditory or visual information about muscle activation or force levels is provided during or after task performance. In an analysis of eight randomized control trials of biofeedback therapy in stroke patients, biofeedback did not restore joint range of motion, but other clinical benefits may have occurred (Glanz et al., 1995). Sunderland et al. (1992) considered the effects of conventional Bobath therapy and enhanced therapy based on Bobath therapy, EMG biofeedback, and other activities. Six months of enhanced therapy resulted in a small but significant improvement in grip strength, range of motion, and manual dexterity. Although therapy clearly enhanced recovery of arm function, the elements of the treatment program responsible for the improvements were not identified. In another study, compared with Bobath treatment, 4 weeks of repetitive wrist extension movements (15 min, twice per day) significantly improved grip strength, peak isometric force, and acceleration of wrist extension (Bütefisch et al., 1995). However, specificity of training may have been responsible for this improvement, and the generalization of this effect to functional improvement was not evaluated. Platz et al. (1994) found little evidence of learning on a 1-day retention test of a simple spatial-motor task after 21 practice trials in stroke patients. However, their group of 20 patients had almost fully recovered function in the arm tested so that comparisons with the healthy control group showed no differences. Similarly, Cushman and Caplan (1987) studied one individual with almost fully recovered function. Evidence thus suggests that specific sensorimotor interventions may diminish specific motor impairments after stroke.

The most promising evidence that arm motor function can be improved is derived from studies in which intensive or prolonged therapy regimens are employed (Kwakkel et al., 1997, 1999; Dean et al., 2000). Indeed, one of the reasons for the equivocal results in previous intervention studies is that the intervention may not have been long enough or intensive enough for the therapeutic effect to be significant. Motor control and motor learning studies suggest that treatment approaches using a small number of trials may not be sufficient for consolidation of an internal representation of movement (internal model) to occur; internal models have been shown to develop slowly, after many trials (Karni et al., 1998; Shadmehr and Holcomb, 1997; cf. Winstein et al., 1999; Cirstea et al., 2000).

The type of practice is an important aspect of arm motor recovery. Despite evidence from studies in healthy subjects that maximal retention occurs when variable training is employed, most studies investigating the effects of repetitive practice have used constant practice regimens (but see Dean and Shepherd, 1997). Volpe et al. (2000) recently showed that, combined with conventional therapy, prolonged practice (5 h/wk for at least 5 wk) of a planar two-joint arm movement using a robot manipulator led to a significantly greater improvement in scores on arm motor impairment scales in a mixed group of stroke patients than conventional therapy alone. However, in this study, no assessment of disability reduction or of retention of training effects was done. In a longitudinal study of arm recovery following stroke, coordination in the affected arm was investigated in tasks requiring different combinations of elbow and shoulder movement (Lough et al., 1984). After training, movements were faster and smoother, and the trajectory was more direct. The authors suggested that better shoulder–elbow coordination may have been responsible for this improvement, but no data were presented to support this suggestion. To address the question of what aspects of motor performance contribute to the recovery of reaching, we conducted a series of studies in which the effects of two types of feedback on performance outcome and movement variables in patients with stroke were tested. Participants practiced a 3D pointing task in which the paretic arm pointed to a target located in the contralateral work space in front of the body at the limit of arm's reach. All participants practiced the pointing movement 75 times per day for 10 consecutive days (constant practice paradigm). Patients with stroke were divided into two groups: One group had summary KR feedback of movement precision and speed after every fifth trial (the nonguided practice group) and the other (the guided practice group) had faded KP in the form of therapist feedback and guidance of motor performance (i.e., the therapist encouraged the patient to use more shoulder horizontal adduction or more elbow extension during specific phases of the movement). Following 10 days of practice, the majority of participants in both groups moved their hemiparetic arms faster and more precisely than before the practice. Of particular interest is that performance improvements were accomplished differently, depending on stroke severity and the type of feedback. In the nonguided practice group, some patients increased joint range (elbow extension, 36% of patients; shoulder flexion, 45% of patients; figure 12.3) and improved interjoint coordination (45%) while decreasing trunk recruitment (anterior trunk displacement, trunk rotation, or both, 36%; figure 12.4). For this group, no correlation between changes in movement patterns and clinical scores, evaluated by the Fugl-Meyer scale, were found. In contrast, in the guided

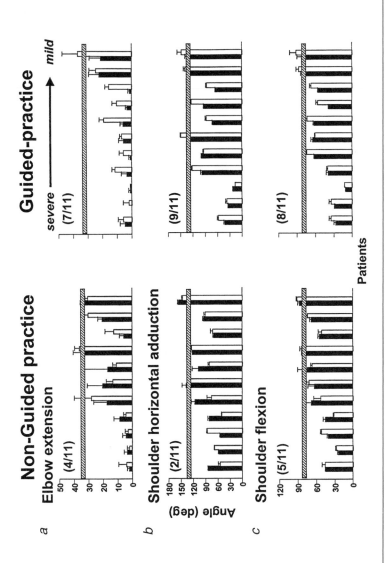

**Figure 12.3** Range of (*a*) elbow extension, (*b*) shoulder horizontal adduction, and (*c*) shoulder flexion for patients practicing a reaching movement before (*black bars*) and after (*white bars*) 10 days of nonguided practice (*left*) or guided practice (*right*). Data are arranged in each graph from left to right by decreasing clinical severity. Numbers in parentheses refer to the number of patients who significantly improved following practice. Horizontal bars indicate mean values obtained from a healthy control group practicing the same task.

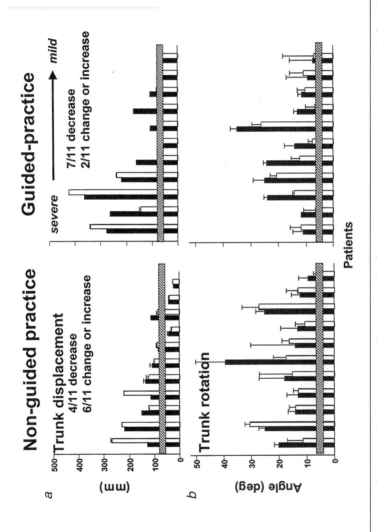

**Figure 12.4** The range of (*a*) trunk displacement and (*b*) trunk rotation for patients practicing a reaching movement before (*black bars*) and after (*white bars*) 10 days of nonguided practice (*left*) or guided practice (*right*). Data is presented as in figure 12.3.

practice group, a larger number of patients improved joint ranges (elbow extension, 64%; shoulder adduction and flexion, 80%) and interjoint coordination (64%) while decreasing trunk movement (64%). In contrast to the nonguided practice group, kinematic improvements were correlated with changes in Fugl-Meyer scores, suggesting that feedback in the form of knowledge of performance may lead to better recovery of lost motor patterns than knowledge of results. In addition, these effects remained significant 1 week following practice in both groups. These early results demonstrate the potential of different practice paradigms to obtain the best gains in arm motor performance in stroke patients.

Some studies have assessed the effect of variable practice training approaches on leg and arm motor recovery. Dean and Shepherd (1997) studied the effect of ten 30-min sessions of variable practice of seated reaching tasks carried out by patients at their homes, compared with a control group who did not practice the tasks. KR in the form of movement time and KP in the form of how to improve submovements of the task were continuously given. After training, the experimental group performed significantly faster and increased maximal reaching distance and weight borne through the affected leg compared with the control group. Carryover effects were not assessed. In another approach, intensive variable practice was assessed through the "forced-use" therapy, in which the unaffected limb is immobilized for several hours a day and the stroke patient is required to employ the paretic limb for all daily life tasks (Taub et al., 1993; Miltner et al., 1999, van der Lee et al., 1999). Effects have been positive for both motor recovery and carryover, but this technique has been largely limited to patients with good motor recovery in the paretic arm. Hanlon (1996) measured the time to complete a functional task involving grasping with the paretic arm in right and left stroke patients. The rate of acquisition and 2- and 7-day retention of the movement sequence were compared between groups ($n = 9$) who did blocked, variable, or no practice. Practice consisted of 10 trials per day until subjects met the criterion of successfully completing 3 consecutive trials. Fewer than 25 practice trials were necessary to meet the criterion in both practice groups. The variable practice group performed better on the mean number of successful trials (out of 5) during retention testing, but no differences in movement time were observed between groups during the acquisition or retention tests. This study provides limited evidence that varied practice may be of more benefit than blocked practice to patients who have had a stroke, but no kinematic analysis was done to determine what aspects of movement improved. These studies add to the increasing evidence that patients with stroke can improve their performance on specific tasks if those tasks are included in training and practiced with sufficient intensity.

To date, few studies have evaluated the capacity for motor learning in patients with stroke. One study evaluated skill learning with the unaffected arm (Winstein et al., 1999), and another with the paretic arm only in well-recovered patients (Hanlon, 1996). Both these studies measured cognitive aspects of learning as well as movement kinematics and concluded that, in their subject groups, no learning deficit existed. However, these studies have limited generalizability to individuals with moderate to severe hemiparesis. More research is needed to assess the effectiveness of enhanced feedback and its timing in the motor retraining of the paretic arms of stroke patients and to address issues related to the type of practice.

## Conclusions

Rehabilitation of stroke patients is aimed at increasing functional ability and improving quality of life. Therapy stresses the importance of movement repetition over days or weeks to improve performance. Studies suggest that improvement in the form of recovery or adaptation of motor output depends on the severity of the motor deficit (Latash and Anson, 1996; Levin, 1996b; Luria et al., 1969). When patients repeatedly practice a single gesture, the functional goals of producing more rapid, smooth, and precise movements are usually met, but how these goals are accomplished depends on the patient's initial level of motor recovery.

Practice and feedback regimens for the acquisition and retention of new motor skills have been extensively studied in healthy subjects, and optimal forms have been described. Optimal learning occurs when subjects practice a variety of related tasks and feedback is given intermittently so that the CNS has time to integrate pertinent sensory information into the production of the movement. It is not known what practice regimen may be optimal for motor learning in patients with stroke-related brain damage or whether the damaged CNS uses sensory information in the same way as in healthy subjects. Indeed, stroke patients may not be able to benefit from variable practice until missing motor elements are relearned. It also appears that motor relearning may occur in different ways for patients with different degrees of stroke severity. The use of fundamental motor learning approaches in the study of motor recovery has already provided some understanding of both the underlying mechanisms of motor control deficits and the processes of learning or relearning lost motor skills in stroke patients. Such an understanding is most urgently needed to maximize the effectiveness of rehabilitation techniques.

## Acknowledgments

The author would like to acknowledge the contributions of colleagues and students to the studies described in this chapter: Alain Ptito, PhD; Numa Dancause, PT, MSc; Philippe Archambault, OT, MSc; Carmen M. Cirstea, MD, MSc; and Danilo Esparza, PT, MSc. Grateful thanks are also extended to the Canadian Institutes of Health Research (CIHR), the National Science and Engineering Research Council of Canada (NSERC), the Fonds de la recherche en santé du Québec (FRSQ), and the FCAR.

# References

Adamovich, S.V., Archambault, P.S., Ghafouri, M., Levin, M.F., Poizner, H., and Feldman, A.G. (2001) Hand trajectory invariance in reaching movements involving the trunk. *Exp Brain Res* 138: 288-303.

Adams, J.A. (1971) A closed-loop theory of motor learning. *J Mot Behav* 3: 111-150.

Andersen, R.A., Snyder, L.H., Bradley, D.C., and Xing, J. (1997) Multimodal representation of space in the posterior parietal cortex and its use in planning movements. *Annu Rev Neurosci* 20: 303-330.

Archambault, P., Pigeon, P., Feldman, A.G., and Levin, M. (1999) Recruitment and sequencing of different degrees of freedom during pointing movements involving the trunk in healthy and hemiparetic subjects. *Exp Brain Res* 126: 55-67.

Asanuma, H., and Keller, A. (1991a) Neurobiological mechanisms of motor learning and memory. *Concepts Neurosci* 2: 1-30.

Asanuma, H., and Keller, A. (1991b) Neuronal mechanisms of motor learning in mammals. *Neuro-Report* 2: 217-224.

Asatryan, D.G., and Feldman, A.G. (1965) Functional tuning of the nervous system with control of movement or maintenance of a steady posture: I. Mechanographic analysis of the work of the joint on execution of a postural task. *Biofizika* 10: 837-846.

Baddeley, A.D., and Hitch, G. (1974) Working memory. In Bower, G.H. (Ed.), *The psychology of learning and motivation,* vol. 8. New York: Academic Press.

Bastian, A.J., Martin, T.A., Keating, J.B., and Thach, W.T. (1996) Cerebellar ataxia: Abnormal control of interaction torques across multiple joints. *J Neurophysiol* 76: 492-509.

Berkinblit, M.B., Feldman, A.G., and Fukson, O.I. (1986) Adaptability of innate motor patterns and motor control. *Behav Brain Sci* 9: 585-638.

Bernstein, N.A. (1967) *The co-ordination and regulation of movements.* Oxford: Pergamon Press.

Bobath, B. (1978) *Adult hemiplegia: Evaluation and treatment.* 2nd ed. London: Heinemann Medical.

Brion, J.-P., Demeurisse, G., and Capon, A. (1989) Evidence of cortical reorganization in hemiparetic patients. *Stroke* 20: 1079-1984.

Brunnstrom, S. (1970) *Movement therapy in hemiplegia: A neurophysiological approach.* New York: Harper and Row.

Bütefisch, C., Hummelsheim, H., Denzler, P., and Mauritz, K.-H. (1995) Repetitive training of isolated movements improves the outcome of motor rehabilitation of the centrally paretic hand. *J Neurol Sci* 130: 59-68.

Carr, J.H., and Shepherd, R.B. (Eds.). (1987) *Movement science: Foundations for physical therapy in rehabilitation.* Aspen: Rockville, MD.

Catalano, J.F., and Kleiner, B.M. (1984) Distant transfer and practice variability. *Percept Mot Skills* 58: 851-856.

Chae, J., Zorowitcz, R.D., and Johnston, M.V. (1996) Functional outcome of hemorrhagic and nonhemorrhagic stroke patients after in-patient rehabilitation. *Am J Phys Med Rehabil* 75: 177-182.

Chollet, F., DiPiero, V., Wise, R.J.S., Brooks, D.J., Dolan, R.J., and Frankowiak, R.S.J. (1991) The functional anatomy of motor recovery after stroke in humans: A study with positron emission tomography. *Ann Neurol* 29: 63-71.

Christina, R.W. (1987) Motor learning: Future lines of research. In Safrit, J.M., and Eckert, H.M. (Eds.), *The cutting edge in physical education and exercise science research,* pp. 26-41. Champaign, IL: Human Kinetics.

Cirstea, M.C., and Levin, M.F. (2000) Compensatory strategies for reaching in stroke. *Brain* 123: 940-953.

Cirstea, M.C., Ptito, A., Forget, R., and Levin, M.F. (2000) Arm motor improvement in stroke patients may depend on the type of training. *Soc Neurosci Abstr* 26: 162.

Colebatch, J.G., Gandevia, S.C., and Spira, P.J. (1986) Voluntary muscle strength in hemiparesis: Distribution of weakness at the elbow. *J Neurol Neurosurg Psychiatr* 49: 1019-1024.

Conrad, B., Benecke, R., and Meinck, H.M., (1985) Gait disturbances in paraspastic patients. In Delwaide, P.J., and Young, R.R. (Eds.), *Restorative neurology: Clinical neurophysiology in spasticity,* vol. 1, pp. 155-174. Amsterdam: Elsevier.

Corcos, D.M., Gottlieb, G.L., Jaric, S., Cromwell, R.L., and Agarwal, G.C. (1990) Organizing principles underlying motor skill acquisition. In Winters, J.M., and Woo, S.L.-Y. (Eds.), *Multiple muscle systems, biomechanics and movement organization,* pp. 195-213. New York: Springer-Verlag.

Cushman, L., and Caplan, B. (1987) Multiple memory systems: Evidence from stroke. *Percept Mot Skills* 64: 571-577.

Dancause, N., Ptito, A., and Levin, M.F. (2002) Error correction strategies for motor behavior after unilateral brain damage: Short-term motor learning processes. *Neuropsychologia* 1359: 1-11.

Dean, D.M., Richards, C.L., and Malouin, F. (2000) Task-related circuit training improves performance of locomotor tasks in chronic stroke: A randomized, controlled pilot trial. *Arch Phys Med Rehabil* 81: 409-417.

Dean, D.M., and Shepherd, R.B. (1997) Task-related training improves performance of seated reaching tasks after stroke. A randomized controlled trial. *Stroke* 28: 722-728.

DeLisa, J., and Gans, B. (1998) *Rehabilitation medicine: Principles and practice.* 3rd ed. Philadelphia: Lippincott-Raven.

DeRenzi, E., Faglioni, P., and Previdi, P. (1977) Spatial memory and hemispheric locus of lesion. *Cortex* 13: 424-433.

Dewald, J.P.A., Pope, P.S., Given, J.D., Buchanan, T.S., and Rymer, W.Z. (1995) Abnormal muscle coactivation patterns during isometric torque generation at the elbow and shoulder in hemiparetic subjects. *Brain* 118: 495-510.

Dombovy, M.L., Basford, J.R., Whisnant, J.P., and Bergstralh, E.J. (1987) Disability and use of rehabilitation services following stroke in Rochester, Minnesota, 1975-1979. *Stroke* 18: 830-836.

Doyon, J., Gaudreau, D., Laforce, R., Castonguay, M., Bedard, P.J., Bedard, F., and Bouchard, J.-P. (1997) Role of the striatum, cerebellum, frontal lobes in the learning of a visuomotor sequence. *Brain Cogn* 34: 218-245.

Duncan, P.W. (1997) Synthesis of intervention trials to improve motor recovery following stroke. *Top Stroke Rehabil* 3: 1-20.

Esparza, D.Y., Archambault, P.S., Winstein, C.J., and Levin, M.F. (2003) Hemispheric specialization in the co-ordination of arm and trunk movements during pointing in patients with unilateral brain damage. *Exp Brain Res* 148: 488-497.

Feldman, A.G., and Levin, M.F. (1995) The origin and use of positional frames of reference in motor control. *Behav Brain Sci* 18: 723-744.

Fitts, P.M., and Posner, M.I. (1967) *Human performance.* Belmont, CA: Brooks-Cole.

Flanagan, R.J., Ostry, D.J., and Feldman, A.G. (1993) Control of trajectory modifications in target-directed reaching. *J Mot Behav* 25: 175-179.

Flash, T., and Henis, E. (1991) Arm trajectory modifications during reaching toward visual targets. *J Cogn Neurosci* 3: 220-230.

Fong, K.N.K., Chan, C.C.H., and Au, D.K.S. (2001) Relationship of motor and cognitive abilities to functional performance in stroke rehabilitation. *Brain Injury* 15: 443-453.

Freund, H.J. (1987) Abnormalities of motor behaviour after cortical lesions in humans. In Plum, F. (Ed.), *Handbook of physiology: The nervous system,* pp. 763-810. Baltimore: Williams and Wilkins.

Fries, W., Danek, A., Bauer, W.M., Witt, T.N., and Leinsinger, G. (1990) Hemiplegia after lacunar stroke with pyramidal degeneration shown in vivo: A model for functional recovery. In von Wild, K., and Janzik, H. (Eds.), *Neurologische Fruhrehabilitation,* pp. 11-17. Munich: Zuchschwerdt.

Fries, W., Danek, A., Scheidtmann, B., and Hamburger, C. (1993) Motor recovery following capsular stroke: Role of descending pathways from multiple motor areas. *Brain* 116: 369-382.

Gelfand, I.M., and Tsetlin, M.L. (1966) On mathematical modeling of the mechanisms of the central nervous system. In Gelfand, I.M., Gurfinkel, V.S., Fomin, S.V., and Tsetlin, M.L. (Eds.), *Models of the structural-functional organization of certain biological systems,* pp. 9-26. Moscow: Nauka. (In Russian; a translation is available in the 1971 edition by MIT Press, Cambridge, MA.)

Gentile, A.M. (1972) A working model of skill acquisition with application to teaching. *Quest* 17: 3-23.

Georgopoulos, A.P. (1990) Neurophysiology of reaching. In Jeannerod, M. (Ed.), *Attention and performance XIII: Motor representation and control,* pp. 227-263. Hillsdale, NJ: Erlbaum.

Ghez, C., Gordon, J., and Ghilardi, M.F. (1995) Impairments of reaching movements in patients without proprioception: II. Effects of visual information on accuracy. *J Neurophysiol* 73: 361-372.

Gielen, C.C.A.M., and Van Zuylen, E.J. (1986) Coordination of arm muscles during flexion and supination: Application of the tensor analysis approach. *Neuroscience* 17: 527-539.

Glanz, M., Klawansky, S., Stason, W., Berkey, C., Shah, N., Phan, H., and Chalmers, T.C. (1995) Biofeedback therapy in poststroke rehabilitation: A meta-analysis of the randomized controlled trials. *Arch Phys Med Rehabil* 76: 508-515.

Gordon, J. (1987) Assumptions underlying physical therapy intervention: Theoretical and historical perspectives. In Carr, J.H., and Shepherd, R.B. (Eds.), *Movement science: Foundations for physical therapy in rehabilitation,* pp. 1-30. Aspen: Rockville, MD.

Gottlieb, G.L., Corcos, D.M., Jaric, S., and Agarwal, G.C. (1988) Practice improves even the simplest movements. *Exp Brain Res* 73: 436-440.

Gowland, C., deBruin, H., Basmajian, J.V., Plews, N., and Burcea, I. (1992) Agonist and antagonist activity during voluntary upper-limb movement in patients with stroke. *Phys Ther* 72: 624-633.

Gribble, P.L., and Ostry, D.J. (2000) Compensation for loads during arm movements using equilibrium-point control. *Exp Brain Res* 135: 474-482.

Grossberg, S., and Kuperstein, M. (1989) *Neural dynamics of adaptive sensory-motor control.* New York: Pergamon.

Haaxma, R., and Kuypers, H.G.J.M. (1974) Role of occipito-frontal and cortico-cortical connections in visual guidance of relatively independent hand and finger movements in the rhesus monkey. *Brain Res* 71: 361-366.

Hallett, M., Wassermann, E.M., Cohen, L.G., Chmielowska, J., and Gerloff, C. (1998) Cortical mechanisms of recovery of function after stroke. *Neurorehabilitation* 10: 131-142.

Halsband, U., and Freund, H.-J. (1993) Motor learning. *Curr Opin Neurobiol* 3: 940-949.

Hammond, M.C., Fitts, S.S., Kraft, G.H., Nutter, P.B., Trotter, M.J., and Robinson, L.M. (1988) Co-contraction in the hemiparetic forearm: Quantitative EMG evaluation. *Arch Phys Med Rehabil* 69: 348-351.

Hammond, M.C., Kraft, G.H., and Fitts, S.S. (1988) Recruitment and termination of electromyographic activity in the hemiparetic forearm. *Arch Phys Med Rehabil* 69: 106-110.

Hanlon, R.E. (1996) Motor learning following unilateral stroke. *Arch Phys Med Rehabil* 77: 811-815.

Haruno, M., Wolpert, D., and Kawato, M. (1999) Multiple paired forward-inverse models for human motor learning and control. In Kearns, M.S., Solla, S.A., and Cohn, D.A. (Eds.), *Advances in neural information processing systems II,* pp. 31-37. Cambridge, MA: MIT Press.

Heald, A., Bates, D., Carlidge, N.E.F., French, J.M., and Miller, S. (1993) Longitudinal study of central motor conduction time following stroke: I. Natural history of central motor conduction. *Brain* 116: 1355-1370.

Hufschmidt, A., and Mauritz, K.-H. (1985) Chronic transformation of muscle in spasticity: A peripheral contribution to increased tone. *J Neurol Neurosurg Psychiatr* 48: 676-685.

Ito, M. (1970) Neurophysiological aspects of the cerebellar motor control system. *Int J Neurol* 7: 162-176.

Jakobsson, F., Grimby, L., and Edstrom, L. (1992) Motoneuron activity and muscle fibre type composition in hemiparesis. *Scand J Rehabil Med* 24: 115-119.

Jordan, M.I., and Rumelhart, D.E. (1992) Forward models: Supervised learning with a distal teacher. *Cogn Sci* 16: 307-354.

Kalaska, J.F. (1991) Parietal cortex area 4: A neuronal representation of movement kinematics for kinaesthetic perception and movement control? In Paillard, J. (Ed.), *Brain and space,* pp. 133-146. Oxford: Oxford University Press.

Kalaska, J.F., and Crammond, D.J. (1992) Cerebral cortical mechanisms of reaching movements. *Science* 255: 1517-1523.

Kaminski, T.R., Bock, C., and Gentile, A.M. (1995) The coordination between trunk and arm motion during pointing movements. *Exp Brain Res* 106: 457-466.

Karni, A., Meyer, G., Rey-Hipolito, C., Jezzard, P., Adams, M.M., Turner, R., and Ungerleider, L.G. (1998) The acquisition of skilled motor performance: Fast and slow experience-driven changes in primary motor cortex. *Proc Nat Acad Sci* 95: 861-868.

Kawato, M. (1999) Internal models for motor control and trajectory planning. *Curr Opin Neurobiol* 9: 718-727.

Kelso, J.A.S., Buchanan, J.J., DeGuzman, G.C., and Ding, M. (1993) Spontaneous recruitment and annihilation of degrees of freedom in biological coordination. *Phys Lett A* 179: 364-371.

Knott, M., and Voss, D.E. (1968) *Proprioceptive neuromuscular facilitation.* 2nd ed. New York: Harper and Row.

Knutsson, E., and Richards, C. (1979) Different types of disturbed motor control in gait of hemiparetic patients. *Brain* 102: 405-430.

Konczak, J., Borutta, M., and Dichgans, J. (1997) The development of goal-directed reaching in infants: II. Learning to produce task-adequate patterns of joint torque. *Exp Brain Res* 113: 465-474.

Koshland, G.F., and Hasan, Z. (1994) Selection of muscles for initiation of planar three joint arm movements with different final orientations of the hand. *Exp Brain Res* 98: 157-162.

Kugler, P.N., Kelso, J.A.S., and Turvey, M.T. (1980) On the concept of coordinative structures as dissipative structures: I. Theoretical lines of convergence. In Stelmach, G.E., and Requin, J. (Eds.), *Tutorials in motor behavior,* pp. 3-45. Amsterdam: North-Holland.

Kwakkel, G., Kollen, B.J., and Wagenaar, R.C. (1999) Therapy impact on functional recovery in stroke rehabilitation: A critical review of the literature. *Physiotherapy* 85: 377-391.

Kwakkel, G., Wagenaar, R.C., Koelman, T.W., Lankhorst, G.J., and Koetsier, J.C. (1997) Effects of intensity of rehabilitation after stroke: A research synthesis. *Stroke* 28: 1550-1556.

LaMotte, R.H., and Acuna, C. (1978) Defects in accuracy of reaching associated with a superior parietal cortex lesion in monkeys. *Brain Res* 139: 309-326.

Lance, J.W. (1980) The control of muscle tone, reflexes, and movement: Robert Wartenberg lecture. *Neurology* 30: 1303-1313.

Latash, M.L., and Anson, J.G. (1996) What are "normal movements" in atypical populations? *Behav Brain Sci* 19: 55-68.

Lavery, J.J. (1962) Retention of simple motor skills as a function of type of knowledge of results. *Can J Psychol* 16: 300-311.

Lawrence, D.G., and Kuypers, H.G.M. (1987) The functional organization of the motor system in the monkey. *Brain* 91: 1-14.

Lee, R.G., and van Donkelaar, P. (1995) Mechanisms underlying functional recovery following stroke. *Can J Neurol Sci* 22: 257-263.

Lee, T.D., Swinnen, S.P., and Serrien, D.J. (1994) Cognitive effort and motor learning. *Quest* 46: 328-344.

Levin, M.F. (1996a) Interjoint coordination during pointing movements is disrupted in spastic hemiparesis. *Brain* 119: 281-294.

Levin, M.F. (1996b) Should stereotypic movement synergies seen in hemiparetic patients be considered adaptive? *Behav Brain Sci* 19: 79-80.

Levin, M.F., and Dimov, M. (1997) Spatial zones for muscle coactivation and the control of postural stability. *Brain Res* 757: 43-59.

Levin, M.F., and Feldman, A.G. (1994) The role of stretch reflex threshold regulation in normal and impaired motor control. *Brain Res* 637: 23-30.

Levin, M.F., Lamarre, Y., and Feldman, A.G. (1995) Control variables and proprioceptive feedback in fast single-joint movement. *Can J Physiol Pharmacol* 73: 316-330.

Levin, M.F., Selles, R.W., Verheul, M.H.G., Meijer, O.G. (2000) Deficits in the coordination of agonist and antagonist muscles in stroke patients: Implications for normal motor control. *Brain Res* 853: 352-369.

Lough, S., Wing, A.M., Fraser, C., and Jenner, J.R. (1984) Measurement of recovery of function in the hemiparetic upper limb following stroke: A preliminary report. *Hum Mov Sci* 3: 247-256.

Luria, A.R., Nayin, V.L., Tsvetkova, L.S., and Vinarskaya, E.N. (1969) Restoration of higher cortical functions following local brain damage. In Vinken, P.J., and Buryn, G.W. (Eds.), *Handbook of clinical neurology.* Amsterdam: North-Holland.

Ma, S., and Feldman, A.G. (1995) Two functionally different synergies during arm reaching movements involving the trunk. *J Neurophysiol* 73: 2120-2122.

Magill, R.A. (1989) *Motor learning concepts and application.* 2nd ed. Dubuque, IA: Brown.

Miller, K.J., Garland, S.J., and Koshland, G.F. (1998) Techniques and efficacy of physiotherapy poststroke. *Phys Med Rehabil State Art Rev* 12: 473-487.

Miltner, W.H., Bauder, H., Sommer, M., Dettmers, C., and Taub, E. (1999) Effects of constraint induced movement therapy on patients with chronic motor deficits after stroke: A replication. *Stroke* 30: 586-592.

Mussa-Ivaldi, F.A., Morasso, P., and Zaccaria, R. (1988) Kinematic networks: A distributed model for representing and regularizing motor redundancy. *Biol Cybern* 60: 1-16.

Newell, K.M. (1985) Coordination, control and skill. In Goodman, D., Wilberg, R.B., and Franks, I.M. (Eds.), *Differing perspectives in motor learning, memory and control*, pp. 295-317. New York: Elsevier.

Newell, K.M. (1991) Motor skill acquisition. *Annu Rev Psychol* 42: 213-237.

Newell, K.M., and McDonald, P.V. (1992) Searching for solutions to the coordination function: Learning as exploratory behavior. In Stelmach, G.E., and Requin, J. (Eds.), *Tutorials in motor behavior II*, pp. 517-532. Amsterdam: Elsevier.

Novack, T.A., Haban, G., Graham, K., and Satterfield, W.T. (1987) Prediction of stroke rehabilitation outcome from psychological screening. *Ann Intern Med* 68: 729-734.

Nudo, R., and Milliken, G. (1996) Reorganization of movement representations in primary motor cortex following focal ischemic infarcts in adult squirrel monkeys. *J Neurophysiol* 75: 2144-2149.

Owen, A.M., Doyon, J., Petrides, M., and Evans, A.C. (1996) Planning and spatial working memory: A positron emission tomography study in humans. *Eur J Neurosci* 8: 353-364.

Owen, A.M., Herrod, J.N., Menon, D.K., Clark, J.C., Downey, S., Carpenter, A.T., Minhas, P.S., Turkheimer, F.E., Williams, E.J., Robbins, W., Saharian, B.J., Petrides, M., and Pickard, J.D. (1999) Redefining the functional organization of working memory processes within human lateral prefrontal cortex. *Eur J Neurosci* 11: 567-574.

Petajan, J.H. (1983) Motor unit control in movement disorders. *Adv Neurol* 39: 897-905.

Petrides, M. (1994) Frontal lobes and working memory: Evidence from investigations of the effects of cortical excisions in nonhuman primates. In Booler, F., and Grafman, J. (Eds.), *Handbook of neuropsychology*, pp. 59-82. New York: Elsevier.

Pigeon, P., Yahia, L.H., Mitnitski, A.B., and Feldman, A.G. (2000) Superposition of independent units of coordination during pointing movements involving the trunk with and without visual feedback. *Exp Brain Res* 131: 336-349.

Platz, T., Denzler, P., Kaden, B., and Mauritz, K.-H. (1994) Motor learning after recovery from hemiparesis. *Neuropsych* 32: 1209-1223.

Pohl, P.S., McDowd, J.M., Filion, D.L., Richards, L.G., and Stiers, W. (2001) Implicit learning of a perceptual-motor skill after stroke. *Phys Ther* 81: 1780-1789.

Posner, M.I., Walker, J.A., Friedrich, F.A., and Rafal, R.D. (1984) Effects of parietal injury on convert orienting of attention. *J Neurosci* 4: 1863-1874.

Proteau, L., Blandin, Y., Alain, C., and Dorion, A. (1994) The effects of the amount and variability of practice on the learning of a multi-segmented motor task. *Acta Psych* 85: 61-74.

Proteau, L., and Marteniuk, R.G. (1993) Static visual information and the learning and control of a manual aiming movement. *Hum Mov Sci* 12: 515-536.

Rapisarda, G., Bastings, E., Maertens de Noordhout, A., Pennisi, G., and Delwaide, P.J. (1996) Can motor recovery in stroke patients be predicted by early transcranial magnetic stimulation? *Stroke* 27: 2191-2196.

Reding, M.J., Gardner, C., and Hainline, B. (1993) Neuropsychiatric problems interfering with inpatient stroke rehabilitation. *J Neurol Rehabil* 7: 1-7.

Reeke, G.N., Finkel, L.H., Sporns, O., and Edelman, G.M. (1990) Synthetic neural modelling: A multi-level approach to the analysis of brain complexity. In Edelman, G., and Gall, W.E. (Eds.), *Signal and senses: Local and global order in perceptual maps*, pp. 232-260. New York: Wiley.

Rood, M.S. (1956) Neurophysiological mechanisms utilized in the treatment of neuromuscular dysfunction. *Am J Occup Ther* 10: 220-225.

Saling, M., Stelmach, G.E., Mescheriakov, S., and Berger, M. (1996) Prehension with trunk assisted reaching. *Behav Brain Res* 80: 753-760.

Salmon, D.P., and Butters, N. (1995) Neurobiology of skill and habit learning. *Curr Opin Neurobiol* 5: 184-190.

Salmoni, A.W., Schmidt, R.A., and Walter, C.B. (1984) Knowledge of results and motor learning: A review and critical reappraisal. *Psychol Bull* 95: 355-386.

Schmidt, R.A. (1975) A schema theory of discrete motor skill learning. *Psychol Rev* 82: 225-260.

Schmidt, R.A. (1988) *Motor and learning: A behavioral emphasis*. Champaign, IL: Human Kinetics.

Schmidt, R.A., and Bjork, R.A. (1992) New conceptualizations of practice: Common principles in three paradigms suggest new concepts for training. *Psychol Sci* 3: 207-217.

Schmidt, R.A., Young, D.E., Swinnen, S., and Shapiro, D.C. (1989) Summary knowledge of results for skill acquisition: Support for the guidance hypothesis. *J Exp Psychol Learn Mem Cogn* 15: 352-359.

Scholz, J.P., and Schöner, G. (1999) The uncontrolled manifold concept: Identifying control variables for a functional task. *Exp Brain Res* 126: 289-306.

Scholz, J.P., Schöner, G., and Latash, M.L. (2000) Identifying the control structure of multijoint coordination during pistol shooting. *Exp Brain Res* 135: 382-404.

Schöner, G. (1995) Recent developments and problems in human movement science and their conceptual implications. *Ecol Psychol* 7: 291-314.

Shadmehr, R., and Holcomb, H.H. (1997) Neural correlates of motor memory consolidation. *Science* 277: 821-825.

Shadmehr, R., and Mussa-Ivaldi, F.A. (1994) Adaptive representation of dynamics during learning of a motor task. *J Neurosci* 14: 3208-3224.

Shea, J.B., and Morgan, R.L. (1979) Contextual interference effects on the acquisition, retention, and transfer of motor skill. *J Exp Psychol Hum Learn Mem* 5: 179-187.

Sunderland, A., Tinson, D.J., Bradley, E.L., Fletcher, D., Langton Hewer, R., and Wade, D.T. (1992) Enhanced physical therapy improves recovery of arm function after stroke: A randomized controlled trial. *J Neurol Neurosurg Psychiatr* 55: 530-535.

Swinnen, S.P., Schmidt, R.A., Nicholson, D.E., and Shapiro, D.C. (1990) Information feedback for skill acquisition: Instantaneous knowledge of results degrades learning. *J Exp Psychol* 16: 706-716.

Tang, A., and Rymer, W.Z. (1981) Abnormal force-EMG relations in paretic limbs of hemiparetic human subjects. *J Neurol Neurosurg Psychiatr* 44: 690-698.

Taub, E., Miller, N.E., Novack, T.A, Cook, E.W., Fleming, W.C., Nepomuceno, C.S., Connel, J.S., and Crago, J.E. (1993) Technique to improve chronic motor deficit after stroke. *Arch Phys Med Rehabil* 74: 347-354.

Thelen, E., and Corbetta, D. (1994) Exploration and selection and the early acquisition of skill. *Int Rev Neurobiol* 37: 75-102.

Traversa, R., Cicinelli, P., Bassi, A., Rossini, P.M., and Bernardi, G. (1997) Mapping of motor cortical reorganization after stroke: A brain stimulation study with focal magnetic pulses. *Stroke* 28: 110-117.

Turton, A., Wroe, S., Trepte, N., Fraser, C., and Lemon, R.N. (1996) Contralateral and ipsilateral EMG responses to transcranial magnetic stimulation during recovery of arm and hand function after stroke. *Electroencephalogr Clin Neurophysiol* 101: 316-328.

Turvey, M.T. (1990) Coordination. *Am Psychol* 45: 938-953.

van der Lee, J., Wagenaar, R.C., Lankhorst, G.J., Vogelaar, T.W., Devillé, W.L., and Bouter, L.M. (1999) Forced use of the upper extremity in chronic stroke patients: Results from a single-blind randomized clinical trial. *Stroke* 30: 2369-2375.

Volpe, B.T., Krebs, H.I., Hogan, N., Edelstein, L., Diels, C., and Aisen, M. (2000) A novel approach to stroke rehabilitation: Robot-aided sensorimotor stimulation. *Neurology* 54: 1938-1944.

Weeks, D.L., Aubert, M.-P., Feldman, A.G., and Levin, M.F. (1996) One-trial adaptation of movement to changes in load. *J Neurophysiol* 75: 60-74.

Weiller, C., Chollet, F., Friston, K.J., Wise, R.J.S., and Frackowiak, R.S.J. (1992) Functional reorganization of the brain in recovery from striatocapsular infarction in man. *Ann Neurol* 31: 463-472.

Weiller, C., Ramsay, S.C., Wise, R.J., Friston, K.J., and Frackowiak, R.S.J. (1993) Individual patterns of functional reorganization in the human cerebral cortex after capsular infarction. *Ann Neurol* 33: 181-189.

Winstein, C.J. (1991) Knowledge of results and motor learning: Implications for physical therapy. *Phys Ther* 71: 140-149.

Winstein, C.J., Grafton, S.T., and Pohl, P.S. (1997) Motor task difficulty and brain activity: Investigation of goal-directed reciprocal aiming using positron emission tomography. *J Neurophysiol* 77: 1581-1594.

Winstein, C.J., Merians, A.L., and Sullivan, K.J. (1999) Motor learning after unilateral brain damage. *Neuropsychologia* 37: 975-987.

Wise, S.P., and Strick, P.L. (1984) Anatomical and physiological organization of the non-primary motor cortex. *Trends Neurosci* 7: 442-446.

Wolpert, D.M., and Kawato, M. (1998) Multiple paired forward and inverse models for motor control. *Neural Netw* 11: 1317-1329.

Wolpert, D.M., Miall, R.C., and Kawato, M. (1998) Internal models in the cerebellum. *Trends Cogn Sci* 2: 338-347.

Yanagisawa, N., and Tanaka, R. (1978) Reciprocal Ia inhibition in spastic paralysis in man. In Cobb, W.A., and van Duijn, H. (Eds.), *Contemporary clinical neurophysiology: EEG,* suppl. 34, pp. 521-526. Amsterdam: Elsevier.

# Index

*Note:* Page numbers followed by an italicized *f* or *t* refer to the figure or table on that page, respectively.

# Contributors

**John H.J. Allum,** Department of Otorhinolaryngology, University Hospital, Basel, Switzerland.

**Hugues Barbeau,** School of Physical and Occupational Therapy, McGill University, Montreal, and Research Center, Jewish Rehabilitation Hospital, Laval, Quebec, Canada.

**Patricia Bate,** Department of Psychology, Indiana University, Bloomington, Indiana.

**Bastiaan R. Bloem,** Department of Neurology, University of Nijmegen, Netherlands.

**Rumpa Boonsinsukh,** School of Physical and Occupational Therapy, McGill University, Montreal, and Research Center, Jewish Rehabilitation Hospital, Laval, Quebec, Canada.

**Mark G. Carpenter,** Department of Otorhinolaryngology, University Hospital, Basel, Switzerland, and Department of Kinesiology, University of Waterloo, Ontario, Canada.

**Frederic Danion,** Mouvement et Perception, Université de la Méditerranée, Marseilles, France.

**Anatol G. Feldman,** Neurological Science Research Center, Department of Physiology, University of Montreal, and Center for Multidisciplinary Studies in Rehabilitation, Rehabilitation Institute of Montreal, Quebec, Canada.

**Tamar Flash,** Department of Computer Science and Applied Mathematics, Weizmann Institute of Science, Rehovot, Israel.

**Joyce Fung,** School of Physical and Occupational Therapy, McGill University, Montreal, and Research Center, Jewish Rehabilitation Hospital, Laval, Quebec, Canada.

**Amir A. Handzel,** Institute for Systems Research, University of Maryland, College Park, Maryland.

**Michel Ladouceur,** Faculty of Applied Health Science, Brock University, St. Catharines, Ontario, Canada.

**Anouk Lamontagne,** School of Physical and Occupational Therapy, McGill University, Montreal, and Research Center, Jewish Rehabilitation Hospital, Laval, Quebec, Canada.

**Francis G. Lestienne,** Laboratoire de Neurosciences de l'Homme en Mouvement, Université de Caen Basse-Normandie, Caen, France.

**Dario G. Liebermann,** Department of Physical Therapy, Sackler Faculty of Medicine, Tel Aviv University, Israel.

**Isabelle Mercier,** Research Center, Jewish Rehabilitation Hospital, Laval, Quebec, Canada.

**Ruud G.J. Meulenbroek,** Nijmegen Institute for Cognition and Information, University of Nijmegen, Netherlands.

**Margherita Rapagna,** School of Physical and Occupational Therapy, McGill University, Montreal, and Research Center, Jewish Rehabilitation Hospital, Laval, Quebec, Canada.

**Magnus E. Richardson,** Laboratoire de Physique Statistique, Ecole Normale Superieure, Paris, France.

**John F. Scholz,** Department of Physical Therapy and Interdisciplinary Neuroscience Program, University of Delaware, Newark, Delaware.

**Gregor Schöner,** Institut für Neuroinformatik, Ruhr-Universität Bochum, Germany.

**Elena Yu. Shapkova,** Children's Surgery Clinic, Institute of Phthisiopulmonology, St. Petersburg, Russia.

**Bert Steenbergen,** Nijmegen Institute for Cognition and Information, University of Nijmegen, Netherlands.

**Esther Thelen,** Department of Psychology, Indiana University, Bloomington, Indiana.

**Francine Thullier,** Laboratoire de Neurosciences de l'Homme en Mouvement, Université de Caen Basse-Normandie, Caen, France.

**Emanuel Todorov,** Department of Cognitive Science, University of California, San Diego, California.

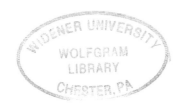

# About the Editors

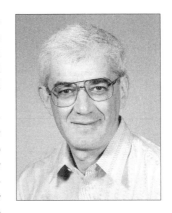

**Mark L. Latash, PhD,** is a professor of kinesiology at The Pennsylvania State University. Since the 1970s, he has worked extensively in normal and disordered motor control. His work has included animal studies, human experiments, modeling, and clinical studies.

The author of *Control of Human Movement* (Human Kinetics 1993) and *Neurophysiological Basis of Movement* (Human Kinetics 1998), Latash also translated Bernstein's classic, *On Dexterity and Its Development* (Erlbaum), in 1996. In addition to serving as editor for both previous volumes of *Progress in Motor Control,* Latash serves as the editor of the academic journal *Motor Control* and was coeditor of *Classics in Movement Science* (Human Kinetics 2001). He also started a series of conferences titled "Progress in Motor Control."

Latash earned a master's degree in physics of living systems from the Moscow Physico-Technical Institute in 1976 and a PhD in physiology from Rush University in 1989. He is president of the International Society of Motor Control and a member of the Society for Neuroscience and the American Society of Biomechanics. He is a fellow of the American Academy of Kinesiology and Physical Education and earned the Pattishall Outstanding Research Achievement Award from The Pennsylvania State University in 2001.

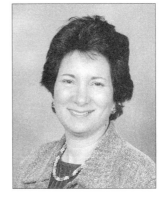

**Mindy Levin, PhD, PT,** teaches physiotherapy at the School of Rehabilitation at the University of Montreal and is director of a research laboratory investigating motor learning and recovery of arm function in adults and children with neurological disorders. For 10 years she has been a practicing physiotherapist, specializing in neurological rehabilitation of patients with spinal cord injuries, Parkinson's disease, neuromuscular disorders, and stroke.

Levin earned a master's degree in clinical sciences from the University of Montreal and a PhD in physiology from McGill University. She is a member of the Order of Physiotherapists of Quebec, the Consortium of Rehabilitation Researchers of Canada, the Canadian Stroke Network, and the Society for Neuroscience and is an executive officer of the International Society of Motor Control. She was recognized by the Heart and Stroke Foundation of Canada in 2002 for excellence in research in preventive cardiology.

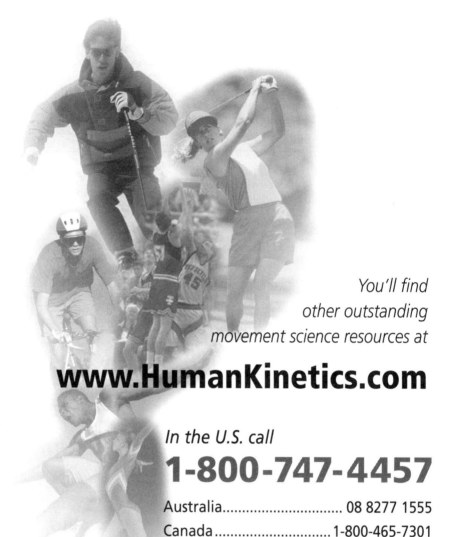

*You'll find
other outstanding
movement science resources at*

# www.HumanKinetics.com

*In the U.S. call*

## 1-800-747-4457

Australia.............................. 08 8277 1555
Canada ............................. 1-800-465-7301
Europe......................+44 (0) 113 255 5665
New Zealand.................. 0064 9 448 1207

**HUMAN KINETICS**
*The Information Leader in Physical Activity*
P.O. Box 5076 • Champaign, IL 61825-5076 USA